Women and Global Health Leadership

Rosemary Morgan • Kate Hawkins
Roopa Dhatt • Mehr Manzoor
Sulzhan Bali • Cheryl Overs
Editors

Women and Global Health Leadership

Power and Transformation

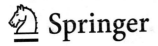 Springer

Editors
Rosemary Morgan
Department of International Health
Johns Hopkins Bloomberg School
of Public Health
Baltimore, Maryland, USA

Roopa Dhatt
Women in Global Health
Washington, District of Columbia, USA

Sulzhan Bali
Women in Global Health
Washington, District of Columbia, USA

Kate Hawkins
Pamoja Communications Ltd.
Research in Gender and Ethics (RinGs)
Brighton, East Sussex, UK

Mehr Manzoor
Department of Health Policy
and Management
Tulane University
New Orleans, Louisiana, USA

Cheryl Overs
Michael Kirby Centre for Public Health
and Human Rights
Monash University
Clayton, Victoria, Australia

ISBN 978-3-030-84500-1   ISBN 978-3-030-84498-1   (eBook)
https://doi.org/10.1007/978-3-030-84498-1

This Springer imprint is published by the registered company Springer Nature Switzerland AG
The registered company address is: Gewerbestrasse 11, 6330 Cham, Switzerland

To all women leaders, and aspiring woman leaders, join us in collective action for a feminist future.

Acknowledgement

The editors would like to thank Molly Sheehan for her proofreading and thorough read through of the book.

Contents

About the Editors

Rosemary Morgan, PhD is an Associate Scientist within the Department of International Health at Johns Hopkins Bloomberg School of Public Health in Baltimore, Maryland, USA. She is an expert in gender, gender analysis, and intersectionality in health and health systems research. She works on a number of global and public health projects as a primary investigator or gender advisor, including the Sex and Gender Analysis Core for the NIH-funded Sex and Age Differences in Immunity to Influenza (SADII) Center; the Gender and COVID-19 Project, Risk and Resilience in the Health Workforce: Understanding and Supporting the Experiences of Women Health Workers during COVID-19, Rapid Mortality Mobile Phone Surveys during COVID-19, the UK Partnerships for Health Systems program (UKPHS); and Learning, Acting and Building for Rehabilitation in Health Systems Consortium (ReLAB-HS). She also coordinated the highly successful Research in Gender and Ethics (RinGs): Building Stronger Health Systems, a project which brought together four research networks encompassing 23 institutions across 26 countries in a partnership to galvanize gender and ethics analysis in health systems research. Prior to joining Johns Hopkins, Rosemary was a Lecturer in Global Health Policy for the Global Public Health Unit at the University of Edinburgh, and a Research and Teaching Fellow at the Nuffield Centre for International Health and Development at the University of Leeds. She holds a PhD in International Health and Development from the University of Leeds, an MSc in Policy Studies from the University of Edinburgh, and a BA in Sociology from the University of British Columbia.

Kate Hawkins is a research communications expert with technical expertise in health, gender, and international development. She is the founder and director of Pamoja Communications Ltd. She has worked in international development and health for over 18 years. She began as a community volunteer delivering HIV prevention interventions to vulnerable groups in her home city of Brighton, UK. This led to paid work in the NGO sector on HIV and sexual and reproductive health internationally with a focus on advocacy. Much of her work was with vulnerable and marginalized groups such as women living with HIV and sex workers. From this she moved into global health more generally and was one of the co-founders of Action for Global Health—a pan-European network of campaigners. Later in her career Kate became interested in the role of evidence in policy and programmatic decision-making. She worked in academia and managed a groundbreaking research collaboration on sexuality in the Global South. Since founding her own company, she has managed the communications of many international research consortia working on health and health systems in low- and middle-income countries. Kate is committed to feminism, international solidarity and support, and the realization of rights.

Roopa Dhatt, MD is a practicing internist in Washington, District of Columbia, USA, trained in international health and a global health and gender advocate. Dr. Dhatt is particularly committed to addressing issues of power, privilege, and intersectionality that keep many women from global health leadership roles and to opening up spaces for the voices of these women to be heard. Dr. Dhatt is the Executive Director and co-founded Women in Global Health (WGH) in 2015. She advises global health institutions on matters of the health workforce, gender equity, and universal health coverage. Dr. Dhatt was recognized in the Gender Equality Top 100, the most influential people in global policy 2019. In 2021, the Lancet featured her work on gender equality. As Co-Chair of the Gender Equity Hub in the Global Health Workforce Network of the WHO, she supported WGH in the "Delivered by Women, Led by Men" report which looked collectively for the first time at issues of leadership, decent work free from all forms of discrimination, harassment including sexual harassment, the gender pay gap, and occupational segregation—across the entire health workforce. Dr. Dhatt has a Bachelor of Arts and a Bachelor of Science from the University of California, Davis; a Master's in Public Affairs from Sciences Po, Paris, France; and a Medical Degree from Temple University School of Medicine. She completed her residency in Internal Medicine and International Health at Case Western Reserve University. She has academic affiliations at Georgetown University and the University of Miami.

Mehr Manzoor is a Fulbright Scholar and a PhD candidate at Tulane University in the Department of Health Policy and Management. Mehr is a strong advocate for gender equality, intersectionality, and women's leadership in global health and beyond. Her research work includes gender and intersectionality analysis of global health organizations and explores issues of diversity, equity, and inclusion in workplaces. She is a co-lead author on the technical report "Delivered by Women, Led by Men: A Gender and Equity Analysis in the Global Health and Social Care Workforce," which explores issues of decent work, organizational segregation, gender pay gap, and leadership in global health workforce and was published by the Gender Equity Hub at the World Health Organization. She taught Social Aspects of Health to incarcerated women in Louisiana in 2020 as part of Newcomb College Institute and Tulane's College in Prison project. She was selected as WLGH Leadership Fellow for the inaugural Women Leaders in Global Health (WLGH) conference in 2017 in Stanford, California, and in 2018 was selected as an Emerging Voice for Global Health (EV4GH) program fellow. She volunteered and served as a research director at Women in Global Health from 2016 to 2019. She has received Changemaker Catalyst Award by Taylor Center at Tulane University for her work on women's leadership in global health, and her social venture on women's leadership in low- and middle-income countries was selected in Taylor Center's Changemaker Institute at Tulane University in 2021. She holds an undergraduate degree in Computer Science from National University of Computer and Emerging Sciences, Lahore, Pakistan, and a Master of Business Administration (MBA) from Lahore University of Management Sciences, Pakistan.

Sulzhan Bali is a health specialist with the World Bank, with over a decade of research and work experience in a variety of public health contexts—including health security, emergency response financing, and disease surveillance and response programs. Sulzhan has a track record of publications in top journals and extensive experience working on low-income and fragile countries across West and Central Africa. Her work includes evaluation of global response efforts for multiple major epidemics. Prior to joining the World Bank, Sulzhan worked with the University of Maryland—University College and the Public Health Foundation of India. In the realm of global health governance, Sulzhan has participated in multilateral dialogues to discuss global health futures for the next decade as a Bosch Global Governance Futures Fellow. She also served as the Director of Production and HR for This Week in Global Health (TWiGH)—an online video and audio podcast on global health. For her work with TWiGH, Sulzhan was featured in the "300 Women Leaders in Global Health" campaign by *The Lancet* and the Graduate Institute of International and Development Studies, Geneva. Sulzhan completed her PhD in Molecular Biology with the Medical Research Council (MRC) in the UK and holds degrees from Duke University (M.Sc., Global Health), the University of Manchester (M.Sc., Virology), and the University of Delhi (B.Sc., Microbiology).

Cheryl Overs joined a group of feminist lawyers lobbying for decriminalization and destigmatization of sex work and protesting violence and discrimination against sex workers in 1981 in Australia. By 1984 that group evolved into a membership-based sex workers group named the Prostitutes Collective of Victoria (PCV). Cheryl led the successful campaign for law reform in Victoria and oversaw the development of innovative programs for sex workers. In 1988 the PCV hosted the Prostitution and the AIDS Debate Conference in Melbourne which led to the formation of the national federation of sex workers' organizations, the Scarlet Alliance. In 1992 Overs met Brazilian sexuality activist Paulo Henrique Longo and they founded the International Network of Sex Worker Projects (NSWP). Cheryl was the first director of the NSWP which was based in France before hubs were established in Brazil and South Africa. Cheryl currently works in academia at Monash University where she contributed to the establishment of the Michael Kirby Centre for Public Health and Human Rights. She also works on human rights and sex work issues at Sussex University and the Institute of Development Studies where she has developed an online resource center on sex work research (PLRI); published a map of sex work law, and several articles about sex work and human rights in the context of public health and development aid; LGBT rights; economic empowerment and poverty reduction for marginalized women and girls; pre-exposure HIV prophylaxis; and sexual citizenship.

Contributors

Yara M. Asi School of Global Health Management and Informatics, College of Community Innovation and Education, University of Central Florida, Orlando, FL, USA

Elizabeth Bakibinga Commonwealth Secretariat, London, UK

Pauline Bakibinga Health and Systems for Health Research Unit, African Population and Health Research Center, Nairobi, Kenya

Stella Bakibinga Örebro University, Örebro, Sweden

Dina Balabanova Department of Global Health and Development, London School of Hygiene & Tropical Medicine, London, UK

Sulzhan Bali Women in Global Health, Washington, DC, USA

Gloria Benny George Institute for Global Health, New Delhi, India

Ivy Lynn Bourgeault School of Sociological and Anthropological Studies, Faculty of Social Sciences, University of Ottawa, Ottawa, ON, Canada

Raquel Pérez Cañal THET (Tropical Health and Education Trust), London, UK

Roopa Dhatt Women in Global Health, Washington, DC, USA

Dilip Ghosh Retired, Department of Health and Family Welfare, Government of West Bengal, Kolkata, India

Kate Hawkins Pamoja Communications Ltd., Research in Gender and Ethics (RinGs), Brighton, East Sussex, UK

John Daniel Ibembe Department of Anthropology, Washington University in St Louis, St. Louis, MO, USA

Barun Kanjilal Retired, IIHMR University, Jaipur, India

Ann Keeling Women in Global Health, Washington, DC, USA

Jamie Lundine Institute of Feminist and Gender Studies, University of Ottawa, Ottawa, ON, Canada

Mehr Manzoor Department of Health Policy and Management, Tulane University, New Orleans, LA, USA

Manasee Mishra IIHMR University, Jaipur, India

Rosemary Morgan Department of International Health, Johns Hopkins Bloomberg School of Public Health, Baltimore, MD, USA

Kui Muraya KEMRI-Wellcome Trust Research Programme, Nairobi, Kenya

Devaki Nambiar George Institute for Global Health, New Delhi, India

Faculty of Medicine, University of New South Wales, Sydney, Australia

Prasanna School of Public Health, Manipal Academy of Higher Education, Manipal, India

Ann Nolan Trinity Centre for Global Health, Trinity College, Dublin, Ireland

Cheryl Overs Michael Kirby Centre for Public Health and Human Rights, Monash University, Clayton, VIC, Australia

Nuzulul Kusuma Putri Research Group for Health and Well-being of Women and Children, Faculty of Public Health, Universitas Airlangga, Surabaya, Indonesia

Hari Sankar George Institute for Global Health, New Delhi, India

Summer Simpson THET (Tropical Health and Education Trust), London, UK

Claire Somerville Gender Centre, Graduate Institute of International and Development Studies, Geneva, Switzerland

Zahra Zeinali Johns Hopkins Bloomberg School of Public Health, Baltimore, MD, USA

Abbreviations

AIDS	Acquired Immunodeficiency Syndrome
ALACITS	Latin American Association Against STDs
AMREF	African Medical and Research Foundation
ANM	Auxiliary Nurse Midwife
APHRC	African Population and Health Research Center
ASHA	Accredited Social Health Activist
AU	African Union
AWCs	Anganwadi Centres
AWW	Anganwadi Workers
AYUSH	Ayurveda, Yoga & Naturopathy, Unani, Siddha, and Homeopathy Therapy
BBC	British Broadcasting Cooperation
BMJ	British Medical Journal
CAM	Complementary and Alternative Streams of Medicine
CECs	County Executives for Health
CEDAW	Convention on Elimination of All Forms of Discrimination Against Women
CEO	Chief Executive Officer
CHE	Current Health Expenditure
CHWs	Community Health Workers
CIRHT	Center for International Reproductive Health Training
CV	Curriculum Vitae
DDP	Deputy Director General of Programs
DFID	Department for International Development
DG	Director General
DMOs	District Medical Officers
EAC	East African Community
EAHRC	East African Health Research Commission
ECCAS	Economic Community of Central African States
ECOWAS	Economic Community of West African States
EEC	European Economic Community

EU	European Union
FGD	Focus Group Discussions
FTAG	Foundation Technical Advisory Group
GB	Great Britain
GBV	Gender-Based Violence
GDP	Gross Domestic Product
GII	Gender Inequality Index
GIL	Gender Innovation Lab
GPI	Global Peace Index
HICs	High-Income Countries
HIV	Human Immunodeficiency Virus
HIV/AIDS	Human Immunodeficiency Virus/Acquired Immunodeficiency Syndrome
HPV	Human Papillomavirus
IAC	Inter-African Committee on Traditional Practices
ICDS	Integrated Child Development Services
ICIPE	International Center of Insect Physiology and Ecology
IMAGE	Intervention with Microfinance for AIDS and Gender Equity
INS	National Institute of Health
IPHS	Indian Public Health Standards
ISM	Department of Indian Systems of Medicine
JAMA	The Journal of the American Medical Association
KII	Key Informant Interviews
KMWA	Kenya Medical Women's Association
KOICA	Korea International Cooperation Agency
LGBT	Lesbian, Gay, Bisexual, and Transgender
LMICs	Low- And Middle-Income Countries
MP	Member of Parliament
MSF	Médecins Sans Frontières
MWASA	Medical Women's Association of South Africa
NDPII	National Development Plan
NEJM	The New England Journal of Medicine
NETLAB	Network of Public Health Laboratories
NGO	Non-Governmental Organization
NRHM	National Rural Health Mission
NSWP	International Network of Sex Worker Projects
NUHM	National Urban Health Mission
OBGYN	Obstetrician-Gynecologist
OECD	Organisation for Economic Co-Operation and Development
PCV	Prostitutes Collective of Victoria
PDPs	Product Development Partnerships
PHC	Primary Health Centre
PPPs	Public-Private Partnerships
SADC	Southern Africa Development Community
SDG	Sustainable Development Goals

SEARO	South-East Asia Region
SIGI	Social Institutions and Gender Index
SMART	Specific, Measurable, Achievable, Realistic, and Timely
SSA	Sub-Saharan Africa
STEM	Science, Technology, Engineering and Mathematics
STI	Science, Technology and Innovations
STIs	Sexually Transmitted Infections
THET	Tropical Health and Education Trust
TICH	Tropical Institute of Community Health and Development in Kisumu
UHC	Universal Health Coverage
UK	United Kingdom
UN	United Nations
UNAIDS	Joint United Nations Programme on HIV/AIDS
UNDP	United Nations Development Programme
UNESCO	United Nations Education, Scientific and Cultural Organization
UNICEF	United Nations Children's Fund
UPCH	Cayetano Heredia University
US	United States
USA	United States of America
WAHO	ECOWAS' West African Health Organization
WEF	World Economic Forum
WHA	World Health Assembly
WHO	World Health Organization
WISH	Women of Integrity, Strength, and Hope
WPS	Women, Peace, and Security

Women and Global Health Leadership: Power and Transformation

Kate Hawkins, Rosemary Morgan, Cheryl Overs, Mehr Manzoor, Roopa Dhatt, and Sulzhan Bali

It is almost obligatory when writing about gender and global health to begin by citing the well-worn statistic that women provide the majority of the health and social care workforce, while comprising 25% of senior leadership roles (WHO, 2019). Similarly, it is well known that women are under-represented in leadership positions within many institutions which make up the health sector. Women from low- and middle-income countries represent less than 5% of executive leadership roles in global health institutions, while low- and middle-income countries (LMICs) represent more than three quarters of the world's population (Global Health 50/50, 2020). Moreover, half of women's contributions in the health sector remain unpaid, equalling approximately $1.5 trillion USD annually (Langer et al., 2015).

While these challenges may feel quite familiar to those working in the global health world, it is only recently that gender parity in health leadership has become a

K. Hawkins (✉)
Pamoja Communications Ltd., Research in Gender and Ethics (RinGs), Brighton,
East Sussex, UK
e-mail: kate@pamoja.uk.com

R. Morgan
Department of International Health, Johns Hopkins Bloomberg School of Public Health,
Baltimore, MD, USA
e-mail: Rosemary.morgan@jhu.edu

C. Overs
Michael Kirby Centre for Public Health and Human Rights, Monash University, Clayton,
VIC, Australia
e-mail: cherylovers@gmail.com

M. Manzoor
Department of Health Policy and Management, Tulane University, New Orleans, LA, USA
e-mail: mmanzoor@tulane.edu

R. Dhatt · S. Bali
Women in Global Health, Washington, DC, USA
e-mail: roopa.dhatt@womeningh.org; sulzhan@gmail.com

© Springer Nature Switzerland AG 2022
R. Morgan et al. (eds.), *Women and Global Health Leadership*,
https://doi.org/10.1007/978-3-030-84498-1_1

1

celebrated cause across a range of global health actors. Arguments about the gendered inequity of global health have been heard among feminist or gender studies scholars for some time. But now women's leadership is clearly a part of mainstream debates in global health. It is now, rightly, difficult to ignore.

This interest in women's position and leadership in global health was undoubtedly catalysed by the creation of Women in Global Health in 2015 and their seminal crowdsourced list of the 300 women in global health (#WGH300). They highlighted the lack of diversity in global health leadership and the glaring need for collective action to address the gender gap (Women in Global Health, 2014). Ensuring parity in terms of the numbers of men and women in leadership positions is a goal which is now supported by many, including the World Health Organization (WHO, 2019). Notably, in 2017 Dr. Tedros Adhanom Ghebreyesus, then incoming Director-General of the WHO, pledged to ensure gender parity in his leadership cabinet, resulting in nearly two-thirds of his cabinet being women among whom there was significant geographical diversity.

Indeed, women's leadership is considered central to the Sustainable Development Goals (SDGs); goal 5.5 aims to "Ensure women's full and effective participation and equal opportunities for leadership at all levels of decision-making in political, economic, and public life" (UN, 2015). Furthermore, the recognition and celebration of women's contributions to health is one that a growing number of woman medics, academics, and practitioners feel a personal commitment to, as evidenced by the creation of 25 Women in Global Health Chapters in many countries with more in the pipeline.

Since 2015, we have seen an influx of new gender equality and women's leadership initiatives in global health. We have better data on the international institutions of global health due to evidence gathering by academics, most notably the Global Health 50/50 project which published its first global report in 2018 and the Gender Equity Hub in the Global Health Workforce Network in 2017. In addition, the inaugural annual Women Leaders in Global Health Conference held at Stanford University in the United States in 2017 and the subsequent WomenLift Health programme started in 2020 have also drawn attention to the importance of women's representation within global health leadership. The initiation of the #LancetWomen Series on women in science, medicine, and global health has drawn significant attention to these issues (Lancet, 2019).

Beyond "Balance" and Parity

Many barriers to entry, progression, and leadership for women within the realm of global health remain. But theorising about women's leadership has always been greater than the counting of bodies within positions of power or balancing out men's and women's involvement (the issue of leadership among non-binary people is rarely raised). There are many questions, still unanswered, about the meaning and purpose of women's leadership.

Both instrumental and social justice arguments have been put forward to justify a focus on women's leadership in global health. Downs et al. (2014) argue that the field of global health exists to reduce health inequalities, and that women have been shown to be more effective than men in this regard. Others have argued that there is a knock-on benefit that would be accrued by changes in governance that place women in the driving seat. When women are in the driving seat, they are more likely to take into account:

> [W]omen's roles in production and reproduction and their dual roles as consumers and providers of health care, which affect all domains of sustainable development - societal, environmental, and economical. [...] when women are valued, enabled, and empowered in each of these domains, gender equality and health can be achieved; and when women are healthy and have equity in all aspects of life, sustainable development will be possible. (Langer et al., 2015, p. 1167)

Equity is a matter of justice, of course, and may even have some cost benefit. However, the fundamental shifts in power dynamics in the health labour market that would be created by gender parity also constitute an opportunity for change in the way that we "do" global health. Conversations about women's leadership have become more critical of models of global leadership which privilege and highlight the role of elite, white women from high-income countries.

In their paper, Downs et al. (2014, p. 3) describe the trajectory of academic women leaders:

> The training pathway for academic global health typically begins with an advanced graduate degree (MD, PhD, MPH, etc.) followed by postdoctoral field work and, ultimately, a career in academia, government, multilateral, or nongovernmental organizations.

This description describes a particular subset of women leaders who occupy the popular imagination. There are many women for whom a tertiary education is unattainable because of socio-economic status and/or the gendered, homophobic, ableist, and racial hierarchies which privilege some scholars over others. This description also underplays the influence of thought leaders outside the formal academe and women leading in spheres of global health where academic qualifications matter less than other skills and knowledge.

The majority of care-giving takes place within the household and the community, particularly in settings where formal health services are physically or financially unattainable—for rural communities living in low-income countries or working-class communities in settings like the United States where free health care is limited.

No country in the world currently remunerates women for this care burden in the home, although some have formalised community-level duties through community health worker programmes which are formally considered part of the health system. It has been argued that these workers play a key interface role between communities and the health sector and are positioned to understand and act on the gendered social determinants of health (Theobald et al., 2015); however, professional hierarchies and social and cultural norms which undermine the importance of women's caring role mean that their contribution is under-reported as a leadership function. There has been a groundswell of research and advocacy on women's unpaid care among feminist economists and those that took a more political economy approach to the topic (Esplen, 2009; Oxfam, 2020). Our understanding of the realms of global health is gradually being expanded to include the household and the community and the women who labour and lead there.

As a field, our notion of who leads or is considered a leader has been influenced by a growing belief in the importance of critical race theory, most notably Crenshaw's theorising about intersectionality (Zeinali et al., 2019), and attempts to decolonise global health (Green, 2019; Pai, 2019). This movement highlights the need for representation from different geographical locations. In 2020 large Black Lives Matter demonstrations, which were spearheaded in the United States but resonated beyond its borders, have led to a racial reckoning in many global health institutions, including those that work on women's empowerment and leadership (Women Deliver, 2020; IWHC, 2020).

The Definition of Global Health Influences How We Consider Leadership

What constitutes women's leadership in global health is dependent on how global health is defined. Beaglehole and Bonita (2010, p. 1) have argued that "global health is collaborative trans-national research and action for promoting health for all". More detail is provided in Kaplan et al.'s theorising:

> Global health is an area for study, research, and practice that places a priority on improving health and achieving equity in health for all people worldwide. Global health emphasises transnational health issues, determinants, and solutions; involves many disciplines within and beyond the health sciences and promotes interdisciplinary collaboration; and is a synthesis of population-based prevention with individual-level clinical care. (Koplan et al., 2009, p. 1995)

The term global health conjures up positive images of nations working together (through research and the provision of services) to tackle common health concerns. Yet the history of global health is far from straightforward, and its mandate remains contested leading to differing priorities and frames for analysing what success or leadership in this realm might look like. Global health's roots stretch back to the field of "Tropical Medicine" with its focus on support to colonial expansion, the health of the invading military and the protection of "trade", or the extraction of resources from the Global South to the Global North.

With the liberation and independence of many former colonies, Tropical Medicine morphed into International Health where there was more of a focus on improving health outcomes in low- and middle-income countries in support of economic development, often underpinned by paternalistic attitudes and the assumption that high-income countries are the sole owners of knowledge (Kickbusch, 2002). However, this movement was often a form of self-interest which reflected the desire of high-income countries to protect themselves from the effects of cross-border movement of ill-health (Brown et al., 2006).

Global health is in part a reaction to the increased interdependence that was wrought through processes of globalisation and became a more common frame for transnational work on health from the early 2000s onwards. It shifted norms of governance to be more representative of all countries and distributed leadership across regions and levels, with a focus on local responses given the transnational nature of ill-health and disease. As Abimbola (2019) puts it:

> It is almost certain that local output is much more consequential, if only because sustainable progress in global health is homegrown, with local processes being responsible for much historical improvements in global health outcomes and equity... (p. 2)

Global health, with its emphasis on interdependencies and equitable systems and institutions, may appear a more fruitful realm for women's leadership which takes class, race, and geography into account. However, global health is a sector still dominated by northern voices and elites who hold disproportionate power to set global agendas on behalf of the majority world (Sheikh et al., 2016).

The institutions of global health are shaped by their historical trajectories where a focus on women's empowerment, gender equity, and equality is a fairly recent phenomenon. Writing in 2014 on the global goal setting exercises related to health, Shiffman (2014, p. 299) notes that the:

> [P]rocess may be privileging some issues whose backers are particularly adept at global lobbying and advocacy, while sidelining other issues whose backers lack such access or capacity. This is not to suggest that these are all examples of illegitimate uses of power - in several respects they may be vast improvements over past priority-setting processes and may offer voice to those who previously lacked expression. It is to suggest that these examples indicate that there is far more to global health decision-making than careful consideration of evidence, and a critical need to investigate how epistemic and normative power gets exercised in the global health field.

Benatar (2016, p. 601) argues that framings within global health are "characterized by an emphasis on individualism, freedom, philanthropy, and an economy dominated by market considerations, all of which give priority to monetary value and short-term interests in all aspects of life". Yet usually these power relations and associated political positions are rendered invisible by those who would rather not debate them (or who would prefer to keep current power structures intact), making contestation taboo (Forman, 2016).

Who Is a Leader? A Focus on Gender and Power

Attention to issues of power is vital in relation to women's leadership. Increasing the number of women in leadership positions, or creating more common acknowledgement of the leadership that they already play, is a laudable goal. However, for many women the idea of being subsumed into institutions and systems that have been created through inequity and perpetuate (however unobtrusively) norms and behaviours that uphold the current status quo is distasteful.

Understanding that global health was not constructed with their equal inclusion in mind, some women leaders decide to conduct their work outside the formal academic, governance, and medical institutions that make up the global health world. Sensibly and yet bravely, they would rather be outside metaphorically throwing stones or building a new way of understanding health and well-being. Others are reshaping these institutions from the inside, or as outsiders offering critical allyship holding powerful actors in the global health sector to account. Still others choose (or are forced) to journey down more traditional leadership paths, conforming to masculine notions and stereotypes of what makes a good leader.

For those of us who aspire to take on leadership, what might this leadership look like? How might women's leadership be of use to the field of global health? And how can current leadership structures be challenged or changed to become more inclusive and sensitive to gender and power relations?

As with the term global health, there are differing definitions of what constitutes leadership. Ford's (2005, p. 245) feminist analysis of leadership definitions found that many definitions associated leadership with traditionally masculine traits such as "individualism, control, assertiveness, and dominance"—logic was lauded and emotion downplayed. Simultaneously, these traits were considered to be gender neutral. Ford notes that over time understandings of leadership have shifted so that they are less about personal qualities and more about transformation and inclusion.

Towards Gender Transformative Leadership

The notion of transformational leadership was first described by James MacGregor Burns in 1978. In the original framework created by Burns, transformational leaders were described as working to change the system, being visionary and inspirational, and working to improve their team's capabilities and work capacities.

Gender transformative leadership is leadership which seeks to address gender inequities in power which perpetuate and reinforce inequities across different systems and structures of oppression. Keeling et al. (2018, p. 2) described it as follows:

> Gender transformative leadership is driven by the vision of gender equality and women's rights embodied in international conventions and agreements including SDG 5 and addresses social and cultural norms, conscious and unconscious bias, and deep-rooted structures of inequality. Rather than expecting women to 'lean in' to professions and organisations that have largely excluded them from leadership and senior roles, gender transformative leadership addresses discrimination, bias, and inequities in the system so women are included on an equal basis to men. The term 'gender transformative' can be applied to decision makers, the institutions they work in, and to the health system itself.

Women in Global Health's conceptualisation of gender transformative leadership contains the following qualities (ibid); it:

- Is grounded in a vision of gender equality and women's rights.
- Challenges privilege and imbalances in power to eliminate gendered inefficiencies and rights deficiencies that undermine global health.
- Is intersectional, addressing social and personal characteristics that intersect with gender (race, ethnicity, etc.) to create multiple disadvantages. In global health, gender transformative leadership would drive equal participation of all genders from all geographies.

- Is imperative for leaders from all genders, not a leadership approach for women only.
- Applies to leadership at all levels in global health from the community to the global.
- Recognises different forms of leadership, such as thought leadership, which are not based on simple hierarchy and people management.
- Allows for different starting points and contexts but prioritises inclusion of the most marginalised and excluded.
- Assumes that gender equality = smarter global health and that gender transformative leadership is necessary for the achievement of all global goals in health, including the SDGs.

Within global health, those who seek to be gender transformative leaders aim to leave no one behind not only in access to health but also in leadership and decision-making.

If women's leadership is characterised, not just as the achievement of parity of numbers of women in decision-making positions, but as a set of normative beliefs and actions which aim to transform the global health sector from the bottom up, then it constitutes an exciting and energising opportunity for positive change. Some authors have argued that having more women in leadership positions will lead to global health solutions which are gender responsive (Dhatt et al., 2017). The desires to both better understand women's leadership in global health and nurture greater gender transformative leadership were the starting point for this book.

About This Book

For all that we currently know about women's leadership in global health, there are many questions that remain unanswered. Why has women's leadership been so elusive in a field that is so heavily reliant on women's labour? What are some of the barriers that prevent women "rising to the top" or being recognised for their endeavours in this field? How can norms, institutions, and systems that prevent equity be changed for the better? How have women made it to leadership positions and what advice can they provide? What does it mean, if anything, to have more women in power? Will women's leadership lead to transformation and the realisation of rights, or will it herald more of the same? How can we foster gender transformative leadership?

This book sheds some light on these issues. The chapters in this book reflect learning from a range of country settings including Ireland, India, Indonesia, Kenya, Somaliland, and Uganda.

This book brings together the experiences and testimonies of a wide range of women leaders in global health from around the world. The interviews we have conducted with women leaders explore the experiences of women from Argentina, Australia, Bangladesh, Botswana, Ethiopia, Germany, India, Kenya, Peru, Saudi Arabia, the United Kingdom, and the United States. In practice, all the women profiled here have had very different trajectories and performed different functions in their global health service.

While it is not possible to reflect the experiences and voices of all women in one book, we have taken some care to ensure that no single region dominates the analysis and that the viewpoints of authors and interviewees from a range of backgrounds, professions, and disciplines are included. Chapters in the book are focused on individuals, institutions, national health systems, and the international architecture of global health; they cover topics as diverse as leadership in a matriarchal context, peace and security, the introduction of comprehensive sex education in schools, and the challenges experienced by community health workers.

Origins of the Book

Inspired by a thought leadership dialogue at the American Public Health Association Annual Conference entitled, "Is leaning in enough?: The role of intersectionality, gender and public health leadership", a lead editor from Springer approached Women in Global Health to consider writing a book on this topic for an audience of academics, researchers, policy-makers, administrators, students, practitioners in public health and global health disciplines. In scoping the field, Women in Global Health was unsurprised to see that there remained a glaring gap in capturing the complexities of women in global health leadership, specifically through a lens of power and privilege. The vision for this book was developed with Research in Gender and Ethics (RinGs): Building Stronger Health Systems, a consortium to stimulate new research on gender and health systems. A range of authors were invited to contribute to this groundbreaking collection that explores the leadership roles of women and unpacks the power dynamics at play in global health at all levels.

The editors of the book are drawn from Australia, Canada, India, Pakistan, the United Kingdom, and the United States.

Rosemary Morgan, PhD, is a gender expert and researcher at Johns Hopkins Bloomberg School of Public Health. She is originally from Canada and identifies as Caucasian, middle class, cis, she/her, and able-bodied. She grew up in a low- to middle-class family and worked from a young age to contribute to the family. She owes a lot of her success to her mother's emphasis on education and determination.

Kate Hawkins is a research communications expert with technical expertise in health, gender, and international development. She is the founder and Director of Pamoja Communications Ltd. She is an atheist, British, bisexual, cis, single, childless, chronically ill, white, middle-aged, and a middle-class homeowner. Class consciousness and internationalism were instilled in her by her parents, who are left-wing organisers, and her grandparents, who were solidly working class.

Sulzhan Bali, PhD, is a public health specialist with the World Bank with technical expertise in health security, and its intersection with one health and gender, and health systems strengthening in low-income and fragile countries. She is a member of Women in Global Health's Washington, DC Chapter. Sulzhan is a woman of colour, cis, she/her, and able-bodied and holds Indian citizenship. Growing up in Northern India—where women still face a multitude of socio-cultural and economic challenges—she has had to defy gender stereotypes at every step of her career.

Sulzhan completed her doctorate in Molecular Biology with the Medical Research Council (MRC) and holds degrees from Duke University (MSc Global Health), the University of Manchester (MSc Virology), and the University of Delhi (BSc Microbiology). In her spare time, Sulzhan likes to paint and write poetry on various development challenges—including women's issues.

Roopa Dhatt, MD, is a practising internist in Washington, DC, USA, trained in international health, and a global health and gender advocate. She is the Executive Director and Co-Founder of Women in Global Health. She grew up with pluralities and identifies as Indian-American immigrant, raised by her grandparents, while her parents worked multiple jobs. She is a woman of colour, cis, she/her, and able-bodied. She is Sikh and Punjabi and considers herself a global citizen, while holding a dual US Citizenship and Non-Resident Indian Citizenship. She grew up in lower socio-economic racially and ethnically diverse lower- to middle-class neighbour-hoods, being exposed to higher socio-economic realities later in life, in higher edu-cation. She was influenced by the civil rights movement in the United States, inspiring her to pursue sociological studies, including majoring in African American and African Studies. She is supported by her family to pursue her advocacy work.

Mehr Manzoor is a Fulbright Scholar from Pakistan and a PhD candidate at Tulane University in the Department of Health Policy and Management. She identi-fies herself as a Muslim, Punjabi, cis, she/her, and able-bodied. Her research focuses on developing a conceptual framework to measure gender inequality regimes in global health organisations. She is passionate about gender equality, intersectional-ity, and women's leadership in global health and beyond and has several publica-tions on these topics. She owes a lot of her success to her parents, whom she lost as a young adult a decade ago, but their teachings and values remain the main pillars of her life.

Cheryl Overs is an Australian woman currently working in academia at Monash University. She is the founder of the Prostitutes Collective of Victoria, the Scarlet Alliance in Australia, and the Global Network of Sex Work Projects. She is a mother, a carer to her own mother, and a prominent leader in the world of HIV. Her contribu-tion to human rights was recognised when her portrait by the Chinese artist Ai Weiwei was exhibited with other prominent Australian human rights activists at the National Gallery of Victoria.

Chapters

A diverse range of chapters within this book highlight different aspects of women's leadership in global health. Claire Somerville uses the feminist concept of gendered institutions to analyse how labour is divided in global health. Her starting position is that global health and its constituent networks and institutions are gendered enti-ties acting within a neoliberal environment, which helps explain why and how they are ordered. Her work helps explain why popular mechanisms to promote gender parity found within gender mainstreaming approaches can become co-opted and defanged by patriarchal institutions.

Yara M. Asi provides an analysis of the relationships between women's empowerment and peace and health. This chapter contributes to the emerging literature base about women leaders in global health and security.

Within academia, publishing in peer-reviewed journals is key to success and promotion and a pathway to leadership. Jamie Lundine, Ivy Lynn Bourgeault, and Dina Balabanova analyse the academic publishing sector, its systems, and the roles of editors and reviewers in supporting or undermining gender equity, and offer recommendations for change.

The chapter by Kui Muraya analyses the use and utility of the two-thirds rule which is applied to governance mechanisms in Kenya. This quota system is intended to support gender parity in decision-making and "no more than two-thirds of the members of public elective or appointive bodies shall be of the same gender". Using research conducted in Coastal Kenya that looked at the career trajectories and experiences of health leaders using a gender lens, she demonstrates that quotas can be a double-edged sword.

The tension between claiming a place in the existing (unjust) power structures, subverting these structures and the vexed nature of leadership are explored by Devaki Nambiar, Gloria Benny, and Hari Sankar in their chapter on Kerala, India. They conclude that there is everyday resistance to playing by the rules but nevertheless this falls short of more radical feminist praxis among women leaders.

The chapter by Ann Nolan gives us a whistle-stop historical overview of the career of Irish politician Mary O'Rourke. O'Rourke rose through the political ranks of the Fianna Fáil party to become Minister of Education. The chapter charts her journey to power and her success in overhauling Ireland's sex education provisions, which were influenced by socio-political transformation in Ireland following membership in the EU, the global AIDS crisis, and the enduring cultural and political influence of the Catholic Church.

Stella Bakibinga, Elizabeth Bakibinga, John Daniel Ibembe, and Pauline Bakibinga reflect on mechanisms to narrow the gender employment and representation gap in global health in sub-Saharan Africa. They call for better laws, policies, and implementation to address inequity, improve mentoring and role modelling for younger women, remove institutional blocks, and have better access to resources and work to address harmful gender norms.

The issue of safeguarding in international development comes under scrutiny in a chapter by Cheryl Overs and Kate Hawkins. They describe the origins of the current push for safeguarding measures and explore (through the lens of sex work) how potential restrictions on women's sexual autonomy in low- and middle-income countries may affect their ability to access leadership positions.

Leadership in health systems is the focus of the chapter by Zahra Zeinali, more specifically at the national level where policy-making and priority setting happens, the sub-national level where policy is implemented, and the operational level among health workers and communities. She identifies gender stereotypes and biases, occupational segregation, pay gaps, dual burdens of professional work and childcare or household chores, and women's lack of access to resources as factors that inhibit gender responsive health systems.

Manasee Mishra and co-authors Barun Kanjilal and Dilip Ghosh provide an exploration of the ways that India's large cadre of mainly female community health or outreach workers are denied access to opportunities for progression to leadership positions. An exploration of the historical, socio-economic, and health system barriers to leadership is counterposed with recommendations for change.

Drawing our attention to the managerial and administrative elements of global health, Nuzulul Kusuma Putri describes how the "glass ceiling" operates in two provinces of the Indonesian health sector—one culturally matriarchal (West Sumatra) and the other patriarchal (East Java). Using position reviews, she analysed promotion processes within District Health Offices and in both provinces found a wide gap in promotion probability between male and female health officers which was not explained by lack of technical competence or merit on the part of women.

In their study from Uganda and Somaliland, Summer Simpson and Raquel Pérez Cañal diagnose how gender discrimination manifests and is experienced among male and female health facility managers, clinical staff, academics, and policy-makers at the personal, institutional, and system level. Their aim is to identify positive stories that might inform strategies for improvement.

For too long the solutions to increasing women in leadership included assertiveness training, mentoring, advice on power dressing, and voice coaching—in short, fixing women to fit into organisations and cultures built by and for men. In the final chapter, Ann Keeling and Roopa Dhatt bring to a close the key themes explored in this book and offer a vision for challenging power and privilege in global health leadership and transforming global health to be gender equitable and, therefore, fit for women.

Interviews

Interspersed with our more traditional chapters, we have included interviews with a range of women leaders in global health from a diversity of backgrounds and settings, to shine a light on the experiences and explore different career trajectories of diverse women leaders. Later on in the book the paths to leadership for these women leaders are summarised.

Soumya Swaminathan, India

Soumya Swaminathan is currently the Chief Scientist at the World Health Organization. She is an Indian paediatrician and clinical scientist recognised for her extensive research on tuberculosis and HIV. From October 2017 to March 2019, she was the Deputy Director-General of Programs at the WHO. She served as the Secretary to the Government of India for Health Research and Director-General of the Indian Council of Medical Research from 2015 to 2017. From 2009 to 2011, she also served as Coordinator of the UNICEF/UNDP/World Bank/WHO Special Programme for Research and Training in Tropical Diseases in Geneva.

Matshidiso Moeti, Botswana

Matshidiso Moeti is the first woman to be elected as WHO Regional Director for Africa. She joined the WHO Regional Office for Africa in 1999 and has served as Deputy Regional Director, Assistant Regional Director, Director of Noncommunicable Diseases, WHO Representative for Malawi, Coordinator of the Inter-Country Support Team for the South and East African countries, and Regional Advisor for HIV/AIDS. Before joining WHO, Moeti worked with the Joint United Nations Programme on HIV/AIDS (UNAIDS) as team leader of the Africa and Middle East desk in Geneva (1997–1999); with the United Nations Children's Fund (UNICEF) as regional health advisor for East and Southern Africa; and with Botswana's Ministry of Health as a clinician and public health specialist. Moeti holds a degree in medicine (MB, BS) and a Master of Public Health degree (MSc in community health for developing countries) from the Royal Free Hospital School of Medicine, the University of London, and the London School of Hygiene & Tropical Medicine, respectively.

Ana Langer, United States

Ana Langer is originally from Argentina and works as a physician specialising in paediatrics and neonatology and in reproductive health. She joined the Harvard T.H. Chan School of Public Health in July 2010 as a Professor of the Practice of Public Health in the Department of Global Health and Population. For more than 30 years, she has been a leading researcher, programmer, and advocate for the improvement of women's health.

Patricia Garcia, Peru

Patricia Garcia is a Professor at the School of Public Health at Cayetano Heredia University (UPCH) in Lima, Peru. She is the former Minister of Health of Peru, Dean of the School of Public Health at UPCH, and former Chief of the Peruvian National Institute of Health (INS). She has been member of the PAHO Foundation Technical Advisory Group (FTAG), board member of the Consortium of Universities for Global Health, and President of the Latin American Association Against STDs (ALACITS).

Sabina Faiz Rashid, Bangladesh

Sabina Faiz Rashid is Bangladeshi and joined the BRAC James P Grant School of Public Health, BRAC University, in 2004 and was appointed as Dean in 2013. She specialises in ethnographic and qualitative research. Her research interests are gender, sexual, and reproductive health and rights; sexuality and the well-being of adolescents, young women, and men; use of social media/digital technology; changing gender relationships; power dynamics; human rights; urban poverty; governance; and health services in urban informal settlements.

Ilona Kickbusch, Germany

Ilona Kickbusch is a German political scientist best known for her contribution to health promotion and global health. Ilona has had a distinguished career with the World Health Organization (WHO), at both regional and global levels, where she led the Global Health Promotion Programme and initiated the Ottawa Charter for Health Promotion. Previously, she served as the Director of the Global Health Centre at the Graduate Institute of International and Development Studies, Geneva, and led Yale University's Global Health Program (1998–2003). She is a member of WHO's Independent High-Level Commission.

Sameera Al Tuwaijri, Saudi Arabia

Sameera Al Tuwaijri is the global lead on population and development at the health, nutrition, and population global practice of the World Bank. She is a board-certified OB/GYN who had over 10 years of experience in clinical practice before she embarked on studying public health. She earned a master's in public health from Harvard University and a doctorate in health policy and completed a post-doctoral fellowship at Johns Hopkins University. Prior to joining the World Bank in 2010, she was the Regional Adviser, Reproductive Health Policy for the United Nations Population Fund, Arab States, and the Director of the International Labour Organization's programme on public health and safety and served as the first Regional Director, Arab States, UN Women.

Juno Roche, Spain

Juno Roche is a writer and campaigner whose work is around gender, sexuality, and trans lives. She studied Fine Art and Philosophy at Brighton and English Literature at Sussex, and writes for a wide range of publications, including *Bitch Magazine*, *Dazed*, *Vice*, *Broadly*, *Cosmopolitan*, the *i*, *i-D*, the *Independent*, the *Tate Magazine*, and *Refinery29*. She co-founded Trans Workers UK and the Trans Teachers Network. She received the National Union of Teacher's Blair Peach Award for outstanding contribution to equality. She was born in the United Kingdom and is now living in the mountains of Andalusia, Spain. Juno's first book, *Queer Sex*, was published in

2018. Her second book, *Trans Power*, was published in 2019. She is a Trustee of the Sophia Forum which promotes and advocates for the rights, health, welfare, and dignity of women living with HIV through research, raising awareness, and influencing policy.

Penina Ochola-Odhiambo, Kenya

Penina Ochola-Odhiambo has over 30 years of extensive cross-cultural public health experience in Eastern and Southern Africa working in diverse socio-cultural settings. She holds a diploma in advanced nursing from the University of Nairobi and a master of Public Health degree from the Harvard T.H. Chan School of Public Health and has received a PhD from Great Lakes University of Kisumu. Previously, she was the Country Director of African Medical and Research Foundation (AMREF) in South Africa; Director of Primary Health Care for AMFREF; Regional Health Advisor for PLAN International for Eastern and Southern Africa; Country Director for FHI/AIDSCAP in Tanzania; and the Dean of the School of Nursing at the Great Lakes University of Kisumu.

Poonam Khetrapal Singh, India

Poonam Khetrapal Singh is the Regional Director of the WHO South-East Asia Region (SEARO). She is currently serving her second 5-year term in office following unanimous reelection by SEARO's 11 member states in September 2018. Khetrapal Singh is an Indian national and the first woman to hold the post. She served as WHO Deputy Regional Director for SEARO from 2000 to 2013 and prior to that was a civil servant in India as a member of the Indian Administrative Services. This included roles as both Joint-Secretary and Secretary of Health in the state of Punjab. She has also served as the WHO Executive Director, Sustainable Development and Healthy Environments Cluster, and a member of the Director-General's Cabinet, and worked with the World Bank as part of the Health, Population, and Nutrition Practice.

Senait Fisseha, Ethiopia/United States

Born in Ethiopia, Senait Fisseha is a leading global health advocate, a reproductive endocrinology and infertility academic at the University of Michigan, and the Director of International Programs at the Susan Buffett Foundation. Senait is known for her work as an advocate for global reproductive health, rights, and gender equality. She is the founder of the Center for International Reproductive Health Training

(CIRHT) at the University of Michigan, and she chaired and led the election campaign of Tedros Adhanom, the first African Director-General of the World Health Organization, from 2016 to 2017.

Cheryl Overs, Australia

Cheryl Overs is a Senior Research Fellow at the Michael Kirby Centre for Public Health and Human Rights at Monash University in Melbourne, Australia. She is known for her work in promoting sex workers' rights. She founded the Prostitutes Collective of Victoria, Scarlet Alliance Australia, and the Global Network of Sex Work Projects. She worked as an early advisor to the Global Program on AIDS at the World Health Organization. In 2011–2012 she was a member of the Technical Advisory Group of the Global Commission on HIV and the Law, and in 2012 she delivered a plenary speech at the International AIDS Conference in Washington, DC.

Conclusion

When we began to develop this book, we were excited that it would be launched in 2020—a year that signified a historic moment for gender equality and women's rights. It would be 25 years since the Beijing Declaration and 10 years since the start of UN Women. But instead we are publishing this book in the midst of the COVID-19 pandemic (our exact immediate and longer-term futures are unknown).

A time that was meant to be spent in contemplation and celebration of progress and challenges on the road to equity has instead been one of emergency, tragedy, and disruption which has hit the poorest and the most marginalised the hardest. The pandemic has not only illuminated and magnified existing inequities—gender and otherwise—it has also made evident the important role of global health leadership and the fact that status quo is no longer working.

The pandemic has proven to be highly gendered, with women, men, and people of other genders impacted disproportionately (Wenham et al., 2020a). Men and women healthcare workers are being predominately impacted by the immediate short-term effects of the pandemic (mortality among men is higher than women, and women healthcare workers are being disproportionately infected) (Baker et al., 2020). However, women are also differentially affected by the secondary, longer-term, social, economic, and health impacts of the pandemic, including financial insecurity, increased domestic violence, increased care-giving responsibilities, and reduction of sexual and reproductive health services, not to mention the long-term negative consequences on women's career progression (Wenham et al., 2020b). The effect of the pandemic on non-binary and trans people is often missing from the discussion altogether.

The pandemic is extremely gendered, and it would make sense that the leadership responsible for responding to the pandemic not only has diverse representation but also takes into account these gendered effects. However, this has not been the case. Men continue to dominate both public and academic discourse and decision-making about COVID-19 (Chatfield et al., 2020). In a widely circulated infographic from Women in Global Health about COVID-19 decision-making, the numbers are stark: women make up only 10% of the representatives on the US Coronavirus Task Force, 20% of the WHO Emergency Committee on COVID-19, and 16% of the WHO-China joint mission on COVID-19, despite women accounting for 70% of the global health workforce on the frontlines (Women in Global Health, 2020). As Wenham et al. (2020a) state:

> Given their front-line interaction with communities, it is concerning that women have not been fully incorporated into global health security surveillance, detection, and prevention mechanisms. Women's socially prescribed care roles typically place them in a prime position to identify trends at the local level that might signal the start of an outbreak and thus improve global health security. Although women should not be further burdened, particularly considering much of their labour during health crises goes underpaid or unpaid, incorporating women's voices and knowledge could be empowering and improve outbreak preparedness and response.

Indeed, when a group is not adequately represented at the table, it less likely that their needs will be prioritised and met (Bali et al., 2020).

How can we expect that the needs of women, non-binary people, and trans people will be met during and after the pandemic if they are not adequately represented within decision-making bodies? COVID-19 has shown us that the need for a gender transformative leadership approach is pressing.

Sometimes moments of radical change provide a shift in the everyday ways of doing things. Perhaps with this pandemic we have a chance to shift global health to become a system that better meets the needs of the poorest and most marginalised and indeed values these people within its decision-making structures. Perhaps it will be less of a shift and more of a rupture brought about by those no longer willing to accept their exclusion and degradation.

We hope that within the pages of this book you will find information, inspiration, and hope for how you can play a part in changing systems that no longer serve us well: information about women's leadership experiences, inspiration from women leaders themselves, and hope for leadership systems and structures which are more equitable and just—leadership which places the most marginalised at the centre and purposefully works towards positive change.

References

Abimbola, S. (2019). The foreign gaze: Authorship in academic global health. *BMJ Global Health, 4*, e002068.

Baker, P., et al. (2020). Men's health: COVID-19 pandemic highlights need for overdue policy action. *Lancet, 395*(10241), 1886–1888.

Bali, S., et al. (2020). Off the back burner: Diverse and gender-inclusive decision-making for COVID-19 response and recovery. *BMJ Global Health, 5*, e002595.

Beaglehole, R., & Bonita, R. (2010). What is global health? *Global Health Action, 3.* https://doi.org/10.3402/gha.v3i0.5142

Benatar, S. (2016). Politics, power, poverty and global health: Systems and frames. *International Journal of Health Policy and Management, 5*(10), 599–604.

Brown, T. M., et al. (2006). The World Health Organization and the transition from "International" to "Global" Public Health. *American Journal of Public Health, 96*(1), 62–72. https://www.ncbi.nlm.nih.gov/pmc/articles/PMC1470434/

Chatfield, C., et al. (2020). Where are the women experts on covid-19? Mostly missing, *BMJ Blogs.* Retrieved from https://blogs.bmj.com/bmj/2020/06/25/where-are-the-women-experts-on-covid-19-mostly-missing/?utm_campaign=shareaholic&utm_medium=twitter&utm_source=socialnetwork

Dhatt, R., et al. (2017). The role of women's leadership and gender equity in leadership and health system strengthening. *Global Health, Epidemiology and Genomics, 2,* E8. https://doi.org/10.1017/gheg.2016.22

Downs, J. A., et al. (2014). Increasing women in leadership in global health. *Academic Medicine, 89*(8), 1103–1107. https://www.ncbi.nlm.nih.gov/pmc/articles/PMC4167801/

Esplen, E. (2009). *Supporting care givers without reinforcing gender roles.* BRIDGE Cutting Edge Pack.

Ford, J. (2005). Examining leadership through critical feminist readings. *Journal of Health Organization and Management, 19*(3), 236–251. https://doi.org/10.1108/14777260510608961

Forman, L. (2016). The Ghost is the machine: How can we visibilize the unseen norms and power of global health? *International Journal of Health Policy and Management, 5*(3), 197–199.

Global Health 50/50. (2020). *Global Health 50/50 Report.* Retrieved from https://globalhealth5050.org/2020Report/

Green A. (2019). *The activists trying to "decolonize" global health.* Retrieved from https://www.devex.com/news/the-activists-trying-to-decolonize-global-health-94904

IWHC. (2020). *IWHC board statement regarding independent reviews.* Retrieved from https://iwhc.org/press-releases/iwhc-board-statement-regarding-independent-reviews/

Keeling, A., et al. (2018). *Gender transformative leadership: A new vision for leadership in global health, women in global health.* Retrieved from https://c8fbe10e-fb87-47e7-844b-4e700959d2d4.filesusr.com/ugd/ffa4bc_5f193fb461714a27a87aafbf3a8828bb.pdf

Kickbusch, I. (2002) *Global health—A definition.* Retrieved from http://www.ilonakickbusch.com/kickbusch-wAssets/docs/global-health.pdf

Koplan, J. L., et al. (2009). Towards a common definition of global health. *Lancet, 373,* 1993–1995. http://www.thelancet.com/journals/lancet/article/PIIS0140-6736(09)60332-9/fulltext

Lancet. (2019). *Launch of The Lancet's theme issue on women in science, medicine, and global health.* Retrieved from https://www.thelancet.com/lancet-women/launch

Langer, A., et al. (2015). Women and Health: The key for sustainable development. *The Lancet, 386*(9999), 1165–1210. http://www.thelancet.com/journals/lancet/article/PIIS0140-6736(15)60497-4/fulltext

Oxfam. (2020). *Time to care: Unpaid and underpaid care work and the global inequality crisis.* Oxford, UK. Retrieved from https://oxfamibis.dk/sites/default/files/media/pdf_global/denmark_pdf/rapport_time-to-care-inequality-200120-embargo-en.pdf

Pai, M. (2019). *Global health still mimics colonial ways: Here's how to break the pattern.* Retrieved from http://theconversation.com/global-health-still-mimics-colonial-ways-heres-how-to-break-the-pattern-121951

Sheikh, K., Bennett, S. C., el Jardali, F., & Gotsadze, G. (2016). Privilege and inclusivity in shaping Global Health agendas. *Health Policy and Planning, 32*(3), 303–304.

Shiffman, J. (2014). Knowledge, moral claims and the exercise of power in global health. *International Journal of Health Policy and Management, 3*(6), 297–299.

Theobald, S., et al. (2015). Close to community health providers post 2015: Realising their role in responsive health systems and addressing gendered social determinants of health. *BMC Proceedings, 9*(Suppl 10), S8. https://bmcproc.biomedcentral.com/articles/10.1186/1753-6561-9-S10-S8#B49

UN. (2015). *Sustainable development goals.* Retrieved from https://sustainabledevelopment. un.org/?menu=1300

Wenham, C., et al. (2020a). COVID-19: The gendered impacts of the outbreak. *The Lancet, 395*(10227), 846–848. https://www.thelancet.com/article/S0140-6736(20)30526-2/fulltext

Wenham, C., et al. (2020b). Women are most affected by pandemics—Lessons from past outbreaks. *Nature, 583,* 194–198.

Women Deliver. (2020). *Statement from board of directors on women deliver's transformation.* Retrieved from https://womendeliver.org/press/statement-from-board-of-directors-on-women-delivers-transformation/

Women in Global Health. (2014). *300 Women Leaders in Global Health (#WGH300). Prof Ilona Kickbusch.* Graduate Institute.

Women in Global Health. (2020). *OPERATION 50/50: Women's perspectives save lives.* Retrieved from https://www.womeningh.org/operation-50-50

World Health Organization. (2019). *Delivered by women, led by men: A gender and equity analysis of the global health and social workforce.* Geneva. Retrieved from https://www.who.int/hrh/resources/health-observer24/en/

Zeinali, Z., et al. (2019). Intersectionality and global health leadership: Parity is not enough. *Human Resources for Health, 17,* 29.

Gendered Institutions in Global Health

Claire Somerville

Introduction

Over-representation of women in the frontline healthcare sector and under-representation in health leadership reflects many gendered drivers, including norms and roles that have shaped the division of labour in the health workforce. But to what extent are the institutions and systems that house these unbalanced representations in themselves gendered?

This chapter adopts a feminist concept of gendered institutions (Acker, 1990, 1992, 2006) to analyse gender stratifications and the division of labour across the global health landscape. Entwined with the gendering of the processes and practices of the work and function of these institutions are pervasive hegemonic masculinities stemming from deep gendered stratifications in the organization of global health. The chapter argues that historically, institutions of international and global health have been organized along lines of gender and also other axes of privilege that have reproduced occupational patterns that have seen women predominate low-status care roles whilst men (of certain privilege) gravitate through "man-agerial" structures to roles of oversight and leadership, sustaining what Acker and others have conceptualized as inequality regimes (Acker, 2006; Risman & Davis, 2013). Being "stuck", as Rosabeth Kanter (1977) describes, at particular levels of large international organizations is a well-recognized phenomenon in organizations across all sectors. It is a known barrier in the United Nations (UN) system, prompting the establishment in 2012 of the UN System-wide Action Plan on Gender Equality and the Empowerment of Women that aims to drive progress with an annual accountability and monitoring framework. However, the question remains: do so-called

C. Somerville (✉)
Gender Centre, Graduate Institute of International and Development Studies,
Geneva, Switzerland
e-mail: claire.somerville@graduateinstitute.ch

© Springer Nature Switzerland AG 2022
R. Morgan et al. (eds.), *Women and Global Health Leadership*,
https://doi.org/10.1007/978-3-030-84498-1_2

enabling environments[1] disrupt the gender regimes, ideologies, practices, and symbols that go far deeper than the fixing of women and men and their unconscious bias at the level of the individual? Gender, argued by scholars of gendered institutions, is not only an individual attribute but also a major organizing system that structures patterns of interactions and expectations throughout and between organizations and their networks.[2]

Taking an institutional perspective facilitates a structural analysis of the gendered making of global health actors—often governed in multilateral or multi-stakeholder arrangements—that make visible the patching and fault lines of post-Beijing[3] approaches to institutional mainstreaming and their somewhat limited impact in transforming the global health workforce beyond its historical patriarchal pyramid.

Gendered Networks and Organizations

Historically, the delivery of health care at the frontline exhibits highly sex-selected divisions of labour with women as nurses and caregivers at the bedside and men as doctors, surgeons, and specialists. The early gendering of nursing as female is illustrated in the writing of Florence Nightingale when she observed, "every woman must at some time, or other of her life, become a nurse" (1860). The nursing role was in many ways seen as an extension of women's gendered social care role beyond the hospital. This care role contrasts with the professionalization of medicine in Europe from the late 1400s which was accompanied, during the nineteenth century, by the introduction of educational qualification, certification, and licensing, which structurally prohibited the entrance of women to the medical field. As such, women have since been clustered at the bottom of the medical hierarchy with lower salaries, precarious social protection, and narrowed career prospects.

The lesser place of women in society throughout the history and in the development of institutions of health care and medicine is an intractable challenge not only at the frontline, but as a pattern reproduced through health systems, processes,

---

[1] Understood here to be constructed through targets, parity goals, quotas, gender trainings, performance indicators, gender budgeting, monitoring, or any number of other gender mainstreaming technologies of governance (Prugl, 2011).

[2] The use of institutions and *their networks* is intentional. The politics and exercise of power in geopolitical constellations are shown in the literature to determine global health agendas and prioritizations (Shiffman et al., 2016; Shiffman & Smith, 2007, etc.), but to date no theorizing or evidence around the gendered dimensions, let alone the place of women, in such networks has been forthcoming. For this reason, I include as global health not only its institutions—old and new—but also the emergence of global health networks and their functioning that politically prioritize the global health agenda (Shiffman et al., 2015, 2016; Heller et al., 2019).

[3] At the Fourth United Nations World Conference on Women, 189 member states unanimously agreed the Beijing Declaration and Platform for Action that prioritized gender mainstreaming as a mechanism to achieve gender equality.

governance, ministries, and all the way through to modern-day global health institutions and networks. Whilst the composition of the medical and allied health professions has shifted in recent decades, the underlying girders of the organization of medicine and health remain gendered along patriarchal axes that typically place women in less well-rewarded care roles, and men in highly compensated and more powerful leadership positions.

More recently, the globalization of health beyond the nation state and towards the emergence of a network of institutions and sectors variously defined as global health actors has exposed the reproduction of the gendered hierarchies that stretch back in this history of health and medicine. The lack of women in the leadership of this new field of global health practice, power, and decision making has long since been observed (Doyal, 2002; Downs et al., 2014; Talib et al., 2017), and many "women-centred" arguments have been proffered to explain why this is the case, many of which perpetuate gendered assumptions around women and work. It is not the intention here to further substantiate these lines of argument but rather to examine the institutions and networks that maintain these gender regimes in global health.

Are Global Health Institutions and Processes Gendered?

During an interview in 2012, a senior member of the executive team of one of the newer global health actors explained how the organization was "gendered", by which was meant that it was gendered male just like medicine and global health. This was despite all number of measures in place across the full spectra of the organization from governance, statutes, policies, and everyday processes that had sought to proactively address gender inequity. Global health is networked, and, as further discussion suggested at the time, there was only so far any single organization in the landscape of actors that could act alone in the chain of global health partnerships. This insight resonates with a large literature on gendered organizations going back to the work of Joan Acker and the launch in 1994 of the journal *Gender, Work and Organization*. As an entry point to the intransigence of gender injustice in global health, this body of thinking enables us to move beyond the "women-centred" arguments that are often used to analyse "the problem of women" in global health, and move towards understanding the gendered dimension of health as a historical, economic, and politically constituted means of organizing and stratifying resources and capabilities.

When we examine global health and its networks and institutions as a priori gendered, we need to also clarify what is meant by the term "gendered". Gender has many meanings, but I argue here the perspective that gender is a concept of power and like all concepts of power—of which there are also many—it operates as a means of organizing, patterning, and ordering the world that is political, historical, economic, and social. As a concept of power, historically and to date, gendered relations of power have fed and sustained hegemonic patriarchal hierarchies.

The gendered hierarchies of global health are well-documented as issues of the sex division of labour, most notably in the (lack of) women leaders in global health, as the title of this book suggests. When we consider organizations as gendered, we seek to get beyond representation. It is an important leap to make that moves us from a corrective measures approach that often accompanies mainstreaming, to viewing the institutions and networks as units of analysis beyond composition of only its human resources. As Mastracci and Arreola (2016) note from a human resource management perspective, norms and practices based on stereotyped male and female workers persist beyond the changing compositions of a workforce and are rather stubbornly rooted in an organization's founding contexts. The history of medicine, international and global health, and its networks is thus significant.

Getting beyond representation towards deeply transformative and perhaps radical feminist thinking may take us beyond the current impasse to challenge the embedded hierarchies of power that are not only gendered but intersectionally stratified across the geopolitical landscape of medicine and global health. Further still, these gendered institutions of global health are not isolated from the wider global post-war economic order in which they are situated, but are entwined through global finance mechanisms, governance structures, and politicized funding streams in the neoliberal paradigm (Keshavjee, 2014). And as Nancy Frazer (2009) pointedly remarked, feminism in an age of neoliberalism is a dangerous liaison[4] where it risks becoming a handmaiden of capitalism.

Principal: Structure and Agency in the Neoliberal Global Health Landscape

There is a well-established literature on the neoliberalization[5] of global health (Keshavjee, 2014; Schrecker, 2016; Shakow et al., 2018; Bell & Green, 2016) that stretches far beyond the scope of this chapter; so too the feminist critiques of these neoliberal forces (Cornwall et al., 2008; Frazer, 2009; Goetz, 1997) that have shaped the post-Washington consensus (Bergeron, 2003) and even the "neoliberalization of feminism" (Prugl, 2014; Frazer, 2009) that promote individualistic solutions to gender oppression and advocate the "business case" of women's economic empowerment.

Whilst these are areas on which I shall reflect, with caution, towards the end of this chapter, I shall begin by re-examining the relevance of gendered organizations against which modern tools and techniques attempting to be gender transformative and even "disruptive" (Hay et al., 2019) are situated. A feminist gendered

---

[4] This line of argument is in reference to Fraser's theorizing on the globalizing financialized capitalism of the third regime of capitalism, the crisis of care, and role of "affective labour" and care work.

[5] The economic, political, and ideological neoliberalization of global health, it is argued, drives inequities.

organization approach renders visible the deep substructures against which neoliberal feminist activists have to function and which in fact may co-opt in producing veneers of non-substantive equality. The agency of actors, individual, and groups of women (and men), feminist or not, is inhibited by gendered structures of power.

Clinton and Sridhar's 2017 book-length case studies of the key global health actors adopt a principal-agent theorizing to examine the complex question of who governs global health. Although their analysis is not one that views organizations as a priori gendered, and nor do they gender the response to their core question, their assembled evidence coupled with my own fieldwork and participant observations of global health in what is so often described as the city of global health, International Geneva, during the past decade suggests that at least two approaches to the challenges of the gendered girders and regimes (Acker, 2006) in global health have evolved. Clinton and Sridhar's dichotomizing of the "traditional" and the "new" players with their very different networks of funding and governance relations to their *principals* (limited in their reading to member states) and *agents* (mainly, in their examples, secretariats) serve here to differentiate how these processes or technical fixes to gender have unfolded in global health institutions. Whilst the discussion in this chapter is not limited to the "old" and the "new" actors split used by Clinton and Sridhar, the different configurations of relations that institutions develop as agents with their principals (e.g. the World Health Organization (WHO) and its UN Member States and Executive Board, or Gavi, the Vaccine Alliance and its multi-stakeholder board) nevertheless determine the scope of gender responses that each organization can reasonably implement.

Transforming Gendered Organizations

The many institutions that comprise the global health landscape lay claim to policies of gender equality, mainstreaming, and other principles of gender audit.

The WHO provides an example of one of the approaches to addressing gender issues in global health. In 1995, the WHO's Director General (DG), Hiroshi Nakajima's Beijing statement focused almost entirely on women's health prioritization and, in particular, committed to addressing women's reproductive health, malnutrition, and violence against women. These priorities were later reflected in the structuring of the WHO with specific programmes to target these issues. As an organization operating by resolutions, a series of member state-agreed initiatives were introduced between 1997 and 2012 that took forward the Beijing agenda. These included the 1997 World Health Assembly (WHA) 50.16 Resolution on recruitment targets that were set to achieve parity by the close of the decade, and the 2003 WHA 60.25 Resolution to integrate gender resulting, the following year, in the publication of the Strategy for Integrating Gender Analysis and Actions into the work of the WHO, followed quickly in 2009 by WHA 62.14 Resolution that cemented gender as part of the new paradigm of thinking developed by the Commission on Social Determinants of Health.

Since 2014, the main activities around gender at the WHO (outside of women's health and human resource mainstreaming) have been housed under the unit for Gender, Equity, and Rights. As noted above with cross-reference to the case studies of Clinton and Sridhar (2017), the governance structure of the only treaty-making global health institution, the WHO, is comprised of member states alone and as such the secretariat (the agent) is a "servant" of those same member states. As a gendered organization it therefore also reflects the varied gender orders of the member state countries under whose governance its resolutions and decision making must operate. And, in this sense, globally, its capacity for transformative gender upheaval—if we think too of gender as a concept of power—is by definition circumscribed and limited to a consensus denominator. Whilst it sits at the global head of norm setting and standards, the operating space for radical disruption of the gendered-masculine history of global health and medicine at the WHO is just that—consensual norms rather than radical power shifting. Its history of passing resolutions and strategies to deal primarily (and until very recently) with gender as a women's health issue is a part of its gendered history.

The WHO is just one of many hundreds of organizations that comprise the landscape of partners that constitute global health, and as such, other new and sometimes quite innovative approaches of analysing (even with data) the gendered dimensions of these institutions have come to fruition. One such recent example is the Global Health 50/50 Report. This advocacy initiative, compiled by a core group of (mainly female) unpaid researchers, monitors and ranks organizations with the intention of advancing institutional transparency and accountability of over 200 global health actors.

The success of the Global Health 50/50 Report of 2019—which saw progress across all ten domains of measurement between 2018 and 2019—as a tool of change based on public ranking of health organizations constitutes a very different strategy from earlier approaches and is one that is embedded in ongoing efforts of gender mainstreaming whilst drawing on neoliberal and feminist technologies of governance and transparency. That it worked in year one is suggestive of the gendered nature of the organizations it measured. As a technology of governance and oversight in the Foucaultian sense, i.e. it seeks to change the conduct of organizations so that they become conducive to advancing gender equality, ranking tools like Report 50/50 gain political traction as a form of public audit, but one that relies on mainly patriarchal leadership to deliver for women.

Despite progress detailed in this first follow-up reporting, the intransigence of gendered divisions of labour in health speaks more to underlying structure and substructures that are, as noted by feminists such as Joan Scott (1986) and Sandra Harding (1986), gendered masculine and are the girders of entire bureaucratic systems and their networks.

Proportional parity has failed to equate with gender equity despite legal and policy initiatives within and between organizations that aimed to achieve just that (Guy & Fenley, 2013). Instead, argues Connell (2019), they have presumed simple dichotomies between women and men based on "loose liberal feminism" (2019) that has tended to celebrate high-achieving individual women in position of power and leadership. In shifting our lens towards the gendered power relations of institutions and their networks, it is possible to elongate beyond any singular moment in time and form an analysis that exposes the deeper structural foundations seeded in the early days of biomedicine, colonialism, and the origins of international global health (Packard, 2016). To foreground the institutions and their networks as gendered hierarchies in global health can further illuminate the ways in which structure and agency and global health governance have evolved in recent years against a changing landscape of traditional and new players, most notably public-private partnerships (PPPs) and product development partnerships (PDPs). The political economy, financing, and governance of global health as detailed in case studies by Clinton and Sridhar (2017) remind us of the centrality of theory that articulate the relations between principals and agents that persist in global health governance. These deep structures are, in part, explicable with a gendered understanding of the operation of power in the relations that constitute neoliberal global health.

The new players in global health, namely but not exclusively forms of PPPs and PDPs, were almost all born post-Beijing and sought in at least their governance structures to address the hegemonic gendered patriarchies from which international public health had grown. But here again, as an approach to addressing gender in global health, these organizations have sought to think of gender as women and gender as an individual rather than an organizational concept of power, as outlined earlier in the Introduction.

In a series of interviews[6] conducted with several PPPs and their partners, respondents regarded policies on gender and equity as means of awareness-raising, to "enlighten people" to "think harder". Policies sought to address only representation (the counting women approach) which in itself exposed underlying gender bias assuming a lack of qualified women in the pipeline, fears of "tokenism", and risk of less capable women replacing better suited men. Such responses speak volumes to the problems associated with individual rather than institutional approaches. Not only do they tell us these institutions are gendered organizations even by Acker's 1990 definition that states "advantage and disadvantage, exploitation and control, meaning and identity, are patterned through and in terms of a distinction between male and female, masculine and feminine" (1990:146), but they get us "stuck", as Rosabeth Kanter might suggest, in gender regimes that perpetuate hierarchies designed to serve the historically constituted patriarchal mode of operation in the practice of medicine and international health.

External pressure among PPP *principals*—often member states and donors with reputations for advancing gender justice and feminist policies—has been nevertheless demonstrated to be entry point to steer more radical organizational change in some organizations. For some, gender ear-marked funding and gender conditionality forces organizations to implement actions, at least at Headquarters. Country-level implementation remains problematic for reasons outlined above related to colonial histories in international health (Packard, 2016; Connell, 2019).

---

[6] Interviews conducted by Somerville during 2017–2018.

A second push, derived from a rights-based approach, typically builds strategic gender equality statements into the organization's mission where it constitutes part of an overall rights-based package, as it is the case with the WHO's Gender, Equity, and Rights team. All these approaches likely chip away at some of the girders that hold in place the processes and practices and gendered hierarchies that result eventually in the highly sex-segregated nature of the global health workforce.

Re-gendering for Global Health Justice

This discussion on the gendered nature of organizations in global health is not in itself intended to suggest that their gendered dimension should be erased or neutralized even if that were possible or desirable. The injustice stems from the hierarchies that are gendered patriarchal rather than that they are gendered per se. As a concept of power, gender operates everywhere; it is pervasive; it is one of the ways by which we organize societies and this is why we need to understand the way it functions in global health through its institutions and networks rather than only its individuals and representations.

Taking an organizational approach, whereby organizations and their networks are the unit of analysis that are gendered, allows us to move away from individuals as enacting and performing gendered norms, roles, and scripts, and rather look at the structures and institutional relations and networks that maintain intersecting forms of discrimination, and also the hegemony of the patriarchal system in which they exist.

In the 1980s BBC comedy show "Yes Minister", an all-white, male cabinet, discussed the merits of promoting women in leadership—then named positive discrimination—across the various government departments. The health minister reports that women are rather well represented in the sector. In fact, he cites the 80:20 ratio of women to men, much as it is today. What the scene illustrates with comical accuracy is the gendered nature of the cabinet office and the civil service as organizations where gender functions as a hierarchical tool of stratification. In the scene, all agreed, in principle, to positive discrimination—the sorts of short-term corrective measures we have come to mainstream as technological fixes to a short-term problem—a moment of "catch-up" to match the liberation and empowerment of women over the past century. To focus on numbers, on representation, rather than the gendered nature of organizations is to assume we know the problem is one of numbers, of balance, of parity and presence at the table. In this fictive comedy sketch, all the men at the table agreed on the principle of equality between women and men but, in a performance of hegemonic masculinity, were rendered incapable of action as each head of government department provided a "rational", mainly "cultural", reason why it was not the time or the place to take such well-principled measures. The culture arguments, frequently still used to describe the status quo of organizations, are dangerous as so often they act to eschew what is in actuality the deeper challenge of gender. After 25 years of gender mainstreaming with limited success using technical fixes, tools, mechanisms, and other such technologies of government that guide conduct (Prugl, 2011), it is perhaps high time that we think again about the nature of the problem we are trying to solve.

The principal-agent theorizing used by Clinton and Sridhar captures inter-organizational types of power relations and governance, but when we view these organizations as also gendered, the simplicity of those apparent relations is compromised by cross-cutting and hierarchical girders. These institutions are able to deliver their outputs within the value systems that underpin their very existence as neoliberal institutions in a global arena. And so too is their approach to addressing gender as institutions that employ human resources as well as deliver programming and health interventions. Typically, the areas that are measurable, or what are often in these institutions called SMART (Specific, Measurable, Achievable, Realistic, and Timely) measures to change, occur in spaces where the problem is easily identifiable—and this is often women themselves. By empowering women through training and mentoring, together with institutional commitments and the use of morally appealing shout-out methods like pledging, these organizations can be seen to deliver on a set group of targets. They are deemed to be successful within the framing that supports them, and if we take a feminist perspective to gendered organizations outlined above, they are co-opted as the very girders of patriarchy. The solution to what becomes constructed in such organizations as the "problem of gender equality" (Prugl, 2016; Bradshaw et al., 2019) is the regulation of processes of inserting women, described also as the neoliberalization of feminism (Prugl, 2016). Solutions to the problem are amenable by intervention with policies that are often couched in efficiencies because they are in themselves measurable. Whilst such interventions may improve outcomes for individual entrepreneurial women, they do little to remove the structural barriers that perpetuate and reconstitute the gendered hegemony.

Some kinds of technologies of gender mainstreaming derive their success and are deemed appropriate and acceptable because they are rolled out in institutions gendered masculine and fit the types of measures that are valued. To "lean-in", to pledge parity goals and publicly rank organizations in a competitive ordering, and to call out "manels" appear to gain traction in what Raewyn Connell might describe as a rather public performance of masculinities that, I would argue, tell us a great deal about the ways in which global health institutions and their networks are organized along axes of gender that sustain and even grow gender orders that are historically patriarchal.

Until we accept that gender is a means by which societies, institutions, and systems organize themselves—that the injustices of gender stem from its patriarchal ordering, not as a gender problem in and of itself—we will never see gender as in need of attention all of the time.

References

Acker, J. (1990). Hierarchies, jobs, bodies: A theory of gendered organizations. *Gender and Society, 4*(2), 139–158.

Acker, J. (1992). From sex roles to gendered institutions. *Contemporary Sociology, 21*(5), 565–567.

Acker, J. (2006). Inequality regimes: Gender, class, and race in organizations. *Gender and Society, 20*(4), 441–464.

Bell, K., & Green, J. (2016). On the perils of invoking neoliberalism in public health critique. *Critical Public Health, 26*(3), 239–243.

Bergeron, S. (2003). The post-Washington consensus and Economic Representations of Women in Development at the World Bank. *International Feminist Journal of Politics, 5*(3), 397–419.

Bradshaw, S., Linneker, B., & Sanders-McDonagh, E. (2019). It's gender Jim, but not as we know it…A critical review of constructions of gendered knowledge of the Global South. *European Journal of Women's Studies,* 1–17.

Clinton, C., & Sridhar, D. (2017). *Governing global health: Who runs the world and why?* Oxford University Press.

Connell, E. (2019). New maps of struggle for gender justice: Rethinking feminist research on organizations and work. *Gender, Work and Organization, 25,* 54–63.

Cornwall, A., Gideon, J., & Wilson, K. (2008). Introduction: Reclaiming feminism: Gender and neoliberalism. *IDS Bulletin, 39*(6), 1–19.

Downs, J., Reif, K., & Fitzgerald, D. (2014). Increasing women in leadership in global health. *Academic Medicine, 89*(8), 1103–1107.

Doyal, L. (2002). Putting gender into health and globalisation debates: New perspectives and old challenges. *Third World Quarterly, 23*(2), 233–250.

Frazer, N. (2009). Feminism, capitalism and the cunning of history. *New Left Review, 56.*

Goetz, A. M. (1997). *Getting institutions right for women.* Zed Books.

Guy, M., & Fenley, V. (2013). Inch by inch: Gender equality since the Civil Rights Act of 1964. *Review of Public Personnel Administration, 34*(1), 40–58.

Harding, S. (1986). *The science question in feminism.* Cornell University Press.

Hay, K., McDougal, V., Henry, S., Wurie, H., et al. (2019). Disrupting gender norms in health systems: Making the case for change. *Lancet, 393*(10190), 2535–2549.

Heller, O., Somerville, C., Suggs, S., Lachat, S., Piper, J., Pastrana, J., Correia, J., Miranda, J., & Beran, D. (2019). The process of prioritization of non-communicable diseases in the global health policy arena. *Health Policy and Planning, 34*(5), 370–383.

Kanter, R. (1977). *Men and women of the corporation.* Basic Books.

Keshavjee, S. (2014). *Blind sport: How neoliberalism infiltrated global health.* University of California Press.

Mastracci, S., & Arreola, V. (2016). Gendered organizations: How human resource management practices produce and reproduce administrative man. *Administrative Theory and Praxis, 38*(2), 137–149.

Nightingale, F. (1860). *Notes on nursing.* D. Appleton & Company. http://digital.library.upenn.edu/women/nightingale/nursing/nursing.html

Packard, R. (2016). *A history of global health: Interventions into the lives of other peoples.* Johns Hopkins University Press.

Prugl, E. (2011). Diversity management and gender mainstreaming as technologies of government. *Politics and Gender, 7*(1), 71–89.

Prugl, E. (2014). Equality means business: Governing gender through public-private partnerships. *Review of International Political Economy, 21*(6), 1137–1167.

Prugl, E. (2016). Neoliberalism with a feminist face: Crafting a new hegemony at the World Bank. *Feminist Economics, 23*(1), 30–53.

Risman, B., & Davis, G. (2013). From sex roles to gender structure. *Current Sociology, 61*(5), 733–755.

Schrecker, T. (2016). Neoliberalism and health: Linkages and the dangers. *Sociology Compass,* *10*(10), 952–971.

Scott, J. (1986). Gender: A useful category of historical analysis. *The American Historical Review,* *91*(5), 1053–1075.

Shakow, A., Yates, R., & Keshavjee, S. (2018). Neoliberalism and global health. In S. Cahill, M. Cooper, M. Kongings, & D. Primose (Eds.), *The Sage handbook of neoliberalism.* SAGE.

Shiffman, J., & Smith, S. (2007). Generation of political priority for global health initiatives: A framework and case study of maternal mortality. *Lancet, 370,* 1370–1379.

Shiffman, J., Quissell, K., Schmitz, H. P., Pelletier, D., Smith, S., Berlan, D., Gneiting, U., Van Slyke, D., Mergel, I., Rodriguez, M., & Walt, G. (2015). A framework on the emergence and effectiveness of global health networks. *Health Policy and Planning, 21*(1), i3–i16.

Shiffman, J., Schmitz, H. P., Berlan, D., Smith, S. L., Quissell, K., Gneiting, U., & Pelletie, D. (2016). The emergence and effectiveness of global health networks: Findings and future research. *Health Policy and Planning, 31*(1), 110–123.

Talib, Z., Burke, K., & Barry, M. (2017). Women leaders in global health. *The Lancet Global Health, 5*(6).

Reports

United Nations. (2017). *System-wide strategy on gender parity.* Retrieved from https://www.un.int/sites/www.un.int/files/Permanent%20Missions/delegate/17-00102b_gender_strategy_report_13_sept_2017.pdf

The Global Health 50/50. (2019). *Report: Equality works.* Retrieved from www.globalhealth5050.org

Interview with Soumya Swaminathan, Chief Scientist at the World Health Organization

Sulzhan Bali and Roopa Dhatt

"Focus on what you want to do, what your passion is. Really work hard, prove yourself, and don't be afraid to speak up or to seek help at any stage."

Soumya Swaminathan is currently the Chief Scientist at the World Health Organization (WHO). She is an Indian pediatrician and clinical scientist recognized for her extensive research on tuberculosis and HIV. From October 2017 to March 2019, she was the Deputy Director General of Programs (DDP) at the WHO. Dr. Swaminathan served as the Secretary to the Government of India for Health Research and Director General of the Indian Council of Medical Research from 2015 to 2017. From 2009 to 2011, she also served as Coordinator of the UNICEF/UNDP/World Bank/WHO Special Programme for Research and Training in Tropical Diseases in Geneva. Soumya is an elected Foreign Fellow of the US National Academy of Medicine and a Fellow of all three science academies in India. She has published more than 350 peer-reviewed publications and book chapters and has been on several WHO and global advisory bodies and committees, including the WHO Expert Panel to Review Global Strategy and Plan of Action on Public Health, Innovation and Intellectual Property, and the Strategic and Technical Advisory Group of the Global TB Department at WHO, and most recently was the Co-Chair of the Lancet Commission on Tuberculosis.

Is There a Gender Equity Gap in Global Health?

Medicine and medical colleges have typically had a good balance in workforce. The global health workforce is made up mostly of women in terms of nurses and midwives and physicians. However, things are still quite different in the biomedical science and research side. There's clearly a gap and inequity there. If you look at membership of the Royal Society, for example, membership of the Science Academies, the proportion of women is less than 10% of overall members. The Academies of Science in the US are younger, but still have a similar gender gap. So,

S. Bali (✉) · R. Dhatt
Women in Global Health, Washington, DC, USA
e-mail: sulzhan@gmail.com; roopa.dhatt@womeningh.org

© Springer Nature Switzerland AG 2022
R. Morgan et al. (eds.), *Women and Global Health Leadership*,
https://doi.org/10.1007/978-3-030-84498-1_3

I would say that I see much more imbalance on the science research side than on the actual medical side.

Also, even though there are a lot of women in the global health workforce, there is still an imbalance. Most of the people who do the bottom rungs of the work are women, but the leadership positions and deans of medical schools are mostly men. There have been efforts in some organizations to change that though. At the level of WHO, for example, there has been a good balance. We've had women Director Generals and we have got a well-balanced senior leadership team with Dr. Tedros [Adhanom Ghebreyesus].

Why Is Gender Equity at the Senior Leadership Level Important for Global Health Governance?

There are quite a few reasons why gender equity is crucial in global health governance. For one, women tend to think differently. They have different perspectives, different ways of looking at issues, and different approach to problem solving. A balance at the senior leadership level and around the table has a positive impact on decision-making. Secondly, it is just logical that when half the world is made up of women, that you should have equal representation of women at all levels and all aspects of life. And thirdly, having a woman in a senior leadership role can prove to be such an inspiration to younger people, both men and women. Women in senior leadership positions bring visibility and voice, set role models, and inspire younger generation that they too can be on the table.

How Did Your Early Experiences Impact Your Career?

Leadership starts from childhood, how you are brought up and what your social circumstances are like. India is a patriarchal society, and in fact many of my extended family members are also very patriarchal in their approach. I was fortunate though that for my parents, my immediate aunts and uncles, and close family friends, there was never any question of difference between boys and girls. We were three sisters. So, of course there was no comparison with a brother, but we were never made to feel that we couldn't do anything that we might have aspired to do. Even mountaineering! My sister allowed to go off on these mountaineering expeditions when she was quite young, which was a departure from the societal rules.

Travel was instrumental too. We got exposed to many different cultural environments when we were growing up. We could travel independently, and our parents took us many different places in India. Travel made us agile. Given that a part of my family was quite orthodox, we learned that patriarchy existed and learned to face it during the few weeks we spent with our extended family. At the same time, we grew up in Delhi, which was quite a cosmopolitan place. So, we learned to adapt and adjust early on. Apart from family, my school was also instrumental in building my self-confidence. I was surrounded by teachers and close family friends who were themselves strong women role models and achievers.

Are There Any Mentors That You Credit with for Your Success?

My parents were the initial influence, which had a big impact on everything that I did later. Some teachers in my school promoted leadership, so school was an important aspect in shaping me. In my working life, I had a Director in an institute that I worked in; he provided me with opportunities and gave me a lot of confidence. He would often send me to meetings in Delhi, where there would be many very senior people, most of them men. Initially, I was very intimidated sitting in those meetings with senior older men. I remember he said to me, "No, you shouldn't think like that. You are not too young. You are the expert in this field, and you need to go and represent the Institute. Why should I go as a Director? You are the one who knows this area well." So, he really gave me the opportunities to speak and to be heard. Initial reactions I faced in such meetings were, "What do you know," but with continued visibility, people started accepting me as an expert and then I got invited in my own right. But it all started with him sending me to represent him.

How Did Gender Impact Your Career Experience?

Well, for one, I had to work harder. One had to try harder. And you had to have had supporting mentors and supervisors to have succeeded. I remember as a young woman who had just finished training in the US and I went back, I was very idealistic, and I really was committed to health research. I wanted to contribute, and I was met with a lot of skepticism and discouragement. Perhaps not so much because I was a woman, but just the field that I wanted to pursue. A lot of people just didn't think that there was any future in medical research in India at that time. I couldn't find anyone at that time who I could go to for advice or support or mentorship or guidance. I eventually met someone who said, "Well, there are organizations in India where you can do research if that's your passion." And he guided me to a place which I ultimately ended up joining, the Tuberculosis Research Center, which is one of the Indian Council of Medical Research (ICMR) Institutes.

Being a young woman in the field wasn't easy though. In my career, I have worked with bosses or colleagues (male and female) who could be patriarchal, bureaucratic, or hierarchical. There was an instance where I was just expected to do what I was asked, and my opinion wasn't valued. I was often told, "You're very junior, your opinion is not important. You just do what I tell you to do." This was a difficult time. So, in my 30s, I did not have the right guidance, supervision, mentorship, to have blossomed. I feel that I lost a lot of years of my professional life due to such an environment and I could have done so much more if the circumstances were different. Good mentors just like bad mentors could be male or female, so just because you have a woman boss doesn't mean it is going to work out well.

Later, when I became the director of the Tuberculosis Research Center, and introduced myself to someone as such, they looked at me and said, "What? They have a woman now?" I let it pass; however, it made me realize that when the institute was founded, the idea of a woman being able to lead anything did not exist. And therefore, I think institutional cultures take time to change.

How Did You Address the Challenge of Unsupportive Bosses?

I guess what I did was to adapt and adjust rather than try to resist. I just didn't know what to do. So, I think it ended up just affecting my psyche and I just changed myself or behaved in a way that would be acceptable to this boss. Though I knew this was not a healthy situation, and neither was I being productive to my capacity. So, in a way I didn't handle it too well. My situation only changed after many years with a new boss who gave me a completely new responsibility and much more independence. By that time, I think I was in my late 30s, maybe approaching 40 so I really felt that that decade had not gone as well as it could have. I suggest, if you have a problem with your boss or with one of your coworkers, you go and talk to the ombudsman; the ombudsman gives you some suggestions and ideas on how to handle the situation.

What Measures Can Institutions Take to Inculcate Greater Representation of Women in Leadership Position?

There are several steps institutions can take. Firstly, they can sensitize senior leadership to promote gender diversity and to encourage young women to seek further opportunities. Johns Hopkins School of Global Health is a good example, I used to work there, and I found that the senior people in the department mentor and actively promote young women to develop their leadership skills. Secondly, they can make sure that there aren't any hidden biases within the interview panels and the committee and interview panel themselves is gender diverse. Thirdly, job adverts can be more tuned to gender biases. Sometimes, when the position is advertised, conditions can be archaic with specific criteria. Women typically have a bit more of an atypical career trajectory than men and can be less confident in applying. There had been many jobs when I looked at advertisement and thought, "Well, this is not for me because I'm not going to fit the criteria." And sometimes when I've discussed it with some senior people, they said, "No, no, of course you fit. You must apply." So, building language in the job advertisement that encourages women (especially with an unusual career pathway) to apply will help.

How Important Are the Peer Networks for Inculcating Leadership?

I wish I had a peer network as they are very important. I did have friends in different parts of the world because I have done some training abroad. But then when I went back to India, I felt that I was in a different world. Peer group in the same socio-cultural context helps because if I was asking for advice from somebody from some other country, they may not even understand the social or cultural context. So, it would have been great to have a peer group of people in a similar career path, culture, and at different levels of career to provide support and peer mentorship. Sometimes it can be difficult with just peer at the same level, as they are all aspiring to go up the ladder, so there is an element of competition there. A network with older and younger women to support each other, to unburden yourself, to guide on handling difficult situations can help.

Is Networking Harder for Women? If Yes, Why?

I think professional networking is certainly harder. I think it is harder because women have many other commitments apart from work, which means your priorities are slightly different. I was fortunate that I had help at home. There are many women who are not so lucky and who must bear both the burdens of career and family care simultaneously. As a woman, you are more responsible for the household, at least in cultures like India, where you must make sure that there is food for the evening, the groceries are done, etc. It makes it more difficult to network. I think women can be good at networking in their own way though because they are used to managing large family and social network and multitask.

How Can We Make It Easier for Women to Professionally Network?

First, we need to ensure that conferences have childcare facilities. Few conferences have that. Once children are looked after, then women are much more relaxed about the networking. Secondly, I think the partners need to recognize that the woman's career is also important, that she needs to be able to do this networking and spend time away from home. So, the partners need to step up and really take over some of those home care, childcare responsibilities and allow her to network.

How Did You and Your Spouse Navigate the Decisions Around Your Career?

I couldn't have done all this, what I've been able to do without a supportive spouse. He took care of the children when I had to travel, and he never said, "Where are you going? Why are you going? Or when will you be back?". He was never resentful of the fact and his job didn't entail a lot of travel so he could take care of the kids and the house. All along he supported my career, my ambition, my goals, absolutely 100%. There's never been any question of having to give up something I want to do because it is inconvenient for him or anything like that. So, I would say the support of the partner is a big reason behind not only my success but for a lot of other women leaders that I know.

Has Your Career Ever Required You to Move Your Country or City? How Did You Navigate That Decision with Your Spouse?

I've done it couple of times. When I became the head of the Indian Council of Medical Research (ICMR), I had to move to Delhi from Chennai. And of course, I could still commute on weekends, but it still meant living away, living in a different city. There was never any question that maybe I should think about it because it will disrupt the family. It was always a question of if it was professionally the right thing to do. When I moved to Geneva, it was an even bigger move. I was not sure whether I really wanted to do this because it was a big disruption for me. However, my family was extremely supportive, including my parents, my in-laws; everybody felt that this was a great opportunity.

Do You Think Perception of Men and Women as Leaders Is Different?

Yes. In fact, in many parts of the world that there is a perception that men can lead better. But I think that is changing and it is changing quite fast among the younger generation. So, there is going to be a big shift in the way people think about these things. In my generation especially, there was a strong perception that men should occupy leadership roles. That is changing.

Do You Think the Reaction to Mistakes Between Men and Women Leaders Is Different?

Yeah, I think very different. You just have to look at the social media. I was looking at the recent report that came out in the Indian media, which said that women politicians and other women who are active on social media, like activists or lawyers, get a lot more hate messages and trolling on social media much than men. This is an example of how society reacts to a woman who are out there and prominent. You are going to face more criticism. I think the same is the case on the professional side. The attitude of criticism toward women is different. However, I also feel the way men and women leaders react to their own mistakes is different. Women are likely to admit to mistakes more often, whereas a man would either defend it, try to deny it, or cover it up with overconfidence. As a result, women leaders get scrutinized more.

What Advice Would You Give to Young Women Who Are Aspiring to Be Future Global Health Leaders?

My advice to young women is to be good at what you do. You must be good at your work. Ambition is good, but ambition without hard work doesn't help. So first, work hard and prove yourself. When you are good at your work, it will help you make a name for yourself. The first 15 years of your career is critical. Once you establish yourself, gain leadership skills, then you are ready to take on a bigger role either within your country or in global health. That's what I did. I was focused on the problem of tuberculosis in India and globally. I wanted to make a mark. Then, when I took on a larger role in India for medical research, I spent my first 2 years just doing advocacy at different levels for medical research because it was so neglected in the country. When Dr. Tedros invited me to take on my role in WHO, it was out of the blue. My first reaction was, "No, I've got a mission and I want to do something here and I've started doing it and I haven't finished my job." There was a lot of thinking before I accepted the position but the reason I was ever even considered for the position was my track record. So, my advice is to focus on what you want to do, what your passion is. Work hard and prove yourself, and don't be afraid to speak up or to seek help at any stage. It is always good to have mentors and advisors of either sex, men or women. So, find somebody who is supportive and who can be a good advisor. It's good to reach out to somebody like that from time to time.

If You Could Have a Billboard for Other Women Leaders, What Would It Say?

It would say "Cultivate a sisterhood." We need to support each other as women leaders.

Gender, Peace, and Health: Promoting Human Security with Women's Leadership

Yara M. Asi

Introduction

Evidence suggests that there is no biological basis of sex differences in risk of contracting Ebola, an infectious disease that has been the cause of several outbreaks in the past few years, particularly in conflict-affected states. Yet, women make up more than half of those who contract Ebola and die from the virus, with fatality rates of up to 75% women in countries like Liberia (United Nations Women (UN Women), 2014), and almost 90% for pregnant women (Bebell et al., 2017). Sociocultural factors such as low prioritization of women's healthcare services and the role of women as primary caretakers of the ill have created these gender disparities that not just threaten women's lives but are a global risk to human security (Menéndez et al., 2015). However, while female family members, nurses, and community health workers perform most of the frontline labor during Ebola outbreaks and other humanitarian crises, much of the leadership—and as a result, the decision making— is led by men. The coordinator of a coalition of local women's groups working to combat the disease in West Africa told the World Health Organization (WHO), "At the start of the outbreak, local women saw these men in jackets doing 'Ebola business' and thought, this doesn't really concern us" (2019b).

This is a clear, and dangerous, illustration of how women often bear the highest burdens in areas of health and security but are routinely excluded from decision making. Existing research suggests that unlike many other social indicators, gender inequality is not linked to a state's gross domestic product (GDP) or level of poverty. This suggests that there are structural forces that keep women from advancing that must be addressed in order to empower women on a global scale (Kim, 2017). The role of these structural forces in maintaining gender inequalities is perhaps best

Y. M. Asi (✉)
School of Global Health Management and Informatics, College of Community Innovation and Education, University of Central Florida, Orlando, FL, USA
e-mail: Yara.Asi@ucf.edu

© Springer Nature Switzerland AG 2022
R. Morgan et al. (eds.), *Women and Global Health Leadership*,
https://doi.org/10.1007/978-3-030-84498-1_4

described by Johan Galtung, who pioneered the concept of structural violence: "When one husband beats his wife there is a clear case of personal violence, but when one million husbands keep one million wives in ignorance there is structural violence" (1969, p. 171).

This chapter will contribute to the emerging literature base about women leaders in global health and security. First, I will define human security and how it relates to gender, followed by a description of the literature that shows how women's empowerment and leadership benefits the security and health sectors in contexts around the world. Second, I will show the relationships between several societal indicators measuring gender equality, health outcomes, and peacefulness. Supported by the human security framework, I will then outline recommendations that will support gender equality, improved health outcomes, and increased peacefulness.

What Is Human Security?

Despite the violence and warfare of the early- to mid-twentieth century, the construct of human security only first emerged in a United Nations Human Development Report in 1994. Prior to the report, "security" was more narrowly defined as state security from military threats. However, the report outlines the deficits in our understanding of conflict based on this rudimentary definition. Mortality is easy to understand and quantify, but human security is less tangible. To address this, the report described security in terms of economic, food, health, environmental, personal, community, and political needs and recognized that these needs often overlap in their causes, symptoms, and outcomes. They famously describe human security as "the child who did not die, a disease that did not spread, a job that was not cut, an ethnic tension that did not explode in violence, a dissident who was not silenced" (UNDP, 1994, p. 22). This same report, however, emphasizes that despite progress in some development and security goals, there persists a "dark shadow of insecurity cast on the majority of the world's population: women" (p. 101). Additionally, the initial definitions of human security have been criticized for being too "gender-blind," missing gendered threats such as targeted violence against women (Parmar et al., 2014). We cannot decouple human security from state security, which are directly linked (Quinn et al., 2017). However, we also cannot ignore the unique role of women in all topics related to human security, which includes facets of human rights and development.

Human security is not just about life without violence—although that is certainly a component—but a life without the fear of threats to the fundamental dimensions of one's livelihood (Gomez & Gasper, 2013). I contend that to achieve greater human security, especially in the overlapping sectors of peace and health, women must be empowered as leaders. While in some ways affirming debated gender stereotypes, the relationship between women and human security is seen in that women "tend to be for the wellbeing of the whole to which they belong" and not in "competing for and defending resources and power" as male counterparts might (Reardon

& Hans, 2010, pp. 17–18). This is not to suggest that women do not actively participate in revolts, armed struggles, and war as combatants, spies, or in support roles like cooks and healthcare providers. Some of these women are coerced or threatened into participation, while others purposefully seek out engagement in warfare (UNDP, 2010a). It is also not accurate to assume that all women in positions of leadership will assume a less "hawkish" perspective of governance, with several prominent examples of women adopting "masculine" approaches to politics, such as Golda Meir from Israel and Margaret Thatcher from the United Kingdom (Jalalzai & Krook, 2010). However, evidence suggests that state gender equality does have a "pacifying effect" on that state's approach to international relations and militarism (Caprioli, 2000) and leads to lower levels of conflict (Melander, 2005).

The fact that women are more likely to experience insecurity does not guarantee that they are uniquely adept at addressing it. However, research and historical perspective suggest that women leaders are more likely to take an approach centered around human security, one that is universal, interdependent, prevention-focused, and people-centered. In both formal and informal ways, women in conflict or post-conflict settings emphasize issues that are typically overlooked in a militarized approach to peacebuilding. These include reintegrating combatants, disarmament, grassroots coordination efforts, and considering a community's social and spiritual needs (Justino et al., 2018). Studies have shown, for example, that when women are permitted adequate access to food, overall food insecurity decreases (Ibnouf, 2009). Including women in humanitarian crises in infrastructure discussions reduces the average amount of time it takes families to walk to accessible drinking water (UN Women, 2015). When women are permitted to serve as police officers, they can more easily interact with and gain the trust of the women in society, increasing safety (Benard et al., 2008). At the expense of more equitable outcomes for whole communities, however, perspectives on human development have followed patriarchal standards of progress that feature two primary limitations. The first is the assumption that a productive economy, dominated by men, is superior to the services of a care economy primarily composed of women, seen as "derivative of nature." Second, efforts to ignore issues related to sexuality and body politics have historically been used to assert a form of power (Truong, 1997). As a result, the roles of women in formal human security work have been limited.

Conflict Actively Disempowers and Hurts Women

Complex relationships between gender, health, and peace are present in wars and conflicts as well as in times of political stability. However, the human security threats made by public health deficits and inequalities mimic the human security threats posed by conflict. In all too many conflicts, it is women who suffer the inordinate burdens of living in an insecure environment. While gender-based inequalities, discrimination, and violence exist everywhere, these factors are exacerbated in environments experiencing conflict and poor access to care services. Men are more likely to die during conflict due to direct violence, but women are more likely to die of indirect causes after periods of violent conflict end (Ormhaug et al., 2009), and make up more than half of the global refugee population (United Nations, 2016). Conflict is especially detrimental to women's reproductive health (Pillai et al., 2017) and mental health (Kastrup, 2006). It is estimated that 61% of all maternal deaths occur in just 35 countries affected by a humanitarian crisis, at a rate more than double the global average (UNFPA, 2015). Additionally, poor healthcare provision in conflict-affected areas, along with restrictions on women's autonomy, may lead to higher birth rates, which strain an entire family's resources (OECD, 2017).

Women also experience a disproportionate amount of the noncombat burdens of insecurity (Aolain, 2011). Women's subjugation and even victimization is a common feature of conflicts of all kinds, from those involving overt physical trauma to those heightening economic deprivation and legislative oppression. As caretakers, it is often women who struggle to feed their families when food is scarce or to clothe them when there is no money. It is women who are expected to tend to the physical and mental suffering of their families but stifle their own distress if they are subject to harassment and sexual violence themselves. Women may experience these traumas as either a weapon of war from opposition forces or as victims of forced prostitution or human trafficking, sometimes coerced by their own needy families. Gender-based violence (GBV) is known to increase in conflict environments, even when recognizing that "conflict simply heightens violence that was already occurring...GBV in armed conflicts should be seen as a continuation of the violence experienced during peacetime" (Manjoo & McRaith, 2011, p. 15). Despite the prevalence of war-related sexual and physical violence, rates of intimate partner violence in conflict-affected settings are even higher, demonstrating risks to a woman's security both in and out of the home (Stark & Ager, 2011). It is ironic, then, that in many post-conflict resolution efforts, the prospect of including gender-based protections, rights, and opportunities is seen as too destabilizing.

The Relationship Between Gender, Conflict, and Health

The Sustainable Development Goals (SDGs) show that the global community understands the importance of these issues: SDG 3 is about good health and well-being, SDG 5 aims to achieve gender equality and empower all women and girls, and SDG 16 calls for peace, justice, and strong institutions. Despite being measured as disparate aims, there are clearly areas of intersection between these issues. Factors like inadequate health services delivery, poverty, social inequalities, and health disparities can lead to state fragility and conflict (Wiist et al., 2014). In turn, conflict disrupts health systems and decreases health outcomes, further reducing human security. Aside from the direct and indirect effects on health, conflict also serves to decrease the available resources to nonmilitary sectors such as healthcare and social services (Levy & Sidel, 2016). All of these factors are connected: a woman in poor health is unable to work; a woman unable to provide basic health care or food to her children is less interested in developing a career; a woman who becomes homeless to pay for the healthcare needs of a family member is less able to enter the workforce. In one study of displaced Kurdish women in Iraq, participants suggested that health support was more important to them than livelihood training (Kaya & Luchtenberg, 2018). As much talk as there is of empowering women economically, there is not enough consideration of the prerequisite conditions needed for these women to be able to take advantage of economic opportunities, including a healthy life and family.

The World Bank estimates that by 2030, 46% of the world's poorest people will live in environments of fragility and conflict (2016). Many of these populations will be in protracted situations with no clear resolution to achieve positive peace, defined as "attitudes, institutions and structures which create and sustain peaceful societies" (IEP, 2017, p.1). From conflicts in Egypt and Israel, to South Africa, Bosnia, and Northern Ireland, most of the world's famous peacekeeping processes were led by men. Yet evidence suggests that post-conflict states are likely to relapse into conflict. Contemporary peace processes report a 45% failure rate within 5 years of the agreement, while violence reappeared after a third of the peace agreements signed between 1950 and 2004. In about half of states with negotiated peace settlements, civil war emerges (Westendorf, 2015). In more than half of states that experience civil war, additional conflict or violence breaks out. This cycle of war has been referred to as the "conflict trap." Either the issues that led to the initial conflict were not adequately resolved, or the conflict itself led to decreased societal stability that provides fertile grounds for more conflict (Collier & Sambanis, 2002). This suggests that there is something lacking in our current approaches to peacemaking and development that may be providing a temporary cessation of warfare as opposed to long-term stability and development.

Considering Women's Leadership in Human Security

Many decades of research have shown that for development of all kinds, gender equality is one of the most significant determinants for positive outcomes. However, in areas of health and human security, women are consistently underrepresented as leaders. Only about a quarter of leadership positions in health care, from global health faculty in universities to positions in state ministries of health, are held by women (Talib et al., 2017). In the last 25 years, just 3% of peace process mediators, witnesses, and signatories have been women. Only two women in history have ever served as chief negotiators in major peace processes, and only one woman has ever signed a final peace accord as a chief negotiator (CFR, 2019). In a study of post-conflict economic reconstruction packages, less than 5% of activities and 3% of budget lines mention women-specific needs or gender equality (UNDP, 2010b).

There are several reasons why women aren't well-represented in leadership despite their obvious work on the ground, stemming from the sociocultural norms regarding the role of women in society. Women are less likely to be afforded opportunities to pursue an education, while even educated women are expected to prioritize caregiving over career aspirations. Lack of schedule flexibility and familial support prevents women from fully participating and advancing in the workplace. When women are prevented from breaking into lower-level leadership roles, there become fewer women candidates to consider for the higher tiers of leaders, perpetuating gender disparities. These issues are, of course, not unique to the health and security sectors. Yet, the remnants of a militarized approach to security issues, dominated by men, still persist. Additionally, the realms of science and medicine, especially in leadership roles, are still widely considered the domain of men (Allotey, 2018).

When women participate in peace processes, prospects for long-term peace increase by 35% (Stone, 2015). Research has shown that including women in post-conflict processes accelerates economic development, allows families to escape poverty, decreases corruption, reduces a country's likelihood of initiating additional conflict, and increases living standards across the society (Benard et al., 2008). When women are excluded from peace and health work, corruption increases, outcomes deteriorate, and the likelihood of additional conflict continues. When women are included, they are more likely to bring up human rights and development issues by recognizing the structural violence in sectors of health and peace that lead to inequalities or inefficiencies in outcomes (O'Reilly et al., 2015). The evidence we have suggests that including women in positions of power and balancing their participation with men (not, as some detractors might fear, manifesting additional gender inequalities by replacing men entirely with women) leads to more stable and healthier societies (Ng & Muntaner, 2018). Regardless of their political affiliation, more representation by women leads to advancement of legislative priorities about issues like pay equity, violence against women, and health care (Wängnerud, 2009). The very process of building a culture that enables women's leadership inherently leads to a more secure society, aside from the outcomes that women leaders may produce.

While not enough evidence exists to establish direct causation between the gender balance of peacemakers and the likelihood of peace, the presence of women or even issues deemed "feminine" are routinely excluded from peace processes at all levels. It is not just due to aspirations for equality and representation that women should be involved in reconciliation and reconstruction efforts. It seems apparent that when all such efforts are skewed almost entirely in one direction, the best outcomes won't be achieved. Feminists have long argued that level of state militarization is inversely correlated with the well-being of women and other vulnerable groups (Enloe, 2016). Aside from women in leadership, high levels of overall gender equity in a state are associated with lower chance of conflict and better societal outcomes (Hudson et al., 2014). Women can see around policy corners that men did not know existed; for example, during conflicts in Angola and Rwanda, women maintained the farmlands while men were engaged in combat. However, post-conflict agricultural initiatives focused primarily on bolstering ex-combatants as farmers and ignored the women who were already doing the work (Zuckerman & Greenberg, 2004).

In 2000, recognizing both the unique role of women in peacekeeping and the unique costs borne by women in conflict, the United Nations put forth the Women, Peace, and Security (WPS) agenda in UN Security Council Resolution 1325. Several additional resolutions in the following years bolstered the core of the WPS initiative: women's full participation in areas of conflict prevention, protection, and relief and recovery. The WPS agenda argues that outcomes of human security and state security are tied—human security and all its components require a peaceful state, and a peaceful state cannot exist if its citizens are not secure. While this has opened the door for women to enter these critical discussions, critics contend that there is no consequence for noncompliance, and a lack of funding for WPS-related initiatives minimizes its effectiveness. Although the WPS framework has empha-sized women's inclusion, their roles may remain marginalized and their work more centered around informal vs. formal participation (Berry & Rana, 2019). We should acknowledge the important work that is currently being done while recognizing that there is still a long road to equality.

Gender, Conflict, and Health: Establishing an Empirical Connection

Despite circumstantial and theoretical relationships between gender, peace, and health, there exists a quantitative gap in the literature connecting these factors, out-side of those assessing specific pilot programs or case studies. There is currently a robust focus on research about gender in global health, and there is a nascent but significant line of study about women in the security sector. However, few studies attempt to measure the relationships between gender, conflict, and health on the macro-level. To add empirical support to the argument of this chapter, I conduct a multiple regression analysis considering three measures. The first is the Global Peace Index (GPI), which ranks 163 states according to level of peacefulness, which is evaluated according to three domains: societal safety and security, ongoing domestic and international conflict, and militarization (IEP, 2019). The lower the score on the index, the higher the level of peace (Iceland, for example, reports a score of 1.072 as the most peaceful nation, while Afghanistan, the least peaceful nation, scores a 3.574). The second is the United Nation's Gender Inequality Index (GII), which accounts for three aspects of gender-focused human development in 161 countries: reproductive health, empowerment, and economic status (UNDP, 2018). The lower the score, the higher the level of gender equality (Switzerland scored the best with 0.039, while Yemen scored the worst at 0.834). Third, Current Health Expenditure (CHE) as % of gross domestic product (GDP) was used to get an understanding of the prioritization of health care in state budgets (WHO, 2018).

Regression analysis was conducted on three models, with each measure serving as the dependent variable as the other measures served as predictor variables. Model

Fig. 1 Relationships between GII, GPI, and CHE

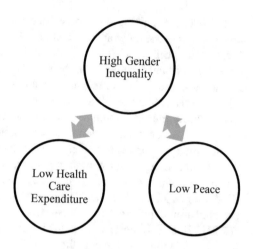

1 (using GPI as the dependent variable and CHE/GII as covariates) demonstrated that a high GII predicted a high GPI, meaning that low gender equality was a predictor for low peace ($b = .690, p = .000$). In Model 2 (dependent variable = GII), higher CHE as a % of GDP predicted lower GII, or higher equality ($b = -.296, p = .000$), while a higher GPI score predicted a higher GII score, reinforcing the relationship between peace and gender. In the third model (dependent variable = CHE), a high GII score predicted lower CHE as a % of GDP ($b = -.796, p = .000$), suggesting that states with lower gender equality spend less on health care. This analysis implies a reciprocal relationship between low peace and high gender inequality as well as between low healthcare spending and high gender inequality (Fig. 1).

Gender, Health, and Peace: Ways Forward

Globally, the largest impediment to women's empowerment is not lack of education or willingness to work, but sociocultural-religious norms that maintain gender inequalities. These norms play out in states, markets, civil society, and communities and within a family (Moussa, 2008). Gender equality efforts must attend to both attitudes and behaviors in each of these environments (Fig. 2). Any successful policy cannot focus solely on changing the behaviors of states or companies or fathers without changing their attitudes about the role of women. On the other hand, we cannot focus solely on outreach and education to change attitudes at the expense of tangible policies and laws that push societies forward as their viewpoints slowly evolve. Disempowered women deserve to have their human rights fully realized, and women's empowerment is essential to facilitate solutions for global stability and development.

The reality is that to change policy and development outcomes, fundamental change first needs to happen at the individual level for both women and men. Long-term increases in health or security outcomes cannot coexist with the patriarchal beliefs that are the root causes of gender inequality. The role of women in a

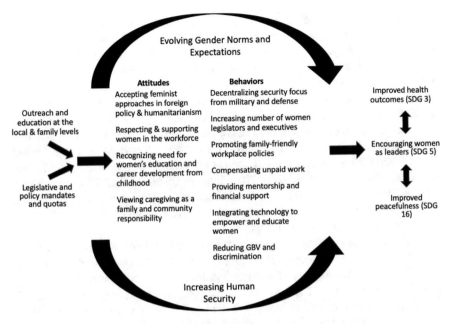

Fig. 2 Framework of increased women's leadership in health and security sectors

household is often broadly representative of a woman's potential role in society. In households that value a woman's chastity and seclusion, where men are considered in control of the household, it may not matter what opportunities may be presented by a local nongovernmental organization (NGO) if a woman's father or husband can prevent her from pursuing them. We also can't forget that women who seek independence outside of what they are expected to achieve are at higher risk for violence (Moussa, 2008). Despite these limitations, there are a few areas of concentration that will make the largest difference in evolving current gender norms and priorities.

Shifting State Priorities

States are responsible for public policies that contribute to poverty and patriarchal systems, such as within reproductive rights and childcare policy. States are also responsible for allocating money and, as a result, the state's priorities. In the traditional patriarchal model, military and defense spending is prioritized over health and peacebuilding activities (Enloe, 2016). Security analysis that takes a feminist viewpoint is often dismissed as primarily academic and pushed aside in favor of the masculine approach to national security. Initiating conversations about the role of the state in achieving human security is the job of elected leaders who represent their populations. To this end, states must have representative governments that can pass laws that end existing structures of inequality while promoting new initiatives and guidelines that promote equality.

Along with shifting the definition of national security from a solely military perspective to one encompassing the totality of human security, states must make an active effort to diversify representation. Women must have free and fair access to voting for representatives, which may include provision of childcare and transportation services. Within legislatures, quotas may be necessary to ensure that government compositions are balanced. Such measures have been discussed as early as 1990 by the United Nations, but few countries have adopted these measures. One reason is debate about their effectiveness; for example, Saudi Arabia reports that women make up 20% of their parliament, the same proportion as in the United States (World Bank, 2018), yet with almost no exceptions, all ministers and other major positions of power are men. The Kingdom appointed their first woman as a cabinet-level member in 2017, as a deputy minister in education. It is clear that the power of the state is still held by men, despite brave and often penalized efforts by Saudi women to achieve equal rights.

However, there are nations where quotas clearly have been successful. Rwanda, one of the few states to adopt a 30% quota for women in elected positions, is now one of the countries with the highest proportion of women in politics, increasing from 18% women in 1991 (shortly before the Rwandan genocide) to 64% in 2013. By comparison, the world average is less than 24% women as parliament members (UN Women, 2018). Rwanda is considered one of the world's global health success stories, with a doubled life expectancy, significantly reduced child mortality, and high vaccination rates, all achieved after one of the worst periods of mass civilian violence in history. Rwandan Health Minister Dr. Agnes Binagwaho said these achievements were only possible because of their focus on social welfare and health equity (Savchuk, 2014).

Promoting Women in the Workplace

Women's economic participation in the market is limited for a variety of reasons outlined earlier in this chapter, despite their massive labor contributions. Gender inequality is not unique to health care or security, but humanitarian initiatives across the spectrum depend on a vibrant, diverse, and well-trained workforce. This interconnectivity is present throughout the framing of the SDGs, which recognize that the success of global development depends on community-level solutions. Women and girls can be encouraged to enter certain fields where they are underrepresented with targeted programs, such as the Women of Integrity, Strength, and Hope (WISH) program in Kenya that trains women in peace education (Zanoni, 2017). Women are also already doing an outsized proportion of the world's caregiving, often unpaid, untrained, and not considered in economic output indicators. Compensating women for the care they are already proving both legitimizes their work and affords them economic autonomy that can allow them to pursue careers in sectors that support human security. Aside from the fact that women, as half the population, should be as equally represented in the workplace, women hold "gender-specific market knowledge" that can contribute to market efficiencies and adequate service delivery (Mercy Corps, 2015). These perspectives can lead to saving lives when applied to health and security sectors.

Providing Support to Future Leaders

In civil society and community circles, women must be supported as early as possible to enable them to achieve their ambitions of leadership. Women who are already doing important grassroots humanitarian work report being unaware of national and international efforts such as the Women, Peace and Security agenda, especially women unaffiliated with organizations (Lorentzen et al., 2019). Leadership grants for women from low- and middle-income countries are one way these women can receive support for schooling, training, and research, while allowing flexible schedules and other considerations for women also acting as caretakers (Downs et al., 2014).

Although the pace and directionality of globalization has led to poor outcomes for some of the world's most marginalized people, it has led to some positive benefits for women and other vulnerable groups. Globalization has led to the development of worldwide women's organizations and networks, especially with the use of the Internet. With a global lens, women's groups can learn from the insecurities that exist for women across cultures, allowing them to better understand the societal structures that maintain women's marginalization (Moussa, 2008). Having all these data points about areas of human security allows women to see how they are affected by security risks but are also active players in maintaining security for themselves and others.

Ultimately, it is not just a matter of empowering women. At the 2018 Women Leaders in Global Health Conference, Médecins Sans Frontières (MSF) President Joanne Liu noted that fully addressing gender disparities in health care will require men to view these disparities as a problem (Watters, 2019). Men raised in patriarchal households may view a woman in their workplace as subordinate, regardless of her position. As a result, it is not just about women being present at the table—women must be able to meaningfully participate in health system strengthening, peace processes, and post-conflict reconstruction. The focus should be not just on the quantity of women's representation but on the quality as well (True, 2013). Men need to serve as allies, mentors, and participants in the process of promoting gender equity in health care.

Using Technology to Measure and Support Women's Empowerment

The SDGs, along with the indices analyzed in this chapter and many other important indicators, are highly dependent on valid and reliable data from all nations. Unfortunately, there are huge gaps in data in all three areas of health, gender, and peace. Most studies assessing gender and global health come from high-income countries. Data on gender-based issues like sexual harassment and the gender pay gap are even more poorly collected across all countries, regardless of income level (WHO, 2019a). In the peace literature, similar issues can be found. Consistent and trustworthy time-series data from fragile states is limited due to the difficulties in the nature of the research. Very few studies address all three areas together. Agencies must find better ways to contend with these data issues, ensuring that consistent data-gathering techniques can be used with adequate funding and training. Forms of information technology, such as tablets and customizable apps, can assist with information gathering and outreach or training for men and women.

Women need spaces where they can safely discuss issues of GBV, discrimination, and harassment, and the independence afforded by technology can play a major role in these aims. Even in the poorest countries, tapping into the worldwide network of smartphones can fulfill women's care needs while remaining affordable, anonymous, and private (Asi & Williams, 2018). For example, in the war-torn Gaza Strip, poverty is high, resources are limited, and many women are expected to shoulder these burdens without support. Seeing this gap in resources, one mother developed an app that provides other Arabic-speaking mothers with free how-to guides on parenting and resources to get support for GBV and other taboo issues. She emphasized that women who need support—or even just someone to listen— may be discouraged from seeking care outside the home by their family or husband (Trew, 2019). Targeted use of customized and affordable educational online platforms could also encourage women to pursue online education and training opportunities from their home on their own schedule. Online resources could also play a role in training men on appropriate workplace behaviors, without the perceived judgment of others.

Conclusion

There is no doubt that much more research needs to be done on connecting gender equality with peace and health outcomes, but what is clear is that women need a seat at the table. There are many context-specific confounding variables present when assessing these relationships and a host of other factors that would be difficult to capture in a large-scale comparison. Such factors include a nation's history, socio-economic status, stage of development, governance structure, level of religious adherence, perspectives on filial piety, and presence of political fragility or conflict. However, the abundance of literature suggesting the direction of these relationships, and the lack of literature suggesting the inverse, indicates that there is reason for policymakers at all levels to more seriously consider how empowering women encourages progress within all of these sectors, especially if SDGs 3, 5, and 16 are to be achieved in some of the world's most challenging environments.

With increased attention to gender-related issues, it is becoming evident that pursuing gender equality is not only a human rights goal in and of itself but is a necessary step to achieving development in all sectors of society. If what we truly want are societies that are peaceful, that are healthy, that allow individuals and communities to flourish to the fullest of their potential, then we need leadership that reflects those aspirations. Existing evidence suggests that elevating and empowering women leaders will only aid in our efforts to become these thriving societies. As we work to induce policy change at the legislative level and behavior change at the individual level, we create the conditions where transformative structural change is possible. When we eliminate the gender disparities that hinder societies from achieving human security, we can divert our full attention to developing solutions for the most vulnerable among us, of any gender, who deserve the whole breadth of our intellectual, creative, and economic potential.

References

Allotey, P. (2018). Out of the shadows: Women in global health leadership. *Global Health, Epidemiology and Genomics, 3*(e16). https://doi.org/10.1017/gheg.2018.15

Aolain, F. (2011). Women, vulnerability, and humanitarian emergencies. *Michigan Journal of Gender & Law, 18*(1). http://scholarship.law.umn.edu/faculty_articles/71

Asi, Y., & Williams, C. (2018). The role of digital health in making progress toward Sustainable Development Goal (SDG) 3 in conflict-affected populations. *International Journal of Medical Informatics, 114*, 114–120.

Bebell, L., Oduyebo, T., & Riley, L. (2017). Ebola virus disease and pregnancy: A review of the current knowledge of Ebola virus pathogenesis, maternal, and neonatal outcomes. *Birth Defects Research, 109*(5), 353–362.

Benard, C., Jones, S., Oliker, O., Thurston, C., Stearns, B., & Cordell, K. (2008). *Women and nation-building.* RAND Corporation. Retrieved from https://www.rand.org/content/dam/rand/pubs/monographs/2008/RAND_MG579.pdf

Berry, M., & Rana, T. (2019). What prevents peace? Women and peacebuilding in Bosnia and Nepal. *Peace & Change: A Journal of Peace Research, 44*(3), 321–349.

Caprioli, M. (2000). Gendered conflict. *Journal of Peace Research, 37*(1), 51–68.

Collier, P., & Sambanis, N. (2002). Understanding civil war: A new agenda. *The Journal of Conflict Resolution, 46*(1), 3–12.

Council on Foreign Relations (CFR). (2019). *Women's participation in peace processes.* Retrieved from https://www.cfr.org/interactive/womens-participation-in-peace-processes

Downs, J., Reif, L., Hokororo, A., & Fitzgerald, D. (2014). Increasing women in leadership in global health. *Academic Medicine, 89*(8), 1103–1107.

Enloe, C. (2016). *Globalization & militarism: Feminists make the link* (2nd ed.). Rowman & Littlefield.

Galtung, J. (1969). Violence, peace, and peace research. *Journal of Peace Research, 6*(3), 167–191.

Gomez, O. & Gasper, D. (2013). *A thematic guidance note for regional and national human development report teams.* United Nations Development Programme. Retrieved from http://hdr.undp.org/sites/default/files/human_security_guidance_note_r-nhdrs.pdf

Hudson, V., Ballif-Spanvill, B., Caprioli, M., & Emmett, C. (2014). *Sex and world peace.* Columbia University Press.

Ibnouf, F. (2009). The role of women in providing and improving household food security in Sudan: Implications for reducing hunger and malnutrition. *Journal of International Women's Studies, 10*(4), 144–167.

IEP. (2019). *Global peace index 2019: Measuring peace in a complex world.* Retrieved from http://www.visionofhumanity.org/reports

Institute for Economics and Peace (IEP). (2017). *Positive peace: The lens to achieve the Sustaining Peace Agenda*. Retrieved from http://visionofhumanity.org/app/uploads/2017/05/IPI-Positive-Peace-Report.pdf

Jalalzai, F., & Krook, M. (2010). Beyond Hillary and Benazir: Women's political leadership worldwide. *International Political Science Review, 31*(1), 5–21.

Justino, P., Mitchell, R., & Müller, C. (2018). Women and peace building: Local perspectives on opportunities and barriers. *Development and Change, 49*(4), 911–929.

Kastrup, M. (2006). Mental health consequences of war: Gender specific issues. *World Psychiatry, 5*(1), 33–34.

Kaya, Z. & Luchtenberg, K. (2018). *Displacement and women's economic empowerment: Voices of displaced women in the Kurdistan Region of Iraq*. LSE Center for Women, Peace and Security. Retrieved from www.lse.ac.uk/women-peace-security/assets/documents/2018/LSE-WPS-DisplacementEcoEmpowerment-Report.pdf

Kim, E. (2017). Gender and the sustainable development goals. *Global Social Policy, 17*(2). https://doi.org/10.1177/1468018117703444

Levy, B., & Sidel, V. (2016). Documenting the effects of armed conflict on population health. *Annual Review of Public Health, 37*, 205–218.

Lorentzen, J., Toure, N., & Gaye, B. (2019). *Women's participation in peace and reconciliation processes in mali*. PRIO Paper. Retrieved from https://www.prio.org/Publications/Publication/?x=11340

Manjoo, R. & McRaith, C. (2011). Gender-based violence and justice in conflict and post-conflict areas. *Cornell International Law Journal, 11*. Retrieved from https://www.lawschool.cornell.edu/research/ILJ/upload/Manjoo-McRaith-final.pdf

Melander, E. (2005). Gender equality and intrastate armed conflict. *International Studies Quarterly, 49*(4), 695–714.

Menéndez, C., Lucas, A., Munguambe, K., & Langer, A. (2015). Ebola crisis: The unequal impact on women and children's health. *The Lancet Global Health, 3*(3), PE130. https://doi.org/10.1016/S2214-109X(15)70009-4

Mercy Corps. (2015). *Gender and Market Development: A framework for strengthening gender integration in market systems development*. Retrieved from https://www.mercycorps.org/research-resources/gender-and-market-development-framework-strengthening-gender-integration-market

Moussa, G. (2008). Gender aspects of human security. *International Social Science Journal, 59*(s1), 81–100.

Ng, E., & Muntaner, C. (2018). The effect of women in government on population health: An ecological analysis among Canadian provinces, 1976–2009. *SSM Population Health, 6*, 141–148.

O'Reilly, M., Suilleabhain, A., & Paffenholz, T. (2015). Reimagining peacemaking: Women's roles in peace processes. In *International Peace Institute*. Retrieved from https://www.ipinst.org/wp-content/uploads/2015/06/IPI-E-pub-Reimagining-Peacemaking.pdf

OECD. (2017). *Gender equality and women's empowerment in fragile and conflict-affected situations: A review of donor support*. OECD Development Policy Papers No. 8. Retrieved from https://www.oecd.org/dac/conflict-fragility-resilience/docs/Gender_equality_in_fragile_situations_2017.pdf

Ormhaug, C., Meier, P., & Hernes, H. (2009). *Armed conflict deaths disaggregated by gender*. PRIO Paper. Retrieved from https://www.prio.org/Publications/Publication/?x=7207

Parmar, P., Agrawal, P., Goyal, R., Scott, J., & Greenough, P. (2014). Need for a gender-sensitive human security framework: Results of a quantitative study of human security and sexual violence in Djohong District, Cameroon. *Conflict and Health, 8*(6). https://doi.org/10.1186/1752-1505-8-6

Pillai, V., Wang, Y., & Maleku, A. (2017). Women, war, and reproductive health in developing countries. *Social Work in Health Care, 56*(1), 28–44.

Quinn, J., Zeleny, T., Subramaniam, R., & Bencko, V. (2017). Public health crisis in war and conflict—Health security in aggregate. *Central European Journal of Public Health, 25*(1), 72–76.

Reardon, B., & Hans, A. (2010). *The gender imperative: Human Security VS State Security.* Routledge.

Savchuk, K. (2014, April 8). *How Rwanda went from genocide to global health model. GlobalPost.* Retrieved from https://www.pri.org/stories/2014-04-08/ how-rwanda-went-genocide-global-health-model

Stark, L., & Ager, A. (2011). A systematic review of prevalence studies of gender-based violence in complex emergencies. *Trauma Violence Abuse, 12*(3), 127–134.

Stone, L. (2015). Annex II: Quantitative analysis of women's participation in peace processes. In M. O'Reilly et al. (Eds.), *Reimagining peacemaking: Women's roles in peace processes.* International Peace Institute.

Talib, Z., Burke, K. K., & Barry, M. (2017). Women leaders in global health. *The Lancet, 5*(6), E565–E566.

Trew, B. (2019, April 27). *'We just want to be heard': Woman in Gaza builds app to help support fellow mothers.* The Independent. Retrieved from https://www.independent.co.uk/news/world/ middle-east/gaza-momy-helper-app-arabic-mothers-parenting-psychology-a8887946.html

True, J. (2013). *Women, peace and security in post-conflict and peacebuilding contexts.* Norwegian Peacebuilding Resource Centre. Retrieved from https://www.peacewomen.org/assets/file/true_ noref_unscr1325_feb_2013_final.pdf

Truong, T. (1997). Gender and human development: A feminist perspective. *Gender, Technology and Development, 1*(3), 349–370.

UN Women. (2015). *Protecting the rights of women and girls in humanitarian settings.* Retrieved from http://wps.unwomen.org/protecting/

UN Women. (2018, August 13). *Revisiting Rwanda five years after record-breaking parliamentary elections.* Retrieved from http://www.unwomen.org/en/news/stories/2018/8/ feature-rwanda-women-in-parliament

UNDP. (2010a). *Price of peace: Financing for gender equality in post-conflict reconstruction.* Retrieved from http://content-ext.undp.org/aplaws_publications/3190612/price-of-peace-financing-for-gender-equality-in-post-conflict-reconstruction.pdf

UNDP. (2010b). *Women in armed conflicts: Inclusion and exclusion.* Asia-Pacific Human Development Report Background Papers Series. Retrieved from https://www.undp.org/content/dam/rbap/docs/Research%20&%20Publications/human_development/RBAP-APHDR-TBP_2010_11.pdf

UNDP. (2018). *Human Development Data (1990–2017) [Gender Inequality Index].* Retrieved from http://hdr.undp.org/en/data

United Nations. (2016). *In safety and dignity: Addressing large movements of refugees and migrants.* Report of the Secretary-General. Retrieved from https://www.un.org/en/ga/search/ view_doc.asp?symbol=A/70/59&=E%20

United Nations Development Programme (UNDP). (1994). Human Development Report 1994. Retrieved from http://hdr.undp.org/sites/default/files/reports/255/hdr_1994_en_complete_ nostats.pdf

United Nations Population Fund (UNFPA). (2015). *Maternal mortality in humanitarian crises and in fragile settings.* Retrieved from https://www.unfpa.org/sites/default/files/resource-pdf/ MMR_in_humanitarian_settings-final4_0.pdf

United Nations Women (UN Women). (2014). *Ebola outbreak takes its toll on women.* Retrieved from https://www.unwomen.org/en/news/stories/2014/9/ebola-outbreak-takes-its-toll-on-women

Wängnerud, L. (2009). Women in parliaments: Descriptive and substantive representation. *Annual Review of Political Science, 12*, 51–69.

Watters, L. (2019, January 11). *How men fit into the quest for more women leaders in global health.* Devex. Retrieved from https://www.devex.com/news/how-men-fit-into-the-quest-for-more-women-leaders-in-global-health-93872

Westendorf, J. (2015). *Why peace processes fail: Negotiating insecurity after civil war.* Lynne Rienner Publishers.

WHO. (2019a). *Delivered by women, led by men: A gender and equity analysis of the global health and social workforce.* Retrieved from https://apps.who.int/iris/bitstream/handle/10665/3 11322/9789241515467-eng.pdf

WHO. (2019b). *Women are key in Ebola response.* Retrieved from https://www.who.int/news-room/facts-in-pictures/detail/women-join-hands-to-oust-ebola-from-drc

Wiist, W., Barker, K., Arya, N., Rohde, J., Donohoe, M., et al. (2014). The role of public health in the prevention of war: Rationale and competencies. *American Journal of Public Health, 104*(6), e34–e47.

World Bank. (2016). *Helping countries navigate a volatile environment.* Retrieved from https://www.worldbank.org/en/topic/fragilityconflictviolence/overview

World Bank. (2018). *Proportion of seats held by women in national parliaments (%).* Retrieved from https://data.worldbank.org/indicator/SG.GEN.PARL.ZS

World Health Organization (WHO). (2018). *Current health expenditure (CHE) as percentage of gross domestic product (GDP) (%).* Data by country. Retrieved from https://apps.who.int/gho/data/view.main.GHEDCHEGDPSHA2011v?lang=en

Zanoni, K. (2017). Kenyan girls as agents of peace: Enhancing the capacity of future women peacebuilders. *Research in Comparative and International Education, 12*(1), 1190–1126.

Zuckerman, E., & Greenberg, M. (2004). The gender dimensions of post-conflict reconstruction: An analytical framework for policymakers. *Gender and Development, 12*(3), 70–82.

Interview with Matshidiso Moeti, WHO Regional Director for Africa

Sulzhan Bali and Roopa Dhatt

"Let's do it for women and girls."

Matshidiso Moeti, from Botswana, is the first woman to be elected as World Health Organization (WHO) Regional Director for Africa. Dr. Moeti is a public health veteran, with almost 40 years of national and international experience. She joined the WHO Regional Office for Africa in 1999 and has served as Deputy Regional Director, Assistant Regional Director, Director of Noncommunicable Diseases, WHO Representative for Malawi, Coordinator of the Inter-Country Support Team for the South and East African countries, and Regional Advisor for HIV/AIDS. Before joining WHO, Dr. Moeti worked with the Joint United Nations Programme on HIV/AIDS (UNAIDS) as team leader of the Africa and Middle East desk in Geneva (1997–1999); with the United Nations Children's Fund (UNICEF) as regional health advisor for East and Southern Africa; and with Botswana's Ministry of Health as a clinician and public health specialist. Dr. Moeti holds a degree in medicine (MB, BS) and a Master of Public Health degree (MSc in community health for developing countries) from the Royal Free Hospital School of Medicine, the University of London, and the London School of Hygiene & Tropical Medicine, respectively. Dr. Moeti was awarded an honorary fellowship of the London School of Hygiene & Tropical Medicine and an honorary doctorate from the University of Health and Allied Sciences, Ghana.

S. Bali (✉) · R. Dhatt
Women in Global Health, Washington, DC, USA
e-mail: sulzhan@gmail.com; roopa.dhatt@womeningh.org

© Springer Nature Switzerland AG 2022
R. Morgan et al. (eds.), *Women and Global Health Leadership*,
https://doi.org/10.1007/978-3-030-84498-1_5

Could You Share with Us Your Early Global Health Journey?

By background, I'm an MD and was trained in the UK. I have a master's degree in public health, also from the UK, from the London School of Hygiene. However, I stumbled into public health almost as a second choice, because, in fact, I wanted to become a clinician specialist. I wanted to study pediatrics, but at the time I was aiming to do that, I had a small child, and there wasn't a medical school in my country. I would have needed to have left my child for several years, so I found that very difficult to contemplate. Having virtually grown up in boarding school myself, I was always clear that if I have a child, I am going to stay with my child. In the end, I opted for a specialty that would take a shorter time to get a qualification in, which is how I decided to study public health.

I had an early interest in public health. I have a family background where both of my parents were doctors who worked a lot in public health. My father was in the WHO Global Smallpox Commission, so he used to make frequent field trips while we were living in Botswana. He was going out into the bush, as we called it, on trips to villages looking for smallpox patients. He used to talk about his work in TB as well, and my mother was the WHO Director of Family and Reproductive and Child Health in the country, so she did a lot of work on family planning and immunizations. I used to listen to discussions of things to do with public health. I acquired the idea of solving problems for people, for a country, as opposed to treating one patient.

Then when I was a medical student in London, my mother used to attend the WHO World Health Assembly in Geneva and ask me to join her. I was very fortunate that my mom was a delegate. She managed to get me in, and I would sit in the gallery listening to discussions, and go to the after-meeting dinners, and had the opportunity to meet prominent WHO leaders.

When I was working as a young doctor in a pediatric ward, many of the children had severe malnutrition. When I asked about the family background, I'd be told, "oh, there is no father." The family structure in Botswana was affected by migrant labor to the South African mines. I found out that there were many young women, teenagers, who had children without any male support. That's what sparked my interest in public health—how social factors like family structure and family income have an impact on severe malnutrition in children.

It was partly family background and partly the experience of understanding my society and seeing the direct impacts of social factors on health—those are the things that got me on my path in public health.

Are There Any Mentors That You Credit for Your Success?

The one person who encouraged me to go for a position in the UN when I was working in my country was the UNICEF representative in Botswana. By then, I had qualified in public health, and I was managing the HIV program in Botswana, which at that time was one of the worst affected countries in the world regarding the prevalence of HIV. I interacted with many people—national and international. The UNICEF representative with whom I worked was very supportive. She was an American who encouraged me to apply for a regional position in UNICEF. At first, I said, "No, I'm happy here. My work is fascinating, and I've got my family here." She said, "Well, think about it. You can build on your experience." She invested time in encouraging me to apply for a position. She was somebody who had a significant influence on me deciding to take a step in my career.

Several others encouraged me. When I worked with UNICEF, Zambia was reforming its health system. The UNICEF representative at that time encouraged me to apply for a position and work with him in the country, and I did, leaving the regional office position, which many people thought was strange. Generally, there is more status in a regional position, but this was somebody with whom I'd had discussions about change, how things could work better, and he invited me to come and join his office and be part of the process of reforming the national health system in Zambia. That was an exceptional experience, which made an essential contribution to my thinking about change and managing change in health systems.

Because of the reform program of the Zambian Ministry of Health, I became the supervisor of Dr. Halfdan Mahler, the former WHO Director-General. He was the team leader of a group of senior consultants who carried out a review of Zambia's pioneering health reform. As a UNICEF program officer in that country office, I was Halfdan Mahler's supervisor. My boss said, "Don't feel intimidated. You have your role, he has his role, and I've got your back. I'm behind you." I have had some very encouraging supervisors.

Why Is Gender Equity in Leadership Important?

It's important because for good global health governance, you need people who bring different perspectives, different experiences, other competencies, and different ways of doing things. If you look at the countries that initially did well in responding to the COVID-19 pandemic, they're all led by women. You need a combination of people with vision, determination, energy, and the ability to be inclusive in ways of working. The ability to provide space for others to voice their opinion and to consider different points of view is essential to leadership. I think it's that diversity of opinions and experience, combined with women's abilities to address the demands and needs in life, that enables a particular outlook and contributes very positively to global health.

So, Do Men and Women Lead Differently?

Yes, I think so. I believe women's style of leadership can be both visionary and transparent in terms of defining a direction, as well as being open to taking into account different points of view and facilitating engagement of other people and opinions. Women can reach a compromise, and find ways to engage different people and ideas, and can find a way forward that works for a range of participants in the process, whereas I think men's style of leadership is very much more authority-based, demanding conformity. Men also have ways of networking among themselves. I think that women's style of supporting each other and including each other are more open, but men tend to use authority more than listening and are less prepared to consider different points of view.

Are Women Perceived Differently as Leaders?

Women are not often recognized as leaders. I've had this experience myself, where you are in a meeting, you say something, and then it's overlooked until a man repeats the same thing and it is remembered as his idea. I've often said, "Well, I said that, and I said it first. How come you didn't recognize it then, and you recognize it because a man said it?" Women must battle for recognition and the endorsement of leadership. As a woman you have to work harder to prove that you are a good leader, that you do know what you are doing, you are competent, you are knowledgeable, and you can work with others, to lead others, to get that recognition. I think with men it's just assumed. Also, when women are very directive, there is resistance; they are regarded as being bossy women, whereas this is considered to be expected for men.

What Obstacles Did You Experience in Your Journey?

One major factor that directed my career was combining the needs of my career and the needs of my family. I think this is very important in many women's careers. I look at the low proportion of women applicants that we have for important jobs. I have a straightforward experience now as the regional director, trying to encourage women to come and join WHO, where women are not mobile due to family responsibilities.

Then, I think in terms of gender, as a woman you need to work exceptionally hard and demonstrate your capabilities in ways that men are not required to do. The people that you find, on the whole, in positions to make decisions, who are making assessments, are men, and men have ways of networking among themselves, supporting each other, which are very well-established because they are in the majority. Those are some of the obstacles that I have had to overcome.

Quite often, when you work to establish that you're competent and you're able to deliver, you get labeled as being "aggressive" or "over-assertive." I've had that kind of comment about myself in the past in a couple of positions. Then there are the obstacles of recognition being a woman from the Global South in the international context; you have to show to people that you are competent, knowledgeable, and experienced. You must always demonstrate that extra capacity.

How Did You Deal with This "Lack of Recognition" and Other Obstacles in Your Career?

I just worked harder. I had to. Initially, it was working harder to show that you are competent, that you can produce the results needed. I was fortunate in the early stages of my career in the UN to work in a regional office of UNICEF, which had a reasonable number of women in senior positions. The female regional director started a program of training for women leaders, making it explicit that it was one of her priorities to develop leadership competencies and support women in the organization to move into leadership positions.

That made a difference at a crucial point in my career. I've been in several positions where I've had to show that I have the competence, can work with people from different backgrounds, and can achieve results and lead teams. I've been fortunate to find supportive peers.

It is also a matter of establishing relationships with people, establishing links with others, and finding common ground with individuals that go beyond me being a woman from the South. It's critical to build the relationship, let people get to know you, to get to know your work, and to invest in getting to know them. Then find common ground with people from diverse backgrounds and show what you believe, what you think is correct, and what you have achieved. Establish links with other people. Be in networks. I think those are some of the cultural differences you have to overcome to gain allies and people who can be supportive of your point of view and your work.

How Important Are Peer Networks?

Peer networks are critical. If I look at a couple of experiences, colleagues can help you find solutions by sharing their own experiences. Both peer networks and structured leadership and networking programs are critical parts of inculcating leadership. Peer networks can help women leverage their strengths and overcome structural and institutional barriers.

I worked with some great women colleagues in Botswana, in UNAIDS, UNICEF, and also in WHO, who have been peers. I've been fortunate to have women colleagues where we supported each other, which made a huge difference. One needs mentors/supervisors who encourage, give you opportunities, and also the chance to exchange with peers who can support you from that perspective of having very similar experiences, with the multiple roles that you have to play, both at work and in families. Networking with other women, and supporting other women, and in turn being supported and mentored by women, and some men, really helped me in my career.

What Advice Would You Give to Young Women Who Are Aspiring to Be Global Health Leaders?

First, it's vital for people to know their strengths and believe in themselves; for women that sometimes does take some effort. Then, having recognized those, to build them up to be ready to learn from others, and to be prepared to be out of their comfort zone. It's important to link up with others and show that you have something to contribute. I think very often women hesitate to build on their strengths for their advantage. Too often, they focus on helping others.

Women are trained to be modest. You are liked because you support others. I think it's important for women to be confident in themselves and show what they can do, of course without boasting. Then, work with others. Support other people. Network. Find connections with women colleagues and with male colleagues. Invite and request others to mentor you and to support you; and indicate that you could benefit from more experienced colleagues sharing their knowledge, their experiences with you, helping you to figure out for yourself how to progress. This is something I am seeing younger women do, which some of us were never taught. We were told, "You cannot be bothering more senior people." I'm delighted to see young women coming forward and asking for support and to be mentored.

Quite often, people who have the competence, the knowledge, the experience, and would be very happy to work with others should also support other younger women coming up. It takes a while to understand that you can progress without necessarily being competitive and that by supporting other people you can gain recognition and support that can help you.

Then, of course, learn things that don't work for you. If you make mistakes or if you feel that something has been a failure, find ways to understand what didn't work, why that happened. Learn from it, and then move on, so that the next time something similar comes along you have built on that experience and do it differently.

What Measures Can Institutions Take to Cultivate a Greater Representation of Women in a Leadership Position?

You have to be very explicit in making it clear that this is your priority. Sometimes it is not clearly stated. Then, I think you need to go looking for women. We need to find networks that will enable us to identify women. Of course, we advertise positions, but I've learned that it's not enough to do that. People won't just bump into the advert and see that they could be suitable. We need to find both direct ways, if you know good people, to encourage them to apply, and we need to invest in finding organizations that go looking for talent on our behalf. In WHO, I do both as an individual, I ask my colleagues to do that, and we have contracted organizations that are dealing with human resources to help us look for good women candidates to apply for positions.

We also need to support women to facilitate their work, such as making sure women have support if they need flexible hours or to be accommodated in terms of their family responsibilities. This is very, very important. Then, to establish specific leadership training for women on gender issues in the workplace, we are putting in place a mentorship program, which has gotten a very enthusiastic response among our women colleagues. We've also reached out to the UN volunteers program, because one of the things that we need to do is to encourage women to come in the early stage of their careers. The intention being that competent young women start applying for positions for the more mainstream professional or even managerial positions in the organization and grow in the organization. Those are some of the things that can be done to support and accommodate women.

Also, being very clear when you are looking at dossiers for recruitment that you look at women candidates, and ask why haven't they ended up on the shortlist? I think there's a certain level of assumption and bias among those people in selection panels as well, and we need to make sure that women don't get screened out at the very first step. See if you can get more women recruited that way.

If You Could Have a Billboard for Other Women Leaders, What Would It Say?

It would say, *let's do it for girls and young women*. One of the things that we have to do as women leaders is make a difference for girls and young women. We need to encourage girls and young women, first of all, to get an education, to gain the life skills that build the confidence to decide the direction of their lives, and then help them to help themselves—to look for mentoring, to look for peer support, to find ways to develop their career. It has to start early, and women need to feel that sense of being encouraged and welcomed, to make progress and to use their talents to their maximum, for global health.

Academic Journal Publishing: A Pathway to Global Health Leadership

Jamie Lundine, Ivy Lynn Bourgeault, and Dina Balabanova

There are myriad paths to leadership in "global health" and the creation of health and well-being more broadly. Academic research is one way to contribute to the global health ecosystem and, thus, to establish oneself as a leader. Academic cultures differ across geographic nations and regions, as well as academic disciplines (e.g. public health, medicine, epidemiology, medical anthropology, etc.). Generally, however, within the context of academia, publishing journal articles is a key metric to establishing oneself as a scientist and, thus, a leader.

The scholarly journal publishing industry provides platforms for researchers to share scientific findings and contribute to scholarly debates. These scholarly debates advance our knowledge about interventions to generate greater health and well-being; furthermore, scholarly journal articles are used as a metric to evaluate an academic's contribution to their chosen field. To publish a scientific finding in a scholarly journal, a researcher must conduct a study, write the findings in the format of a journal article, and submit the article for review by peers. Peers are generally scholars with the requisite knowledge in the same or similar specific area (geographic, discipline, methodological area, etc.). Funding organizations and institutional hiring and promotion committees, thus, use the quality and quantity of publications to evaluate an academic's contributions and make funding or hiring

J. Lundine (✉)
Institute of Feminist and Gender Studies, University of Ottawa, Ottawa, ON, Canada
e-mail: jlund037@uottawa.ca

I. L. Bourgeault
School of Sociological and Anthropological Studies, Faculty of Social Sciences, University of Ottawa, Ottawa, ON, Canada
e-mail: ivy.bourgeault@uOttawa.ca

D. Balabanova
Department of Global Health and Development, London School of Hygiene & Tropical Medicine, London, UK
e-mail: Dina.Balabanova@lshtm.ac.uk

© Springer Nature Switzerland AG 2022
R. Morgan et al. (eds.), *Women and Global Health Leadership*,
https://doi.org/10.1007/978-3-030-84498-1_6

and promotion decisions. As such, an academic's publication record is arguably the most important factor for her career success.

Despite its "global" nature, global health research does not occur on a level playing field. The health research ecosystem is influenced by what Patricia Hill Collins, bell hooks, and others have described as a matrix of domination (Hill Collins, 2002), namely, intersecting structures of patriarchy, imperialism, colonialism, and capitalism. Decades after the end of direct colonial rule, the influence of inequitable systems is reflected at all levels of the research ecosystem. Researchers from high-income countries (HICs) (many of which are imperial nations in North America and Europe) have greater access to resources than their colleagues from low- and middle-income countries (LMICs) (Abimbola, 2019). Global health funding, for example, is more likely to be given to HIC researchers, in part because of their closer proximity to global health funders (Walsh et al., 2016).

At the other end of the research cycle, high-impact academic health journals are also concentrated in HICs (or imperial nations). The "big five" high-impact weekly medical journals (Allotey et al., 2017), for example, are all located in either London, England, or cities in the United States. Namely, *The British Medical Journal* (BMJ) and *The Lancet* are published in London, England. The *Annals of Internal Medicine*, the journal of the American College of Physicians, is located in Philadelphia, USA. *The New England Journal of Medicine* (NEJM) is published in Boston, USA, and *JAMA: The Journal of the American Medical Association* is published in Chicago, USA. In 2018, Publons reported that 96.1% of journal editors worked in countries with "established" research infrastructure (Publons, 2018). In addition to geographical disparities, gender influences access to resources. Women in all contexts (HICs and LMICs) are less likely to be authors, peer reviewers, and editors. A recent study demonstrated that women from low-income countries are the least likely population to be published (Morgan et al., 2019).

Despite the seemingly global or international nature of journal publishing (JAMA's Twitter handle reads "JAMA is an international peer-reviewed general medical journal published weekly online and in print, and a member of the @ JAMANetwork family of journals" and NEJM's Twitter handle reads "The New England Journal of Medicine is the world's leading medical journal and website"), journals are concentrated in particular nations and even within particular regions and cities. In 2018, Wei and Lei reported that nearly a quarter of the research articles (23.89%) published in the *NEJM* between 1997 and 2016 had an author affiliated with Harvard University (Wei & Lei, 2018). The geographic concentration of authors is attributed to research collaborations and institutional bias which favours "prestigious" universities. Despite claims of universal access and reach, studies of influential journals can highlight the importance of proximity to a journal's headquarters in terms of accessing opportunities to publish (both Harvard University and NEJM are located in Boston, USA).

Within this highly unequal (let's call it inequitable) system of global health research, how do we strive towards equity? In this chapter, we will consider this main question, but first, we ask: What is academic journal publishing? How does it function? What do editors think about nationality and gender as factors influencing knowledge production within the journal publishing process? What would a consideration of equity in academic publishing look like?

First, we will consider how academic publishing works, including how it is organized. Second, we will explore both the literature and the editors' perspectives on gender and nationality in publishing. Finally, we will think about some ways in which publishing can provide greater visibility and support for a diversity of knowledge.

The Social Organization of Academic Journal Publishing

Scientific journals originated out of learned societies in Europe in the 1700s, exclusively for men and in particular white men from the "leisure" class (Harding, 1991). One of the earliest medical journals was *Medical Essays and Observations*, which began circulating shortly after the Royal Society of Edinburgh was established in 1731 (Farrell et al., 2017). These journals were initially organized like a magazine or a newspaper written, edited, and published by members of the society which acted as gatekeepers to the content (Farrell et al., 2017).

From these exclusive origins, journals have evolved to become an integral player within the academic ecosystem. This is in part because, in academia, one of the critical metrics for staff performance and career progression is an individual's publication record (Moher et al., 2016; van Dalen & Henkens, 2012). Publishing in high-profile and high-impact peer review journals is key to any academic's success and recognition in their chosen field (Moher et al., 2016; Sidhu et al., 2009; Van Dalen & Henkens, 2012). It is also key to visibility achieving an impact on policies and agendas. It is, therefore, concerning that research across various disciplines shows how women, particularly black women, Indigenous women, and women of colour, are underrepresented in various parts of the peer review process, as authors, peer reviewers, and editors. Looking back at the history of academia and journal publishing, it is not surprising that men are overrepresented in science journals; however, several large-scale studies suggest that increasing the numbers of women authors is insufficient to counteract the effect of gender bias (Helmer et al., 2017). We are all exposed to the structures of domination (Hill Collins, 2002) (sexism, racism, imperialism, etc.) and must therefore actively learn and practise anti-racism and anti-imperialism, which includes women challenging their own assumptions about gender, sex, race, class, ability, and nationality.

Why We Chose to Examine Academic Publishing?

Our own journey into the world of academic publishing is instructive. Interest in the topic of inequities in publishing was sparked by a conversation at the fourth annual Health Systems Symposium in Vancouver, Canada, in 2016. At one of the sessions, one of the editors at BioMed Central presented data showing the representation of women and LMIC authors on panels at the Symposium. The presentation generated wide interest. Dr. Balabanova and Dr. Bourgeault both independently had conversations with the publisher BioMed Central about if and how these types of analyses would be relevant to publishing. Dr. Balabanova has been serving on the editorial board of BMC *Health Systems Research* and Dr. Bourgeault had been involved as a peer reviewer and would later join the editorial board of *Human Resources for Health*. In 2016, Dr. Balabanova sought colleagues to work on the project at the London School of Hygiene & Tropical Medicine (LSHTM). This is when Jamie Lundine, a Canadian student who had worked in Kenya before joining LSHTM, joined the team. Through their shared interest in gender and various paths to health leadership, Jamie, Dina, and Ivy began collaborating on this project.

A Pathway to Leadership

Both Dr. Balabanova and Dr. Bourgeault had experienced the typical academic imperative to publish. They realized how large the influence of publications was on their own careers. They recognized that well-known adage "publish or perish" as a truism for those seeking a path to global health leadership in academia. For a global health researcher, one's publication record (the quantity and quality of the journals you publish in) is the main criteria used to make promotion and salary decisions, as well as consideration for awards and other recognitions. Critically, this is also essential for attracting funding and achieving credibility and recognitions by peers.

The power of publishing also influences leadership beyond the sphere of academia. Peer-reviewed publications influence health decision-making and are used to support particular programmatic and policy actions. The media often follows scientific discovery through the publication of articles as a "gold standard" of academic evidence (Smith, 2006). Government agencies make policy decisions that can be informed by evidence from peer-reviewed articles.

Knowledge is power, and in relation to academic careers, we could also understand power as the ability to inform or influence decisions about policies and funding priorities that directly impact people's lives. Academic articles become the knowledge or the "evidence" which can be used to inform policy decisions. How do governments deliver pre-natal care in different cities, countries, and regions? Who can access (and regulate) safe and legal abortions? Should we regulate and fund midwifery care? At what age do children receive vaccines? Which vaccines are made freely available? Which healthcare providers administer the vaccines? What type of health knowledge do we teach in elementary schools? What is an appropriate sexual education curriculum? The answers to these questions are informed, to a certain degree, by research conducted in academic institutions and published in peer-reviewed journals. We believe that the question of who does this research (if it even gets done at all), who frames the questions, what is the funding source for the research, and ultimately, how it is written up, reviewed, evaluated, communicated, and attributed (or cited) is wrapped up in questions of power and privilege, which includes important considerations of gender and location. We believe it is important to scrutinize the research processes, including its communication.

How Does Peer Review Work?

Editorial peer review in biomedical and scientific journals began in the mid-twentieth century and evolved in different forms across journals (Burnham, 1990). It was only later that a formal peer review process as a means to judge and suggest improvements to submitted manuscripts was established (Smith, 2006). Notable health science journals, such as *The Lancet*, did not institutionalize peer review until the 1970s (Farrell et al., 2017). In peer review, experts in a particular discipline or field (often identified from an existing pool of authors) are invited to review the work of other colleagues in the same discipline or field (Lee et al., 2013). Subjecting an article to peer review lends credibility to a piece of research and communicates research findings to the wider academic community, as well as policy makers and practitioners in the field (Ali & Watson, 2016; Smith, 2006). Peer-reviewed journal articles document new knowledge and, in some cases, scientific discovery (Ali & Watson, 2016). In this way, journals play a key role in the advancement of knowledge and subsequently influence policy and practice in the field of public health (Ali & Watson, 2016). The involvement of a diversity of voices is thus vital to producing innovation and knowledge (Lee et al., 2013).

Briefly, a typical peer review process at the majority of public health journals starts with the author (or group of authors), who develops a manuscript, selects a suitable journal, and submits the manuscript (Ali & Watson, 2016). The manuscript is received by an editor, who reviews the document and makes an initial assessment of its suitability for the journal and its readership, as well as its scientific quality (Ali & Watson, 2016; Manchikanti et al., 2015; Wall et al., 2006). A manuscript may be rejected at this point (i.e. desk reject) or proceed for full review. Depending on the size and organizational structure of the journal, the article may then be sent to a designated editor who takes it through the peer review process (Manchikanti et al., 2015). The designated editor seeks one to three independent peer reviewers, to provide an expert review of its content (Manchikanti et al., 2015; Molassiotis & Richardson, 2004). The manuscript may undergo several rounds of review and revision before a decision is taken on its fate—to accept or reject (see Fig. 1) (Molassiotis & Richardson, 2004).

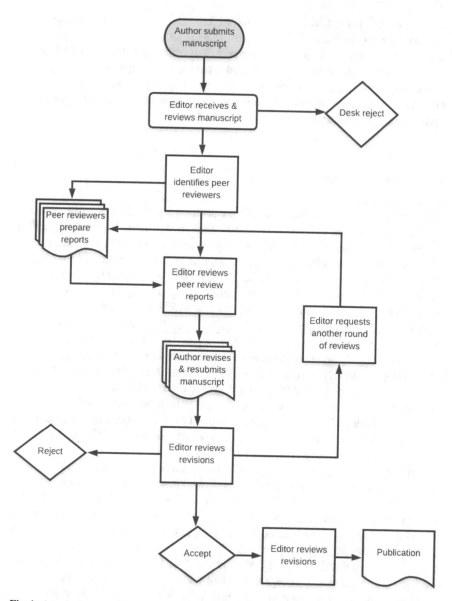

Fig. 1 A typical peer review process (Wiley.com, n.d.). (Source: The peer review process, adapted with permission from Wiley.com. ©John Wiley & Sons. Please see original figure at: https://aut-horservices.wiley.com/Reviewers/journal-reviewers/what-is-peer-review/the-peer-review-process.html)

Roles in Peer Review

The Role of Editors in the Peer Review Process

Editors act as important "gatekeepers" to the production of scientific knowledge (Heidari et al., 2016; Hojat et al., 2003). The leading editor at a journal is usually called the Editor-in-Chief (Galipeau et al., 2016; Wall et al., 2006). The Editor-in-Chief receives and can review all manuscripts submitted to the journal (Wall et al., 2006; Wiley.com, n.d.). Other types of editors include managing editors, editors in specialist topics, and associate editors (Ali & Watson, 2016; Galipeau et al., 2016; Wall et al., 2006; Wiley.com, n.d.). Most editors operate on a part-time, volunteer basis and are employed at academic or research institutions (Borsuk et al., 2009), although some journals employ full-time, in-house editors (Lee et al., 2013). Each editor has a different role and responsibilities. The number and type of editorial roles vary between disciplines, journals, and publishers (Elsevier, n.d.; Wiley.com, n.d.).

The primary editorial role is to receive a scientific manuscript and provide an assessment of its suitability for academic peer review (Ali & Watson, 2016; Galipeau et al., 2016). The editor uses his/her expertise in the field to determine whether or not the manuscript fits with the scope of the journal, for example, its relevance to the field of public health (Galipeau et al., 2016; Wall et al., 2006). An assessment of the methodological rigour and quality of the document is also undertaken. In some instances, the editor "desk rejects" the manuscript (without sending it out for peer review) (Lee & Schunn, 2011). In other instances, he/she will request revisions before sending the manuscript out for peer review (Ali & Watson, 2016). If the manuscript is deemed suitable, it can be sent straightaway for peer review (Ali & Watson, 2016). In this case, the editor may search for one, two, or three peer reviewers or send the manuscript to an associate or junior editors to carry out the search for reviewers (Ali & Watson, 2016; Wiley.com, n.d.). The search for reviewers usually involves searching a series of databases for those with relevant expertise and contacting several potential reviewers to secure one to three reviews (Borja, 2015). Peer reviewers work voluntarily and in many cases do not benefit from reviewing in terms of promotion, which contributes to the challenge of finding peer reviewers for manuscripts (Ali & Watson, 2016). Other editorial roles and responsibilities include involvement in editing and the final publishing of manuscripts (Galipeau et al., 2016).

Beyond handling manuscripts, senior editors play an important role in setting the direction and strategy for a journal, including what type of content the journal will publish and how to promote submissions to the journal (Galipeau et al., 2016). In this way, editors are integral to defining and upholding standards for what is considered relevant and high-quality public health research (Galipeau et al., 2016; Smith, 2006; Wall et al., 2006). Furthermore, the Editor-in-Chief and senior editors will decide on best practices and guidelines and monitor their implementation in the peer review process (Galipeau et al., 2016).

The Role of Peer Reviewers in the Peer Review Process

Peer reviewers are recognized experts in their field of study, who are asked to volunteer their time to contribute to the advancement of knowledge through reviewing and providing feedback on the work of authors (Ali & Watson, 2016). Reviewers' expertise can be defined through different criteria, but predominantly falls within the subject-area expertise, for example, in adolescent health or water and sanitation, and areas of methodological expertise, for example, randomized controlled trials or quasi-experimental methods (Ali & Watson, 2016; Smith, 2006). These criteria are typically assessed through their publication record. The peer reviewers conduct an expert assessment of a manuscript and provide feedback to the authors. Peer reviewers also make a recommendation to the editor, usually for "acceptance, acceptance subject to minor revisions, major revisions and reconsideration by the reviewers, or rejection"(Molassiotis & Richardson, 2004).

The basic principle behind peer review is that reviewers can act with impartiality, which is "the ability for any reviewer to interpret and apply evaluative criteria in the same way in the assessment of a submission" (Lee et al., 2013). There are several common approaches to peer review to attempt to ensure impartial judgement of a manuscript: single-blind, double-blind, and open peer review (Ali & Watson, 2016; Ford, 2015; Lee et al., 2013).

The Role of Authors in the Peer Review Process

Authors have been described as some of the main beneficiaries of peer review (Ali & Watson, 2016). This is because it is their work that is being assessed, potentially improved, and disseminated (Ali & Watson, 2016). Authors have the responsibility to ensure their manuscript addresses an important research question, uses rigorous and well-described methodology, and is clear and transparent in its documentation (Dixon, 2001). They must also follow standard academic writing guidelines, as well as those of the specific journals (Dixon, 2001). Authors are responsible for selecting an appropriate journal for their manuscript, a process which should help to minimize the number of desk rejections on grounds of relevance (Dixon, 2001). During the process, authors must respond to requests for changes and modifications to their manuscript or any requests for data or further information to support their findings (Dixon, 2001).

Gender Perspectives on the Editorial Process

Given the central role that editors play in shaping the scientific record, we wanted to speak to editors regarding their knowledge of and views on gender in academic publishing. We have noticed an increasing interest in quantitative research into women in publishing, studies of women's representation on editorial boards and as authors or peer reviewers in discipline-specific journals, or length and quality of peer review reports by women and men. There remains, however, little qualitative research on this topic. As documented elsewhere (Lundine et al., 2019), we began our research with a focus on the representation of women in publishing, as well as concerns over gender bias. Our work has since evolved to become much more broadly focused on power and privilege in publishing, examining structures of domination. We recognize that work on gender must look beyond the binary of women and men, which the research reported on in this chapter does not. We recognize that current approaches to quantifying participation in publishing contribute to the erasure of non-binary and transgender researchers in global health and beyond.

In the rest of this chapter, we report findings from interviews with 15 editors working in a range of health science editorial roles. Editors were recruited through partnership with a publisher, worked mostly for open access journals (10 out of the 15), are based in high-income countries, and come from health science fields (see Lundine et al., 2019). During in-depth interviews, editors were asked (amongst other topics) about their perspectives on gender balance and any policies or targets related to equality at the journal. We report our findings on this theme in the next section.

Gender-Balanced Approach to Gender Equality in Publishing

Gender of Authors, Peer Reviewers, and Editors

When asked, editors seemed relatively comfortable discussing gender balance in publishing. They were aware of gender issues within academia more broadly. They knew of initiatives within their own academic institutions seeking to create a more gender-balanced faculty. A few were aware of the literature on gender in peer review. The general perception amongst most editors was that participation in the peer review editorial process amongst authors, peer reviewers, and editors was balanced in terms of gender.

> …It would be interesting to see the metrics, from my perspective it does seem fairly balanced, you know, maybe a bit more male contributions, but especially … I mean, yeah, they're more or less fairly balanced. (Participant 6, Man)

There was no consistent articulation of what constitutes gender balance and how to measure it. Editors interpreted gender balance differently—some spoke of balance, referring to a third female as being representative of women in that discipline (e.g. women comprise about 30% of the workforce in dentistry, and therefore, a third of women on dentistry editorial boards would be "balanced"); others spoke of "fifty-fifty" or "a good balance" of men and women. Others wondered about gender balance being equal numbers of men and women acting as peer reviewers and in positions such as senior author, or the presence of women or men writing influential pieces, such as editorials. Moreover, most were not collecting the data necessary to measure or track change over time. One editor remarked:

> Really—we don't collect any information at this point about gender, despite having lots of papers and lots of supplements around the topic of gender equality, and having lots of great reviewers in this area, we don't collect that information at this point in time. (Participant 12, Woman)

As gender indicators were not systematically captured by any of the journals, one editor who was interested in gender in peer review, but who had not specifically done work on the topic, expressed hesitancy to comment on the gender break-down of her fellow editors, authors, and peer reviewers at the journal. She wanted more information before reaching a conclusion; she was sensitive to gender issues and their implications and seemed not to want to draw inaccurate conclusions.

Table 1 outlines the varied perceptions of gender of the different editor participants and in this case on the gender "balance" on their own editorial boards. The quotes presented here relate to the particular masthead or editorial board that the journal editor was referring to. We collected these data in July 2017 and used names of editorial board members as a proxy for gender. Where gender was not clear from a name, the authors conducted a Google search of the editorial board member and searched their biographies for pronouns. This approach is an established method within work on journals and gender representation.

Some editors held the opinion that their journal's editorial staff was gender balanced (Table 1). In one case, this was informed by the editor having done work to actively recruit women to the board (e.g. journal 4) or editors taking explicitly feminist perspectives (see Table 1, journals 8 and 9). In other cases, the view that the board was balanced was based on gender representation in his/her own discipline more broadly:

> We're now at a point where 50 percent of our trainees are female, in general surgery, and because of that, the composition of authorship, in my opinion, is pretty close to that. (Participant 10, Man)

For one journal, the Editor-in-Chief was highly aware that his editorial board needed to make improvements:

> But we have, apart from me…we have five male editors. So, the ratio is five-to-one, which is completely um embarrassing. Um… And I've been looking for female editors, I haven't found [any]. (Participant 14, Man)

On the other hand, some editors reported that their journal had more women on the board (5 men and 21 women) (see Table 1):

> …we are a very feminist journal as well, so we are a little bit on the other side of the spectrum, where we have mostly female editorial board members, all female editorial team, and all female associate editors. And I'm really looking into changing that as well. (Participant 13, Woman)

Regarding reviewing Table 1, please note that the journals in this study are diverse and cannot be easily compared to one another. The functions and roles of editors varied widely, as did the size and level of responsibility or engagement with the

Table 1 Gender composition of editorial boards of journals and editors' perceptions of gender composition of the board

Journal	Male/female representation on editorial board	Participant(s) perceptions regarding gender composition on editorial boards
Journal 1	123:27[a]	I don't know what percentage of our editorial board is female, but it's fifty-fifty and...it's pretty close. Maybe it's 52/48, but I've never even looked at this (Participant 10, Man)
Journal 2	8:1	But we have, apart from me...we have five male editors. So the ratio is five-to-one, which is completely um embarrassing. Um... And I've been looking for female editors, I haven't found (Participant 14, Man)
Journal 3	8:3	...in the position of Editor-in-Chief, that are generally men. Even if there are lots of female editors, the Editor-in-Chief are generally men (Participant 7, Woman)
Journal 4	35:20	Our Editorial Board is one third female which isn't half but it's better than any other journal [in this specialty], I haven't checked, but I bet if you looked you would know (Participant 9, Woman)
Journal 5	202:131	What I see is I think there are more women than men with this position, and it takes a lot of time (Participant 1, Woman)
Journal 6	149:103	I think that maybe three out of ten are female. ...You know what, I'm going to have to say it's probably fifty-fifty female now that I look at it. (Participant 8, Man) I mean, it seems fairly balanced to me in terms of when I'm assigning to. Again, I don't know any of them, but based on what the names seem like, it seems like a fair balance. (Participant 6, Man) I haven't really picked up on that at all with a lot of the editors that are male or female (Participant 2, Man)
Journal 7	6:9	I don't know whether you're at all interested in that, but we have, probably, about 60 to 70% women on our editorial team (Participant 12, Woman)
Journal 8	5:21	...we are a very feminist journal as well, so we are a little bit on the other side of the spectrum, where we have mostly female editorial board members, all female editorial team, and all female associate editors, and I'm really looking into changing that as well (Participant 13, Woman)
Journal 9	3:15	I mean it's ... we are very much a female-dominated journal which is amazing. Including some very senior members that ... you know, of the top five or six senior members of the editorial staff...three of them are women (Participant 3, Woman)

[a]Gender could not be determined for three board members so they were excluded

journal. With the high-impact journals, smaller full-time mastheads may be supported by larger editorial boards that function in an advisory capacity. In other cases, editorial boards function in both an advisory capacity and as a pool of peer reviewers. In other cases, boards and EIC are volunteer positions, while editors work full-time in academic institutions.

Positioning Gender Imbalance as a Problem

Not all editors thought that women's participation in journal processes was gender balanced. Some editors referred to changes over time or a changing landscape in academia more broadly and journals specifically:

> So, you're seeing those trends change, but I think traditionally, a lot of EICs [Editors-in-Chief] at other journals have been more male, versus a managing editor, which is more of a staff editor, where you may see more people that are female. (Participant 5, Man)

There were also discussions about certain roles that were more likely to be occupied by men. This included the position of Editor-in-Chief and senior author—first or last author. Some participants observed that there were more women than men in terms of graduate students than in public health institutions, but that women of colour and white women tend to not occupy as many senior roles as men in journals and/or at their own academic institutions. Some recognized pipeline issues and were working to change the situation (see Lundine et al., 2018). Others chose not to problematize gender inequality to avoid challenging the status quo:

> If you just looked at the top department chair and deans, that's not balanced but it's hard to say … That doesn't necessarily mean that there's a problem. (Participant 8, Man)

Some editors observed that there are more women in full-time editorial positions. Two full-time, women editors in this study spoke about the full-time academic publishing field as "female-dominated". They spoke of "female-friendly" policies, such as working hours and maternity leave, in the publishing industry as a possible explanation for this.

It is interesting to note that several editors expressed greater concern with author representation in terms of nationality than with gender. As one editor explained:

> … we always ask the question about representation from low- and middle-income countries … we actually stipulated the proportion of papers that had to be either led, or the corresponding author, first of all, had to be from low- and middle-income countries, so there were quite specific things around that.

Another editor described the challenge of processing the large volume of papers from Chinese authors. He spoke candidly about what he perceived to be bias at the level of Editor-in-Chief regarding processing of papers:

> So, I think in terms of bias, this is probably the thing that bothers me every day the most, and it is primarily Chinese articles because we get so many of them, but there are some European investigators who also suffer from the same problem. They come from institutions that don't have a good enough infrastructure to compete in terms of how they do clinical research, and so you have to sort of take that into context when you're making a decision about whether to review an article or not.
>
> So, to me, the real place where bias could come into play is at the Editor-in-Chief level; it's not at the review level. If you went around and asked a lot of the EICs who have international journals that question, I think if they're fair about it, this is a place where you'll find people starting to admit that there could be a problem. (Participant 10, Man)

Most editors, however, described how gender and nationality data are not collected during the article submission process:

> For gender, we don't collect any information at this point. So, for example, when you told me about this discussion that we were going to have, I contacted our team; I tried to find out more—basically, we don't. And it's very hard for me to even search for. We haven't collected that information on submission. I can't even really tell from looking at our running sheets who's male, who's female. (Participant 12, Woman)

Editors must therefore rely on best guesses using the data to which they have access (i.e. names and institutional affiliations). As reported elsewhere (Lundine et al., 2019), editors spoke about how the lack of familiarity with naming conventions made it difficult to infer gender from names.

> Some of them are Asian, for whom I cannot... I don't know their gender because I can't decode their names and with that person it's all been online. The same is true for some of the Arabic or Middle Eastern names like we had some from Turkey, for example, so I couldn't tell you. (Participant 8, Man)

Some editors were working to promote equity in terms of gender and nationality amongst authors and peer reviewers.

Editorial Action

All of the editors interviewed for this study were interested in further research regarding gender, nationality, and participation of authors, peer reviewers, and editors at the journals where they work. Of the 15 editors, 5 were aware of gender issues in relation to the publishing process and actively working to manage any gender inequalities or biases in the peer review process. All five editors working on gender in peer review were women. They came to believe there was a problem in peer review for various reasons: through training in feminist theory, consciousness raising by colleagues, or through the realization that authors were not reporting sex and gender in the journal articles she was receiving. The editors were promoting a greater focus on the importance of sex and gender reporting in research, as well as gender representation in peer review within and outside of the journal where they work.

Of those already acting, one of the strategies was positive discrimination or affirmative action. Positive discrimination "is the specific recognition of certain characteristics (typically sex, race/ethnicity, disability, religion, sexual orientation, and age) considered to have disadvantaged a group of people through no direct fault of their own. It brings consideration of the disadvantage into the formal decision-making process by making these characteristics legitimate criteria for evaluating candidates" (Noon, 2010). Another was the active recruitment of women and LMIC researchers through their own networks. This was aimed to increase the number of women editors on the editorial board and to increase the number of women conducting of peer reviews.

> I just know from my career in global health that if you want an alternative perspective, if you want a perspective from the ground, if you want women instead of the usual suspect men, you can get them, you just sometimes have to be more strategic, spend more time, be more devoted to the cause. (Participant 3, Woman)

As mentioned earlier, editors are also working to support authors from LMICs. Some have started to institute journal policies in this regard; for example, papers that don't include authors from the countries where research is conducted will not be accepted for publication.

Conclusion

How do editors understand gender and nationality as influencing knowledge production within the publishing process? Health science journals function as transnational collaborations (Razack, 2000). At all levels—authors, peer reviewers, and editors—people work across national borders. Journal publishers, however, operate within imperial research systems and respond to capitalist market incentives (Striphas, 2012). Discrimination against research coming from countries or institutions is a concern that the academic publishing community should explicitly address.

Journal editors are increasingly aware and critical of unethical practices regarding research conducted in LMICs. A recent editorial in *The Lancet Global Health* said that the journal's editors "look extremely unfavourably" on papers conducted in the global south that do not include LMIC authors. They go on to question the exclusion of LMIC authors: "Perhaps, as events played out, none of those individuals additionally fulfilled the criteria of a substantial contribution to the design of the study or writing of the report, but then perhaps they were not given the opportunity" (The Lancet Global Health, 2018). The editorial goes even further, questioning the use of secondary data, such as the Demographic and Health Survey (DHS) without LMIC authors who were either involved in data collection or as authors providing the context required for analysis (The Lancet Global Health, 2018). Editors shape the scientific record and can institute policies that support LMIC authors. Editors and publisher can also increase the visibility of LMIC women (Lundine et al., 2019) and a diversity of research from around the world. We support editors who are challenging entrenched systems of power and privilege and providing greater visibility and support for authors from the Global South.

What specific actions can editors take to increase the representation of women from LMICs as authors, peer reviewers, and editors? The following recommendations were explored in a workshop we held in London in November 2017, and a short version is published in a commentary (Lundine et al., 2018).

First, editors can conduct an internal audit of their journal's data. Journals can, thus, establish a baseline and track progress towards more equitable participation of authors, peer reviewers, and editors. Editors can communicate the need to collect this data to their publishers. Publishers must be involved, as system-level change is necessary. Voicing your concerns may contribute to change.

Second, editors can institute quotas and set up recruitment processes to meet those quotas. In terms of recruitment processes, editors may continue to expand their social networks, for example, through participation in women's or LMIC organizations. Editors may ask for authors to recommend reviewers and remind authors that LMIC women are underrepresented in peer review.

Third, editors can make their commitments and/or quotas public, which has been demonstrated to increase accountability in other contexts (European Institute for Gender Equality, 2016). Some journals are now making public commitments. In 2017, responding to a report on diversity within the leadership of the American Society of Anesthesiologists, Leslie and colleagues published ten recommendations for improving diversity in leadership. They amplified the report's message that "the leadership [of an organization] should model gender and racial diversity rather than just reflect it" (Leslie et al., 2017). The American Medical Women's Association has launched the #NeedHerScience Campaign, calling on scientists to pledge to "address journal level gender bias" (https://www.surveymonkey.com/r/KNV2TQZ). In August 2019, *The Lancet* launched its Diversity Pledge, as well as a No All Manel Panel Policy (The Editors of the Lancet Group, 2019).

Fourth, editors and other gatekeepers can undertake a commitment to continuing education in equity and ethics. This may start with unconscious bias training, as the basis for conversation and change (Devine et al., 2017). How can we recognize and examine the wider structures of domination that act upon the editorial processes? What does it mean to hold a discriminatory viewpoint? How can you recognize and challenge your own preconceptions?

Fifth, scientists, editors, journals, and publishers can continue to conduct both qualitative and quantitative data on the impact of their interventions. We have too little evidence about how to build and sustain political will and effective interventions in this area.

Although there is currently a lack of consensus around what constitutes "gender balance" in publishing, some journals are making commitments to equity more broadly. We can learn to recognize when discussions about quotas and targets overshadow discussions about historical and ongoing injustice within research processes. A focus instead on equity and social justice leads us to question how and why imperial nations continue to dominate the publishing industry. Academic publishing can be a more equitable pathway to global health leadership only if editors and publishers recognize their role in the systems of domination.

References

Abimbola, S. (2019). The foreign gaze: Authorship in academic global health. *BMJ Global Health, 4*(5). https://doi.org/10.1136/bmjgh-2019-002068

Ali, P. A., & Watson, R. (2016). Peer review and the publication process. *Nursing Open, 3*(4), 193–202. https://doi.org/10.1002/nop2.51

Allotey, P., Allotey-Reidpath, C., & Reidpath, D. D. (2017). Gender bias in clinical case reports: A cross-sectional study of the "big five" medical journals. *PLoS One, 12*(5), e0177386. https://doi.org/10.1371/journal.pone.0177386

Borja, A. (2015). Is there gender bias in the peer-review process in several Elsevier's marine journals? *Marine Pollution Bulletin, 96*(1–2), 1–2. https://doi.org/10.1016/j.marpolbul.2015.05.046

Borsuk, R. M., Aarssen, L. W., Budden, A. E., Koricheva, J., Leimu, R., Tregenza, T., & Lortie, C. J. (2009). To name or not to name: The effect of changing author gender on peer review. *Bioscience, 59*(11), 985–989. https://doi.org/10.1525/bio.2009.59.11.10

Burnham, J. C. (1990). The evolution of editorial peer review. *JAMA: The Journal of the American Medical Association, 263*(10), 1323–1329. https://doi.org/10.1001/jama.1990.03440100023003

Devine, P. G., Forscher, P. S., Cox, W. T. L., Kaatz, A., Sheridan, J., & Carnes, M. (2017). A gender bias habit-breaking intervention led to increased hiring of female faculty in STEMM Departments. *Journal of Experimental Social Psychology, 73*, 211–215. https://doi.org/10.1016/j.jesp.2017.07.002

Dixon, N. (2001). Writing for publication—A guide for new authors. *International Journal for Quality in Health Care, 13*(5), 417–421. https://doi.org/10.1093/intqhc/13.5.417

Elsevier. (n.d.). *What is peer review?* Retrieved September 5, 2017, from https://www.elsevier.com/reviewers/what-is-peer-review

European Institute for Gender Equality. (2016). *Gender Equality in Academia and Research (GEAR) tool* (p. 60). Publications Office of the European Union. Retrieved from http://eige.europa.eu/gender-mainstreaming

Farrell, P. R., Magida Farrell, L., & Farrell, M. K. (2017). Ancient texts to PubMed: A brief history of the peer-review process. *Journal of Perinatology, 37*(1), 13–15. https://doi.org/10.1038/jp.2016.209

Ford, E. (2015). Open peer review at four STEM journals: An observational overview. *F1000Research, 6*, 1–15. https://doi.org/10.12688/f1000research.6005.2

Galipeau, J., Barbour, V., Baskin, P., Bell-Syer, S., Cobey, K., Cumpston, M., Deeks, J., Garner, P., MacLehose, H., Shamseer, L., Straus, S., Tugwell, P., Wager, E., Winker, M., & Moher, D. (2016). A scoping review of competencies for scientific editors of biomedical journals. *BMC Medicine, 14*(1), 16. https://doi.org/10.1186/s12916-016-0561-2

Harding, S. G. (1991). *Whose science? Whose knowledge? Thinking from women's lives.* Cornell University Press.

Heidari, S., Babor, T. F., De Castro, P., Tort, S., & Curno, M. (2016). Sex and gender equity in research: Rationale for the SAGER guidelines and recommended use. *Research Integrity and Peer Review, 1*(2), 1–9. https://doi.org/10.1186/s41073-016-0007-6

Helmer, M., Schottdorf, M., Neef, A., & Battaglia, D. (2017). Gender bias in scholarly peer review. *eLife, 6*, 1–18. https://doi.org/10.7554/eLife.21718

Hill Collins, P. (2002). *Black feminist thought: Knowledge, consciousness, and the politics of empowerment* (2nd ed.). Routledge. https://doi.org/10.4324/9780203900055

Hojat, M., Gonnella, J. S., & Caelleigh, A. S. (2003). Impartial judgment by the "gatekeepers" of science: Fallibility and accountability in the peer review process. *Advances in Health Sciences Education, 8*(1), 75–96. https://doi.org/10.1023/A:1022670432373

Lee, C. J., & Schunn, C. D. (2011). Social biases and solutions for procedural objectivity. *Hypatia, 26*(2), 352–373. https://doi.org/10.1111/j.1527-2001.2011.01178.x

Lee, C. J., Sugimoto, C. R., Zhang, G., & Cronin, B. (2013). Bias in peer review. *Journal of the American Society for Information Science and Technology, 64*(1), 2–17. https://doi.org/10.1002/asi.22784

Leslie, K., Hopf, H. W., Houston, P., & O'Sullivan, E. (2017). Women, minorities, and leadership in anesthesiology: Take the pledge. *Anesthesia & Analgesia, 124*(5), 1394–1396. https://doi.org/10.1213/ANE.0000000000001967

Lundine, J., Bourgeault, I. L., Clark, J., Heidari, S., & Balabanova, D. (2018). The gendered system of academic publishing. *The Lancet, 391*(10132), 1754–1756. https://doi.org/10.1016/S0140-6736(18)30950-4

Lundine, J., Bourgeault, I. L., Glonti, K., Hutchinson, E., & Balabanova, D. (2019). "I don't see gender": Conceptualizing a gendered system of academic publishing. *Social Science & Medicine, 235*(August), 112388. https://doi.org/10.1016/j.socscimed.2019.112388

Manchikanti, L., Kaye, A. D., Boswell, M. V., & Hirsch, J. A. (2015). Medical journal peer review: Process and bias. *Pain Physician, 18*(1), E1–E14.

Moher, D., Goodman, S. N., & Ioannidis, J. P. A. (2016). Academic criteria for appointment, promotion and rewards in medical research: Where's the evidence? *European Journal of Clinical Investigation, 46*(5), 383–385. https://doi.org/10.1111/eci.12612

Molassiotis, A., & Richardson, A. (2004). The peer review process in an academic journal. *European Journal of Oncology Nursing, 8*(4), 359–362. https://doi.org/10.1016/j.ejon.2003.11.005

Morgan, R., Lundine, J., Irwin, B., & Grépin, K. A. (2019). Gendered geography: An analysis of authors in The Lancet Global Health. *The Lancet Global Health, 7*(12), e1619–e1620. https://doi.org/10.1016/S2214-109X(19)30342-0

Noon, M. (2010). The shackled runner: Time to rethink positive discrimination? *Work, Employment and Society, 24*(4), 728–739. https://doi.org/10.1177/0950017010380648

Publons. (2018). *Global State Of Peer Review 2018.* https://doi.org/10.14322/publons.GSPR2018

Razack, S. (2000). Your place or mine? Transnational feminist collaboration. In *Anti-racist feminism: Critical race and gender studies* (pp. 39–53). Fernwood.

Sidhu, R., Rajashekhar, P., Lavin, V. L., Parry, J., Attwood, J., Holdcroft, A., & Sanders, D. S. (2009). The gender imbalance in academic medicine: A study of female authorship in the United Kingdom. *Journal of the Royal Society of Medicine, 102*(8), 337–342. https://doi.org/10.1258/jrsm.2009.080378

Smith, R. (2006). Peer review: A flawed process at the heart of science and journals. *Journals of the Royal Society of Medicine, 99*, 178–182. https://doi.org/10.1258/jrsm.99.4.178

Striphas, T. (2012). Performing Scholarly Communication. *Text and Performance Quarterly, 32*(1), 78–84. https://doi.org/10.1080/10462937.2011.631405

The Editors of the Lancet Group. (2019). The Lancet Group's commitments to gender equity and diversity. *The Lancet, 394*(10197), 452–453. https://doi.org/10.1016/S0140-6736(19)31797-0

The Lancet Global Health. (2018). Closing the door on parachutes and parasites. *The Lancet Global Health, 6*(6), e593. https://doi.org/10.1016/s2214-109x(18)30239-0

van Dalen, H. P., & Henkens, K. (2012). Intended and unintended consequences of a publish-or-perish culture: A worldwide survey. *Journal of the American Society for Information Science and Technology, 63*(7), 1282–1293. https://doi.org/10.1002/asi.22636

Wall, S., Emmelin, M., Janlert, U., Mustonen, L., & Skog, B. (2006). Who submits to and publishes in this journal? A peer-review study of 772 manuscripts 2000–2004. *Scandinavian Journal of Public Health, 34*(4), 337–341. https://doi.org/10.1080/14034940600811465

Walsh, A., Brugha, R., & Byrne, E. (2016). "The way the country has been carved up by researchers": Ethics and power in north-south public health research. *International Journal for Equity in Health, 15*(1), 1–11. https://doi.org/10.1186/s12939-016-0488-4

Wei, Y., & Lei, L. (2018). Institution bias in the New England Journal of Medicine? A bibliometric analysis of publications (1997–2016). *Scientometrics, 117*(3), 1771–1775. https://doi.org/10.1007/s11192-018-2948-7

Wiley.com. (n.d.). *The Peer Review Process | Wiley.* Retrieved September 5, 2017, from https://authorservices.wiley.com/Reviewers/journal-reviewers/what-is-peer-review/the-peer-review-process.html

Interview with Ana Langer, Professor of the Practice of Public Health, Harvard T.H. Chan School of Public Health

Mehr Manzoor

"We need to do a better job of demonstrating that women's leadership and the advancement of women is a legitimate and critical issue that we need to tackle as a community and as a society".

Ana Langer is originally from Argentina. She trained as a physician specializing in paediatrics and neonatology and is a reproductive and maternal health expert. She joined the Harvard T.H. Chan School of Public Health in 2010 as a Professor of the Practice of Public Health in the Department of Global Health and Population. For more than 30 years, she has been a leading researcher, programmer, and advocate for the improvement of women's health.

Early Years

I'm originally from Argentina in South America although I lived for many years in Mexico. My husband and my kids are from Mexico, so I have both citizenships and I feel that I come from both countries. I've been living in the USA now for almost 15 years. I would say that I'm from a developing country or from two developing countries and am, in fact, "global" as we understand it now.

I'm a physician and I come from a family of Austrian Jewish physicians, who left Europe right before the Second World War. I'm mentioning my parents only because they were always very supportive of me and my career, and my mother was an important role model. I always thought I would study medicine and serve the most vulnerable, which is ultimately what I did.

At the beginning of my career I trained as a paediatrician and then as a neonatologist, I didn't have global health in mind. But at some point, I switched from clinical work to research and public health in other countries in my region, Latin America. I joined the Population Council and I was the regional director for Latin America and the Caribbean. As a part of my work, I interacted a lot with my peers in other regions and also with people doing global work in the Population Council

M. Manzoor (✉)
Department of Health Policy and Management, Tulane University, New Orleans, LA, USA
e-mail: mmanzoor@tulane.edu

© Springer Nature Switzerland AG 2022
R. Morgan et al. (eds.), *Women and Global Health Leadership*,
https://doi.org/10.1007/978-3-030-84498-1_7

headquarters office in New York. That got me interested in global health and learning more about both challenges and opportunities, and differences across regions and across countries.

After 12 years with the Population Council I thought that I really wanted to go from regional to global, and I applied and got the position of president and CEO of EngenderHealth and I was in that position for 5 years. I joined the Harvard T.H. Chan School of Public Health in 2010 as a professor of the practice of public health.

A Focus on Sexual and Reproductive Health and Rights

The reproductive health situation, domestically and globally, is not good for women. The expanded global gag rule that the Trump administration endorsed and adopted has put a lot of pressure on NGOs [non-governmental organisations] working internationally in other countries. It has made them lose a large proportion of the financial support they were getting, so this is definitely a dark time for sexual reproductive health internationally. Domestically, there are many states that are introducing new restrictive legislation for access to abortion and to a great extent to family planning too. The Affordable Care Act includes access to free contraceptives as one of its key features. So, these are challenging times. People are fighting against those trends, but it's not easy.

Maternal health has been at the centre of my work for a long time, and we have a focus on women in conflict settings and women facing particularly difficult challenges, such as refugees. I am also working on gender and noncommunicable diseases and sex differences, an area that I'm becoming increasingly interested in, which I think is fascinating.

We recently launched an 18-month fellowship programme that allows women leaders from low- and middle-income countries to come to Harvard for a semester to take courses and participate in leadership skill building activities. We hope to create a network of alumni from that programme.

Challenges in Achieving Leadership

I have not faced significant personal experiences of bias and discrimination, much less of sexual harassment or other situations that so many women suffer from and have to deal with. I come from a family that was very, very supportive. I'm very aware of how lucky I've been.

At Harvard Chan I'm a member of the committee for the advancement of women faculty, and I hear a lot about the challenges that my younger colleagues face: the lack of supportive policies that would allow them to better integrate their professional and personal life, the evaluation system, and all the policies that were designed with men in mind. It's much more difficult for women. Just to give you an example, clinical medicine and residency programmes are not designed for women with young kids or women who are breastfeeding, and that contributes to women lagging behind or dropping out of academic programmes or the tenure ladder.

I was affected by, and very clearly felt, the conflict between the demands of a young family and the demands of my professional work. It was difficult for me to balance them. For example, I very much wanted to enrol in a doctoral programme after I had studied medicine. But I couldn't because I had two small children at the time. It's not only the expectations of other people regarding my role as a mother. It was what I wanted to do because I wanted to spend more time with my children. I don't know, a man would probably have done things differently and to some extent that affected my career. But I want to emphasise the different perceptions you can have about that situation. I wouldn't want to feature it as a negative thing that I had a young family. Being a mother and having kids has always been something I love and treasure. Now I have a granddaughter, a toddler, and I want to spend so much time with her too. Having access to childcare is completely essential, as is maternity leave and other policies that make it easier to care for your children while you get ready to go back to work or when you are already working.

Something else that has supported me or enabled me in my work are the mentors I had throughout my career, very often men. Working with men who are champions of women is incredibly important. We need to make an effort not to perpetrate or even deepen the gaps between men and women and to try to create a shared agenda. We are not doing enough to give younger women an opportunity to be mentored; it's something that is usually not in your job description, but it should be there very explicitly.

What Is Leadership?

Leadership means many things and brings responsibilities and opportunities. I think that being a leader involves the obligation to inspire and create opportunities for colleagues that might be in a more disadvantaged situation than you, due to lack of opportunities in the country they come from. I think that as a leader you're also expected to share your experience and draw some lesson from it that will be helpful to younger people. You also have to come up with new and innovative ideas, interventions, or approaches and lead intellectually.

As a leader you have more opportunities to be heard, to be listened to, to be paid attention to. I have worked with men and women, and I think women are more prone to be consensus builders in that we are more horizontal or we feel more comfortable working with or in horizontal structures, and not in a hierarchical way. I wouldn't say that this applies to all women because I've seen women who think or behave very differently. But I think that as women we are more interested in considering personal situations that may be affecting our colleagues' performance. I have spent a considerable amount of time with colleagues who are going through a rough period in their lives, and I always try to make them feel comfortable enough to tell me about those situations at the level of detail they want. I think that sometimes it's important for us as leaders to be able to also speak about the difficulties that we might be facing or faced in the past in our efforts to balance our personal and professional lives. In public health, in global health, having empathy and being caring and having solidarity with women with whom you work or seek to serve is an asset.

Looking to the Future

I think we need to do a better job of demonstrating that women's leadership and the advancement of women is a legitimate and critical issue that we need to tackle as a community and as a society. There are studies that show the economic impact of fully engaging women and giving them the opportunities to thrive and have parity with men. There are some people who come at the issue from a human rights perspective. When women are enabled and valued, they care better for other people's health. We need to connect the roles that women play both as providers and leaders and the needs they have as users of the health system.

I think we can learn more about other sectors and potentially join forces with other movements that are further ahead in terms of raising the visibility of these issues, providing evidence and finding solutions. It's very important to include men, because there are so many wonderful men who are fully aware of these gaps and are ready to do whatever is needed to make them disappear or at least narrow them. We should avoid siloing the issue. We should make it societal or institutional, not just an individual, one or an issue that only affects women.

It is very important to generate more evidence about the types of situations that we face and the solutions that some groups or people have found. We need more case studies and quantitative information that can be analysed to illustrate the issues that we talk about now on a more anecdotal basis. We often talk generically about the proportion of women in leadership positions, but you could drill down deeper and look at tenured women in particular departments and the time it took women to get to a tenure position compared to men and the difference that having a mentor or not has made for women in particular academic institutions. There's so much research still to do. We should keep trying to interest funders and liaise with influential organisations and people to raise the visibility of these issues.

Gender Quotas, the *'Two-Thirds Gender Rule'* and Health Leadership: The Case of Kenya

Kui Muraya

Gender equity is crucial to attaining the 2030 Agenda for Sustainable Development and has been asserted as a basic human right and a prerequisite to a prosperous, peaceful, and sustainable world (United Nations Development Programme, 2016). Addressing gender inequity is, therefore, integrated throughout the Sustainable Development Goals (SDGs) more broadly and is the focus of SDG 5 with a specific target, 'to ensure women's full and effective participation and equal opportunities for leadership at all levels of decision-making in political, economic, and public life' (target 5.5). The indicators for this particular target include (1) proportion of seats held by women in national parliaments and local governments and (2) proportion of women in managerial positions (https://sustainabledevelopment.un.org/sdg5).

Beyond equity, literature on women in politics and the development sector suggests that when empowered, women have a higher likelihood to make decisions that positively impact children and families. Futhermore, investment in women has been shown to result in long-term benefits including reduced poverty, greater economic growth, more resilient communities, and improved nutrition, health, and education of children (Beaman et al., 2007; Bhalotra & Clots-Figueras, 2014; Downs et al., 2014; Powley & Peace, 2006; United Nations Development Programme, 2016). In India, for example, randomized trials investigating the impact of increased female leadership in local government structures indicate that women are more likely to implement policies that are supportive of children and women, and more favourable for achieving universal health coverage (UHC), compared to men occupying the same positions (Bhalotra & Clots-Figueras, 2014; Chattopadhyay & Duflo, 2004). Specifically, female elected officials were more likely to support health facilities, antenatal care, and immunizations (ibid.). The research by Bhalotra and Clots-Figueras (2014) found that for every one standard deviation increase in the number of female-held seats in the district council of their study areas in India, neonatal

K. Muraya (✉)
KEMRI-Wellcome Trust Research Programme, Nairobi, Kenya
e-mail: KMuraya@kemri-wellcome.org

© Springer Nature Switzerland AG 2022
R. Morgan et al. (eds.), *Women and Global Health Leadership*,
https://doi.org/10.1007/978-3-030-84498-1_8

mortality dropped by 1.5%. Literature from business and the corporate world also suggests that having increased female leadership—and specifically the presence of a female CEO—is associated with stronger business and equity practices, greater investments in corporate social responsibility, and potentially better organizational performance (Glass & Cook, 2018; Hoobler et al., 2018).

One common strategy that governments and institutions put in place to increase the proportion of women in leadership spaces is adoption of quota systems (Ballington, 2004). In addition to raising gender consciousness of female representation and engagement in leadership spaces (Burnet, 2011), quota systems have been observed to have additional positive societal benefits, including in low- and middle-income countries (LMICs). A study in rural Afghanistan, for example, demonstrated that women residing in villages that had been randomly assigned to a programme requiring 50% female council representation were more likely to generate their own income compared to villages without a similar requirement (Beath et al., 2013). In Rwanda, a constitutional gender quota including reserved seats combined with voluntary party quotas for women have resulted in a majority female lower house of parliament—the only one of its kind globally (Bauer & Burnet, 2013; Burnet, 2011). Women in Rwanda also make up at least 30% of local elected or nominated leaders at local government levels (cell, sector, or district levels) and in the community (Burnet, 2011). Qualitative research from Rwanda suggests slow but steady gains as a result of increased female representation in the legislature, with women parliamentarians viewed as foremost champions and advocates on matters relating to children and families in terms of budgeting, legislation, and government oversight (Powley & Peace, 2006). Another study by Burnet found that although Rwandan women had made few legislative advances even with the increased female participation in local and national governments, they had gained other benefits including a societal shift in attitudes around women generally and specifically their ability to lead, increased economic and career opportunities including in female entrepreneurship, greater respect from family and community members, increased ability to voice their opinions and be heard in public forums, greater autonomy in decision-making within the family, and improved access to education (Burnet, 2011).

Notwithstanding the possible gains of quota systems, they can also potentially deflect from more nuanced examination of gender barriers such as social and structural factors that impede equity, as the focus is primarily on gender parity in terms of numbers. Furthermore, whilst increased representation of women may lead to symbolic representation effects (shifting of gendered ideas about the roles of women and men including in leadership) as observed in the case of Rwanda, it does not necessarily lead to substantive representation impacts (progressing women's interests through the policy-making process and measured in terms of policy agendas or legislative items that enhance or protect women's rights and interests) (Bauer & Burnet, 2013; Burnet, 2011). Gender quotas can also result in unanticipated adverse social consequences as seen in Rwanda which included tensions with male siblings as a result of extension of inheritance rights to women, which was granted following concerted lobbying by women in government and civil society organisations; male withdrawal from politics; increased marital disharmony; and a view that marriage as an institution has been brought into disharmony by the 'disruption of gender roles' (Burnet, 2011). Furthermore, women in elected local government positions in Rwanda provided unpaid services. Whilst this was highly advantageous to urban and rural elite women who earned salaries, ran businesses, or supported their husbands' careers, mainly using the government role to accrue social capital, rural peasant women saw their workload increase and their economic security undermined with a sense that the role was purely exploitative (Burnet, 2011), highlighting the importance of applying an intersectional lens even to 'well-intended' policies.

The Case of Kenya

In 2010, Kenya promulgated a new 'gender-sensitive' constitution that moved the country from a centralized to a devolved system of government with 47 semi-autonomous counties, and the decentralization of many functions to county level including some health functions. The new constitution explicitly references gender representation in leadership spaces stating that 'no more than two-thirds of the members of public elective or appointive bodies shall be of the same gender' (henceforth referred to as the 'two-thirds gender rule') and emphasizes the role of the state in taking legislative and other measures to implement this principle (National Council For Law Reporting (Kenya Law), 2018). Although the law does not make explicit reference to women, given the prevailing dearth of women in leadership positions both in the legislature and in the public service, in effect, it has been interpreted to mean that there should be at least 33% female representation in the various government leadership bodies and agencies.

This law applies to all sectors and directly impacts on all national ministries, counties, and sub-counties. It has also been embedded in the human resource policies of the Public Service Act, 2016 (Public Service Commission, 2016a, b), which in turn impacts on the public workforce including in the health sector. Specifically, the Gender Diversity Policy of the Public Service Act, 2016, states that,

> 'Every public service institution shall implement the [constitutional] principle that not more than two-thirds (2/3) of its employees shall be of the same gender at all levels; ensure that gender issues are mainstreamed at the workplace and take appropriate measures including affirmative action to ensure gender equality; and uphold, observe and protect the right of women to health and safety in working conditions, including the safeguarding of the function of reproduction,' (Public Service Commission, 2016a, p. 12–13)

A survey conducted by the Public Service Commission in 2013–2014 showed that the ratio of men to women in the public service stood at 70:30 with the ratio of women at policy-making levels reducing to 23% (Public Service Commission, 2016a). This, together with the new legislative requirements, has resulted in added impetus and concerted efforts to increase the number of women in leadership positions in the entire public sector (Public Service Commission, 2016a).

Across the board, female leadership in Kenya has progressively increased. However, the implementation of the 'two-thirds gender rule' has been marred by political interference and the country is still yet to achieve the required constitutional representation in the majority of sectors. Furthermore, the focus of the implementation of the 'two-thirds gender policy' has largely been on the political space and legislative representation (Ali & Begisen, 2017), with much less work undertaken to explore its application in other areas such as the public health sector. In the absence of systematic work documenting the current gender landscape of appointed governing bodies in the public sector at national and sub-national level (post the 2010 Constitution), this chapter briefly reflects on the influence of the 'two-thirds gender rule' in the health sector based on findings from a qualitative study undertaken in two counties of Coastal Kenya, examining career trajectories and experiences of health leaders using a gender lens.

Gender, Health Leadership, and the Case of Kenya

Women comprise the majority of the global health workforce (Dhatt et al., 2017; Hoss et al., 2011). They are, however, significantly under-represented in higher professional categories including leadership and decision-making spaces. Even in countries with established gender equity polices (Downs et al., 2014; World Health Organization, 2008). A study in 2017 by Kuhlmann et al. on cross-country comparison of women in management and leadership in academic health centres in the European Union showed that even in countries with robust policies and strategies in place and high Gender Equality Indices, such as Sweden, Austria, Germany, and the United Kingdom, gender inequalities still persist in top- and mid-level leadership of health institutions (Kuhlmann et al., 2017). In these countries, for example, although 40–60% of medical school matriculants were female, there were far fewer women specialists and senior doctors or in leadership positions such as heads of hospital departments or chiefs of division (Kuhlmann et al., 2017). We also know from literature that in their progression to leadership positions—and once in leadership—women face a varied and complex set of gendered challenges including discriminatory attitudes based on cultural norms and prejudices, gendered societal expectations around domestic roles and responsibilities including childcare, gender-based leadership stereotyping, and sexual harassment (Branin, 2009; Eagly, 2013; Eagly & Carli, 2007; Foundation of the American College of Healthcare Executives, 2006; Lantz, 2008; McDonagh, 2010; Muraya et al., 2019; Shung-King et al., 2018; Tlaiss, 2013). Phenomena commonly referred to as 'the glass ceiling', i.e. barriers faced by women in climbing to top leadership positions, and 'the glass cliff' meaning that women frequently face an enduring uphill battle once in leadership, placing them in situations where they are likely to fail. All of these challenges could, in turn, impact on their ability to undertake their leadership roles and responsibilities and limit their capacity for influence.

Few studies have been conducted in LMICs investigating the role of gender in healthcare leadership, with existing research largely focusing on high-income countries (Branin, 2009; Foundation of the American College of Healthcare Executives, 2006; Lantz, 2008). A 2013 study undertaken in Lebanon, a middle-income country, to explore barriers and facilitators of Middle Eastern women's career advancement in the health sector showed that prejudicial cultural values and gendered social roles and expectations hindered the career advancement of women in this context (Tlaiss, 2013). It also highlighted how women's agency at an individual level acted as an enabler in navigating meso- and macro-level factors such as patriarchal cultural norms and intrinsic discrimination in their organizations, supporting their career move upwards and their negotiation into management positions (Tlaiss, 2013). A more recent study in South Africa, using a gender lens to explore leadership experiences of health managers, found that women have a significantly slower progression into health management and senior positions compared to their male counterparts (Shung-King et al., 2018). This study also found strong intersections between gender, race, and professional categories which influenced the experiences and career pathways of black female (and male) managers (Shung-King et al., 2018). Similarly, in Nigeria work exploring inequities in senior healthcare leadership found that gender beliefs and stereotypes influence how men and women are perceived as leaders, with women less accepted as leaders than men, including by fellow women (Mbachu & Uguru, 2018). As with the South African study, gender intersected with professional categories and formal and informal networks often to the advantage and upward mobility of male doctors into health leadership positions compared to other health worker cadres including female doctors (Mbachu & Uguru, 2018).

In Kenya, the author and colleagues conducted a qualitative study in two counties of Coastal Kenya exploring gendered leadership experiences and career progression in view of the new constitutional dispensation (Muraya et al., 2019). Twenty-five (13 female and 12 male) senior and mid-level healthcare managers were interviewed drawing on a life history approach. The study found that gender was not explicitly considered—by either men or women—as an influencing factor in their upward career progression or experience of leadership. To quote one of the respondents, a senior healthcare manager:

> [Gender] is not even a side issue…it's a non-issue. Both our CECs [county executives for health] so far have been ladies…I do not think it's an issue for our department. If you look for example at the balance of our [management] team, we have about 5-6 females from a team of about seventeen. (R005, male manager)

However, was gender really a non-issue? Even the implication that having approximately one-third representation of one sex within health management bodies means that gender equity has been achieved is in itself problematic, as it suggests an inference that gender equity is solely about having a certain proportion of each sex represented. This perception was not entirely surprising given the 'two-thirds gender rule' cited in the new Kenyan Constitution (National Council For Law Reporting (Kenya Law), 2018) and which, as earlier stated, directly impacts on public service diversity and human resource policies. Thus, in this case, having achieved this quota was viewed as having attained gender equity and consequently gender issues as being irrelevant and insignificant in the context of the particular health management team, potentially diminishing the existence of other gendered influences that may impact on career paths and leadership experience.

Although gender did not spontaneously emerge as an influencing factor in the Kenya study, further exploration of responses revealed that gendered factors played an important role. Most fundamentally, women's role as child bearers and gendered societal expectations including child nurturing and other domestic responsibilities can limit their ability to assume leadership positions and their selection and appointment as leaders. As one of the female mid-level managers stated:

> [When appointing a health manager]…if she is female, you have to consider if she has kids or not. That makes a difference. You will find that you select someone, train them and invest so much in them, then after working for only a few months they fall pregnant and go off on maternity leave. Also, once they have a child, the women tend to become irregular with work, there isn't that commitment…. (R016, female manager)

Additionally, concerns around maintaining a work-life balance were mainly raised by female respondents, with many stating that it was sometimes a challenge to juggle full-time work and domestic responsibilities. This was often pegged to prescribed cultural and societal expectations of the role of women (and men) and was further exacerbated by the fact that many of the female respondents were also undertaking part-time studies to augment their educational qualifications, which could then lead to job promotions. All of which could have impacted on their ability to take up, and effectively perform when in, leadership roles. Nonetheless, many of the female respondents stated that having good support systems at home—usually supportive husbands and/or domestic help—assisted them in coping with the demands of their work and personal lives; and thus facilitated their career progression and contributed to a more positive experience of their leadership role. This suggests that women without such support may not have had the same opportunities to progress.

The Kenya study also found that women's selection and appointment as leaders may potentially be influenced by perceptions of women and men as having different leadership styles (against women, who some described as more emotive and reactive or unduly authoritative in an attempt to assert their leadership). The quotes below illustrate this notion of women as having less-than-optimal leadership traits.

> …men as much as whatever stress they are in, they don't express it the way women do…We tend to have more outbursts than men. I guess it's just the way women are made, that whatever stress that you are going through you tend to express it…you can start shouting, you get grumpy, you can start crying…It definitely affects leadership…I have seen it even with our leaders [here]. (R021, female manager)

> This is a society where women have been depressed for a long time. This leadership has very much been a male domain unless something like nursing…Therefore at times, because of asserting their authority, the women go to the extreme. They end up being dictators…Women want to prove that they can be leaders…even to include here where we are…many of the women who have access to leadership positions right away, because it

was not a normalcy for women to climb up the ladder to that level, they want to be known that they are the leaders. (R004, male manager)

Findings from the Kenya study (Muraya et al., 2019) and other contexts such as Rwanda (Bauer & Burnet, 2013; Burnet, 2011; Powley & Peace, 2006) illustrate that gender quotas can be a double-edged sword. As earlier described, they play an important role, for example, in symbolic representation effects and should be cautiously encouraged. Nonetheless, their focus on numbers has the potential of crowding out recognition of, and discussion around, other important barriers that hinder gender equity. As such, implementation of quotas should be done in tandem with other strategies that, for instance, enable women to take up leadership positions whilst still managing domestic 'obligations'. These strategies can include family-friendly policies that, for example, institutionalize adequate maternity and paternity leave, flexible working hours and breastfeeding-friendly spaces that enable a smooth transition back to work post-maternity leave, requirements for on-site or subsidized child day care, allowing work away from the worksite such as working from home, and so on. Beyond these practical strategies, there is need for gender-transformative approaches using culturally appropriate strategies that critically examine and challenge harmful gender norms for sustainable change. Indeed, unintended adverse social consequences of gender quotas such as those observed in Rwanda suggest that a gender-transformative approach is required if we are to achieve equity.

Although not related to health leadership, an example of a gender-transformative approach is the Intervention with Microfinance for AIDS and Gender Equity (IMAGE) in Limpopo, South Africa (Kim et al., 2007). This programme evaluated the impact of combining microfinance for women, with participatory approaches for raising awareness and challenging behaviours in relation to intimate partner violence and HIV transmission. A significant reduction in the risk of physical and sexual violence by an intimate partner was observed 2 years after introduction of the intervention. This reduction was linked to a range of empowerment indicators and attributed to various responses enabling women to contest the tolerability of violence, leave abusive relationships, have expectations of and receive better treatment from intimate partners, and promote public awareness of intimate partner violence (Kim et al., 2007). More recently, similar observations have been seen in Uganda through a transformative approach known as *SASA!* which uses trained community activists to engage community members in dialogue about power relations. This intervention has reported changes in gender norms contributing to gender-based violence, a significant increase in men's likelihood to report greater participation in household tasks, and greater appreciation of their partner's work inside and outside the home over a 5-year period (Kyegombe et al., 2014; http://raisingvoices.org/sasa/).

In addition to gender-transformative approaches, an intersectional lens is also required recognizing that gender does not operate in isolation but interacts with other social axes to create unique positionalities and experiences for individuals (Hankivsky, 2014; Larson et al., 2016). In the Kenya study, for example, gendered influences were observed to intersect in relatively invisible ways with other factors such as professional categories that were more readily identified by respondents as influencing their career progression and leadership experience (Muraya et al., 2019). As in Nigeria and South Africa (Mbachu & Uguru, 2018; Shung-King et al., 2018), medical doctors in Kenya were viewed as a 'favoured cadre' who were preferentially appointed to leadership positions and whose career progression was well-defined and distinct from other health cadres. Preferential selection of medical doctors could result in unintended gender inequity in health leadership, given that the medical profession in Kenya was *historically* a male-dominated field, with women mostly being in health professions such as nursing (Kitulu, J., personal communication, September 17, 2015). In fact, a working paper on the labour market for human resources for health in Kenya by Kiambati et al. (2013) showed that men made up 70% of medical officers in the country (Kiambati et al., 2013). Such inequity underscores how gender is shaped by other hierarchies, in this case professional categories. Although there was a sense amongst respondents in the Kenya study that this pattern is gradually shifting, it was still viewed as a major issue by many, potentially 'crowding out' obvious recognition of, and discussion around, gender influences. These findings and the broader literature highlight the need for an intersectional lens in future work. In a recent literature review on the intersectionality of gender and health systems' leadership in LMICs led by Zeinali et al. (2019) and which this author was a part of, we did not find any studies that explicitly used an intersectionality lens (Zeinali et al., 2019). This is an important gap: better understanding of the ways in which societal and political structures of power are imbued into organizational structures, processes, and daily life is important to inform more equitable practice and policies that tackle and address gender and its complex interactions with other social stratifications.

References

Ali, N., & Begisen, J. A. L. (2017). *Women strongly emerge as political leaders in Kenya.* Retrieved from https://www.ke.undp.org/content/kenya/en/home/blog/2017/9/14/Kenyan-women-emerge-in-political-leadership-and-governance.html

Ballington, J. (2004). *The implementation of quotas: African experiences quota report series.*

Bauer, G., & Burnet, J. E. (2013). Gender quotas, democracy, and women's representation in Africa: Some insights from democratic Botswana and autocratic Rwanda. *Women's Studies International Forum, 41*, 103–112. https://doi.org/10.1016/j.wsif.2013.05.012

Beaman, L., Duflo, E., Pande, R., & Topalova, P. (2007). *Women politicians, gender bias, and policy-making in rural India.* The State of the World's Children.

Beath, A., Christia, F., & Enikolopov, R. (2013). Empowering women through development aid: Evidence from a field experiment in Afghanistan. *American Political Science Review, 107*(3), 540–558. https://doi.org/10.1017/S0003055413000270

Bhalotra, S., & Clots-Figueras, I. (2014). Health and the political agency of women. *American Economic Journal: Economic Policy, 6*(2), 164–197.

Branin, J. J. (2009). Career attainment among healthcare executives: Is the gender gap narrowing? *Forum on Public Policy Online, 2009*(2), 11. http://search.proquest.com.acces.bibl.ulaval.ca/eric/docview/61808176/529814B4AA2C4A37PQ/3?accountid=12008

Burnet, J. E. (2011). Women have found respect: Gender quotas, symbolic representation, and female empowerment in Rwanda. *Politics and Gender, 7*(3), 303–334. https://doi.org/10.1017/S1743923X11000250

Chattopadhyay, R., & Duflo, E. (2004). Women as policy makers: Evidence from a randomized policy experiment in India. *Econometrica, 72*(5), 1409–1443.

Dhatt, R., Theobald, S., Buzuzi, S., Ros, B., Vong, S., Muraya, K., et al. (2017). The role of women's leadership and gender equity in leadership and health system strengthening. *Global Health, Epidemiology and Genomics, 2*, e8. https://doi.org/10.1017/gheg.2016.22

Downs, J., Reif, L. K., Hokororo, A., & Fitzgerald, D. W. (2014). Increasing women in leadership in global health. *Academic Medicine, 89*(8), 1103–1107. https://doi.org/10.1097/ACM.0000000000000369.Increasing

Eagly, A. H. (2013). Women as leaders: Leadership style versus leaders' values and attitudes. In *Gender and work: Challenging conventional wisdom*. Harvard Business School Press.

Eagly, A. H., & Carli, L. L. (2007). *Through the labyrinth: The truth about how women become leaders*. Harvard Business Press.

Foundation of the American College of Healthcare Executives. (2006). *A comparison of the career attainments of men and women healthcare executives*. Retrieved on June (Vol. 11). Retrieved from https://www.ache.org/pubs/research/gender_study_full_report.pdf

Glass, C., & Cook, A. (2018). Do women leaders promote positive change? Analyzing the effect of gender on business practices and diversity initiatives. *Human Resource Management, 57*, 823–837. https://doi.org/10.1002/hrm.21838

Hankivsky, O. (2014). *Intersectionality 101*. The Institute for Intersectionality Research and Policy, SFU.

Hoobler, J. M., Masterson, C. R., Nkomo, S. M., & Michel, E. J. (2018). The business case for women leaders: Meta-analysis, research critique and path forward. *Journal of Management, 44*(6), 2473–2499. https://doi.org/10.1177/0149206316628643

Hoss, M. A. K., Bobrowski, P., McDonagh, K. J., & Paris, N. M. (2011). How gender disparities drive imbalances in health care leadership. *Journal of Healthcare Leadership, 3*, 59–68. https://doi.org/10.2147/JHL.S16315

Kiambati, H., Kiio, C., & Toweett, J. (2013). *Understanding the labour market of human resources for health in Kenya*.

Kim, J., Watts, C., Hargreaves, J., & Al, E. (2007). Understanding the impact of a micro-finance based intervention on women's empowerment and the reduction of intimate partner violence in South Africa. *American Journal of Public Health, 97*(10), 1794–1802.

Kuhlmann, E., Ovseiko, P. V., Kurmeyer, C., Gutiérrez-Lobos, K., Steinböck, S., Von Knorring, M., et al. (2017). Closing the gender leadership gap: A multi-centre cross-country comparison of women in management and leadership in academic health centres in the European Union. *Human Resources for Health, 15*(2), 1–7. https://doi.org/10.1186/s12960-016-0175-y

Kyegombe, N., Abramsky, T., Devries, K., Starmann, E., Michau, L., Nakuti, J., et al. (2014). The impact of SASA! A community-based mobilization intervention, on reported HIV-related risk behaviour and relationship dynamics in Kampala Uganda. *Journal of the International AIDS Society, 17*(1).

Lantz, P. M. (2008). Gender and leadership in healthcare administration: 21st century progress and challenges. *Journal of Healthcare Management/American College of Healthcare Executives, 53*(5), 291–301. https://www.ncbi.nlm.nih.gov/pubmed/18856135

Larson, E., George, A., Morgan, R., & Poteat, T. (2016). 10 Best resources on... intersectionality with an emphasis on low- and middle-income countries. *Health Policy and Planning, 31*(8), 964–969. https://doi.org/10.1093/heapol/czw020

Mbachu, C., & Uguru, N. (2018). *Gender stereotypes and inequities in health care leadership perceptions and experiences of senior managers in Nigeria*. RESYST Consortium. Retrieved from https://resyst.lshtm.ac.uk/resources/gender-stereotypes-and-inequities-in-health-care-leadership-perceptions-and-experiences-of

McDonagh, K. J. (2010). Secrets of the labyrinth: Insights into career advancement for women. *Nurse Leader, 8*(4), 41–43. https://doi.org/10.1016/j.mnl.2010.05.010

Muraya, K. W., Govender, V., Mbachu, C., Uguru, N. P., & Molyneux, S. (2019). 'Gender is not even a side issue…it's a non-issue': Career trajectories and experiences from the perspective of male and female healthcare managers in Kenya. *Health Policy and Planning, 34*(4), 249–256. https://doi.org/10.1093/heapol/czz019

National Council For Law Reporting (Kenya Law). (2018). *The Constitution of Kenya.* Retrieved May 3, 2018, from http://kenyalaw.org/kl/index.php?id=398

Powley, E., & Peace, W. W. (2006). *Rwanda: The impact of women legislators on policy outcomes affecting children and families.*

Public Service Commission. (2016a). *Diversity policy for the public service.* Retrieved from http://www.publicservice.go.ke/images/guidlines/PSC_DIVERSITY_POLICY_MAY_2016.pdf

Public Service Commission. (2016b). *Human resource policies and procedures manual for the public service.* Retrieved from http://www.publicservice.go.ke/images/guidlines/PSC_HR_POLICIES_MAY_2016.pdf

Shung-King, M., Gilson, L., Mbachu, C., Molyneux, S., Muraya, K. W., Uguru, N., & Govender, V. (2018). Leadership experiences and practices of South African health managers: What is the influence of gender? A qualitative, exploratory study. *International Journal for Equity in Health, 17*(148), 1–12. https://doi.org/10.1186/s12939-018-0859-0

Tlaiss, H. A. (2013). Women in healthcare: Barriers and enablers from a developing country perspective. *International Journal of Health Policy and Management, 1*(1), 23–33. https://doi.org/10.15171/ijhpm.2013.05

United Nations Development Programme. (2016). *UNDP support to the integration of gender equality across the SDGs including Goal 5.*

World Health Organization. (2008). Gender and health workforce statistics. *Spotlight on Statistics, 2*, 2. www.who.int/hrh/statistics/en/

Zeinali, Z., Muraya, K., Govender, V., Molyneux, S., & Morgan, R. (2019). Intersectionality and global health leadership: Parity is not enough. *Human Resources for Health, 17*(1), 4–6. https://doi.org/10.1186/s12960-019-0367-3

Interview with Patricia J. Garcia, Professor, School of Public Health at Cayetano Heredia University (UPCH), Former Minister of Health of Peru, and Former Dean of the School of Public Health at UPCH, Lima

Mehr Manzoor

"Everyone can be a leader in their own space. You do not need a title or a rank for that. I believe everybody can lead change and whoever leads change is a leader".

Patty Garcia is a recognized name in global health. She served as a Minister of Health of Peru from July 2016 to September 2017. During her term, she introduced new public health policies in sexual and reproductive health, HPV vaccination, food labelling, cervical cancer, electronic medical records, and telemedicine. Dr. Garcia was a Menschel Senior Leadership Fellow at the Harvard T.H. Chan School of Public Health during the Fall 2018 academic term. In this capacity, she taught an 8-session, weekly course titled, "Leadership development in global health: Strategies for effective public health policy implementation, the view of a researcher in politics". Dr. Garcia was recently appointed as a member of the United States' National Academy of Medicine, the first Peruvian to earn such a distinction. She is actively engaged in research, training, reproductive health, global health, and medical informatics. As a chief of the Peruvian National Institute of Health from 2006 to 2008, she introduced the first information system for the National Network of Public Health Laboratories in Peru (NETLAB). Dr Garcia also served as the Dean at the School of Public Health at Cayetano Heredia University in Lima, Peru, from 2011 to 2016, and where she continues to serve as Research Professor.

M. Manzoor (✉)
Department of Health Policy and Management, Tulane University, New Orleans, LA, USA
e-mail: mmanzoor@tulane.edu

© Springer Nature Switzerland AG 2022
R. Morgan et al. (eds.), *Women and Global Health Leadership*,
https://doi.org/10.1007/978-3-030-84498-1_9

Early Years

I will start by telling my personal story. When I was around 7 years old, I got very, very sick. Doctors could not diagnose what I had. They initially thought I had lymphoma. But my initial diagnosis was wrong. I had an infectious disease called brucellosis instead of lymphoma, a disease that, at that point, was very prevalent in Peru. I stayed in bed for a long time, about 5 months in hospital and other time at home. I almost missed the entire year of school. But all these doctors really treated me well and I felt so good. I felt so secure with them. This experience changed my life and developed my interest in becoming a doctor, so that I could treat people just like these doctors were treating me and make people feel good.

I pursued medicine in Peru, and I was the first one in my family to earn a university degree. There were no doctors around. At that time, I never planned to travel to the United States or to pursue global health. But then my father fell very sick with lung cancer. I was looking for better options for him, and one of my professors advised me to apply for international residency programs and ask them if I could bring my father there for treatment. I got lucky as several American universities were looking in Lima for residents at that time. I applied to five programs and got selected in all of them. I chose the one that would offer the best treatment option for my father. But unfortunately, my father died several weeks before my departure to the United States. I was committed to study medicine from the very beginning, but now I had added responsibility of sustaining my family and financially supporting my mother and sister, who was only in school at the time. So, I embarked on the journey to the United States to pursue my residency program. This experience allowed me to view a different world. I started an internal medicine residency at the University of Miami. The first years were not easy at all, but I worked hard and learnt a lot and enjoyed it. By then, I had completed 8 years of medical school, and 4 years of internal medicine, including one as chief resident. I met my mentor Dr. King Holmes at the University of Washington (UW) where I did my infectious diseases residency. He was an expert in sexually transmitted diseases. He is the one who really introduced me to research and public health and eventually global health. While I was a resident at UW, Dr. Holmes convinced me to pursue an MPH and I have never regretted that! He told me that public health is very important as with one action you can change the lives of thousands of people. He made me see how research played an integral role in answering critical questions about people's health, and he is the one from whom I heard from the first time the term "global health".

I am from a generation when the term global health was still relatively new as before that international health was more often used to refer to the health beyond geographic boundaries, i.e. the health in developing countries. I always wanted to return to Peru, to serve my people to the best of my capability. And that is what I have done. So, in short, personal moments in my life such as being sick at an early age and my dad's health, but also my mentor's guidance, triggered me into entering the field of global health.

Challenges in Achieving Leadership

During my life in academia, I realized that in most of the meetings and activities I was one of the very few women in the room. In the beginning, I was also the youngest woman and sometimes the only woman from Latin America. But I never felt discriminated against until I entered politics. The first time I really felt discrimination was when I became minister of health in Peru. I realized the higher women climb on the leadership ladder, the higher the discrimination they face. I faced discrimination from the other politicians within congress. One time, I was presenting to congress the law regarding labelling of processed food to raise more awareness among the people regarding intake of salt, sugar, and processed fat, which is a prevalent issue among many developing countries like Peru. While I was presenting, one of the congressmen raised his hand to ask me a question. And guess what he asked me: whether I was single or married. I felt this question had nothing to do with my presentation. But then he went on to comment that single women never had good nights. While I felt very angry at him, I had to keep my composure as I was so close to getting this law approved. Luckily, there were some journalists present including some female journalists. So, the next day his disrespectful behaviour was reported in the media and he later apologized. This is just one example and I can narrate many more.

The other group I have faced a lot of discrimination from is the medical group. Especially male physicians (not all, there are feminist male physicians too!), who could not accept females in leadership roles. This group turned against me as I was trying to bring women from otherwise traditional roles such as nursing and midwifery into leadership roles. They were very upset at me. They even approached me and shared if I were to appoint women as leaders, then I could choose female doctors, but female nurses or midwives were not acceptable to them as leaders. Other major challenges I faced as a minister of health were corruption and difficulty in getting things implemented. Public-private partnerships have the capacity to implement better population health policies. But making the public sector work with the private sector can be very challenging.

Several times it is much harder for women to get things done as compared to men, especially in leadership roles. For example, when I was head of the National Institute of Health in Peru, while addressing an issue related to corruption I was accused of having a lover, but not only that, of hiring him as well. Of course, that was not true. But that was a way of trying to stop me from what I was doing. There are many tactics used to sabotage women's careers as well as personal lives especially when they are handling difficult situations. However, those tools do not affect men that much, e.g. character assassinations, sexual harassment, etc. So, women need to be prepared to handle such situations and they need to take their families, especially their husbands and children, in confidence to be able to fight through this system.

So, while I have not felt that gender affected my career choices, I did have to deal with a lot of gender-related issues at workplaces and policy forums especially in higher leadership positions.

Enabling Factors

The biggest support in my life is my feminist husband. I was extremely lucky to pick the right person. Because I had never planned to get married or to have children. But eventually you reach a point in life, where if you meet the right person, then you start thinking about living together or even planning a family. My husband has always been supportive of me and my career. I have also been able to share the division of labour at home with him including childcare which has been wonderful. I have a son and a daughter, and I raised my kids to be feminists. They are both doctors now.

Key people in my life that have always been supportive and instrumental in my success include my parents, my grandmother, my academic mentor Dr. King Holmes, and my family and husband. Their support allowed me to achieve what I have been able to achieve so far. My grandmother was one of my earliest mentors, she was from an Andean town and she was a "Chamana" (traditional healer), and she taught me a lot about traditional medicine, but more importantly, how to listen to people, especially those who are sick.

The other important thing is to create networks and try to identify your champions. You need to be nurturing these networks from the beginning of your career. This is something I learnt from the beginning. So, I had champions within the civil society, non-governmental organizations, and even congress, who helped me during different situations. For example, when I wanted to address the issue of corruption in the health sector during my term as the minister, I had the support from the civil society especially that had been working together before.

Another thing I learnt is to be patient and to be able to turn people who are initially against you to turn to your side. For this you need to create a sense of ownership, so that people can be transformed by what you are doing. This takes time but with patience it can be achieved.

Future Directions

There are things that need to change at the societal level to enable more women to enter leadership roles. It will take a long time. For example, starting from the issue of motherhood. When I was a chief resident, I got pregnant. My pregnancy made me so guilty that I would give my job 200% just to prove myself. After having my baby, I was able to re-join my work with the support of my husband. This is something I am trying to change in the minds of my students: that women should never feel guilty about being mothers.

Moreover, we need to be more aware of our biases at the institutional level. We need to change mindsets and norms regarding women's leadership and career choices. For example, women are evaluated more strictly without considering that they also need to take care of their homes and children. Therefore, as a minister of health, I was offering leadership positions to women, because they are smart and capable. Women tend to hold themselves back and they don't fight to take the space. This needs to change. Women need to be bold to take up roles and decision-making spaces, instead of holding themselves back. Women tend to be too harsh on themselves and conscious of their limitations, sometimes too conscious, whereas men think differently. Women tend to be more reflective naturally, maybe because they have to keep their offspring alive. But women need to reclaim their space as leaders and challenge themselves to take on leadership roles. Sometimes women turn against other women more than men. I have seen women being worse towards other women than men. This is perhaps because women compete for the fewer leadership roles that exist for women. I think women can understand each other better and should help each other. There is enough space for all of us! So, they need to be more aware of this and work more in harmony with each other. Men tend to coach other men, as well as advocate for each other. At times men support other women. Both men and women need to work on this together.

Advice for Emerging Women Leaders

The first advice I would give young women is to be well prepared. I was lucky to have had a supportive father who provided me good opportunities to educate myself. I realize that many women in my country would not have had similar opportunities. But I used the opportunities I was given. So, women need to aim high to be able to achieve high. And use every single opportunity to learn and be very well prepared. Another thing is when someone offers you an opportunity to work with them, like I was offering to people to come work with me, then take those opportunities. Never shy away or underestimate yourself. Give your 100% and take your chances.

Also try to reach out to other women who are in positions you aspire to be in and ask them to be your mentors. They can be very good mentors. Every woman should find a time and opportunity to mentor other women. Also start creating your support groups or networks and start sharing within that group about the strategies that work and don't work. Learn from each other. Develop a work-life balance, as that is a very important aspect of life. And lastly, choose your partners very carefully. Choose a feminist husband. And never let anybody tell you that you are less than anybody. Listen to others but raise your voice when you need to. I remember one of my students asking me: how do I know that what I have to say is correct or not? Everybody has great ideas, but women tend to be too strict on themselves. Women should not hold themselves back because they feel ashamed to say something. All voices matter and women bring different perspectives to the table. So, it is important to hear everyone and give everyone a chance to speak.

Well, we talked about the importance of training, the importance of networking, the importance of raising the voice, and the importance of mentoring other women. We need change at the societal level as well as the institutional, but more importantly we also need change at the personal level because in the end, individuals are the ones that are going to change institutions and eventually society. Both men and women have a role to play. I do not think there is any one kind of leadership style. Everyone can be a leader in their own space. You do not need a title or a rank for that. I believe everybody can lead change and whoever leads change is a leader.

Women Health Leaders in Kerala: Respectability and Resistance

Devaki Nambiar, Gloria Benny, and Hari Sankar

Introduction

Women's leadership in India—whether in the context of the women's rights movements or more broadly—has for a long time involved a tension and negotiation between resistance and respectability. There are many examples of this within the country since the post-independence era within India but also in relation to global movements and perspectives (Jain, 2012). As Jain has pointed out, speaking of the heyday of the international women's movement:

> …we asked, '…do we want to sit at the table with generals?' This was in the context of the fact that many nations had military governments. 'Do we want to eat part of the poisoned cake?' was another, when it came to extremely unjust economic policies. 'Let us set our own table…' was the reply…. Leadership is also linked to power; feminist claims on the political are not just to share power, but to change the nature of power, not just to govern, but to change the nature of governance. (Jain, 2012, p. 2)

The tension Jain speaks of—between claiming a seat in the existing (unjust) power structures and subverting these structures altogether—is one long seen not

D. Nambiar (✉)
George Institute for Global Health, New Delhi, India

Faculty of Medicine, University of New South Wales, Sydney, Australia

Prasanna School of Public Health, Manipal Academy of Higher Education, Manipal, India
e-mail: dnambiar@georgeinstitute.org.in

G. Benny · H. Sankar
George Institute for Global Health, New Delhi, India
e-mail: hsankar@georgeinstitute.org.in

© Springer Nature Switzerland AG 2022
R. Morgan et al. (eds.), *Women and Global Health Leadership*,
https://doi.org/10.1007/978-3-030-84498-1_10

just in the women's movement in India but also in the vexed nature of leadership across sectors in even the most progressive of Indian states.[1]

In the southern Indian state of Kerala, considered one of the most progressive from the standpoint of health and development, this holds true as well (Jeffrey, 1992b; Nandraj & Nambiar, 2018). The contributions of women to the development of the health sector are substantial, just as the specific motivations and contexts in which women have made these contributions are typified by certain kinds of class or community privilege on the one hand and intransigent patriarchal norms on the other (Jeffrey, 1992b, 2004).

It is this legacy that has led to Kerala having the highest female health workforce (64.5%) in India (Anand & Fan, 2016) and eight times the female doctor density than other Indian states like Uttar Pradesh and Bihar (Rao et al., 2012). In 2019, apart from having a female Health Minister, all the Technical Directors of Kerala's health-related departments—Allopathic medicine, Ayurveda, Homeopathy, and Medical Education—were female. We were informed by the Director of Health Services—herself a woman—that half of the heads of administration (at the Additional Director level), two-thirds of the District Medical Officers (DMOs), and half of nearly 6000 allopathic doctors working in the government health department were female (personal communication 5/06/2019; see Fig. 1). Kerala's nurse cadre has made major contributions to the global nursing workforce, particularly in high-income countries (Kodoth & Jacob, 2013).

While it is perhaps premature and out of scope for us to reflect on the impact this representation of women has had on the functioning of the health system in the state, we nonetheless found the phenomenon in general to be unprecedented and worthy of study. How did such a situation arise? Was it intended? How did this many women achieve these positions of power? What were their struggles? What have been their achievements in their eyes? Our growing understanding of the Kerala health system as part of a 5-year health systems and policy research project on health equity drew us to want to "illuminate the special qualities and ethics of women" (Jain, 2012, p. 11) as they inhabit and negotiate positions of leadership in the state.

In this chapter, adapting the approach used by Dhatt et al. (2017), we seek to more deeply understand the representation and leadership of women in the Kerala health sector, with an emphasis on the public sector. First, we present the most up-to-date estimates of women's participation in the health workforce, comparing Kerala to national estimates. Second, we provide historical context for women's entry into the health sector in leadership positions, and contributions to the "Kerala model", mindful of broader political and policy evolutions in the state. Finally, we present themes from a small study covering 6 of the state's 14 districts, where we interviewed a respondent-driven sample of 15 women leaders working in health about their professional and personal trajectories; their style and vision of

---

[1] This tension can also be seen in the political arena, exemplified quite plainly in the case of the Women's Reservation Bill, an affirmative action measure which reserves quotas for women in legislative bodies. The Bill was introduced as early as 1996, just 2 years after the International Conference on Population and Development, but lack of political consensus has meant that the Bill has never been passed, even as the Indian Constitution, and various commissions have sought to create a more enabling environment for women's political participation (Chadha, 2014).

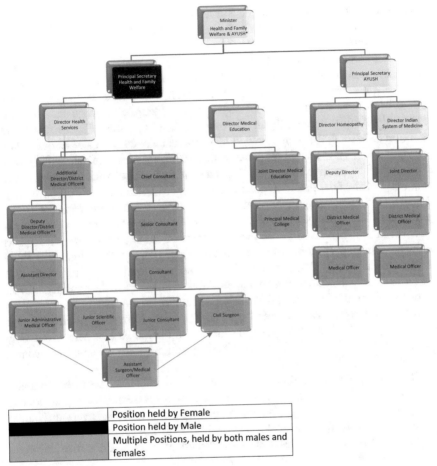

	Position held by Female
	Position held by Male
	Multiple Positions, held by both males and females

Fig. 1 Organisational chart representing gender distribution of major decision-making positions in public health sector of Kerala. Notes: *The AYUSH department in Kerala was formed as a separate department by delinking the Complementary and Alternative Medicine (CAM) from the existing Health and Family Welfare Department, to ensure a more focused approach towards issues relating to the healthcare, research, and education sector of Ayurveda, Yoga and Naturopathy, Unani, Siddha, and Homeopathy (AYUSH) therapy practices in the State. This department is further divided into the Department of Indian Systems of Medicine (ISM) (Ayurveda, Yoga, Unani, Siddha) and the Department of Homeopathy. #Additional Director and District Medical Officer level posts have a preponderance of women candidates

leadership; challenges, enablers, and lessons learnt on their paths; and their visions for the Kerala health system.

Health Workforce Participation in Kerala

The National Sample Survey data from 2011/2012 applied to make projections for 2016 conclude that Kerala had among one of the highest concentrations of health workers in the country in overall terms (Karan et al., 2019). While drawing upon the National Sample Survey data for leadership positions is relatively more difficult to do, the sex-disaggregated distribution of the workforce is worth mentioning (see Table 1).

Several points are noteworthy here. First, while the representation of women in the health professional group of allopathic and Ayurveda, Yoga and Naturopathy, Unani, Siddha, and Homeopathy therapy (AYUSH) doctors and dentists is roughly a third of the whole cadre, once we consider the nursing, midwifery, and associate cadres, the relative representation of women shifts to upwards of four-fifths of the workforce. Second, the representation of women in Kerala is greater across cadres in relation to what is seen in India nationally. Third, as is the case nationally, moreover, the representation of women is greater in positions considered lower in the hierarchy of medical practice (in ancillary, supportive, and supervised positions). Finally, it is noteworthy that women are well represented in the cadre of health associates. The health sector appears to be a viable employment prospect across genders in the state, even as the overall pattern of employment is gendered. This compares favourably to trends in the country more broadly. The cumulative effect of this gender distribution is that while at the national level women represent 42% of the core cadres of the health system, in Kerala women are in the majority at 67%. It bears mentioning, however, that this representation is sequestered in lower-level and frontline positions. This trend holds for political leadership positions in the state, where in 2017 only 7 of the 140 members of the Kerala Legislative Assembly were women, while 54% of all local body positions were occupied by women (Ameerudheen, 2017).

It is not clear whether such trends hold in the private sector, which dominates healthcare provisioning in the state (Thresia, 2018). Research on this nationally suggests likely not, although data on the private sector in India is very difficult to access (notwithstanding the analysis in Table 1, which includes the private sector). Sundar (2012), in the context of women's participation in the corporate sector

Table 1 Sex-disaggregated estimates of health human resources in Kerala and India, 2016

Cadre	Male	Female	Total	Males	Females	Total
	Kerala			India		
Health professional[a]	35,203 (66%)	18,255 (34%)	53,457	1,163,961 (79%)	304,515 (21%)	1,468,475
Nursing professional	989 (3%)	31,530 (97%)	32,519	42,560 (17%)	207,403 (83%)	249,963
ANM and midwife	20,831 (19%)	87,753 (81%)	108,584	220,659 (22%)	771,099 (78%)	991,758
Health associate[b]	24,589 (50%)	24,902 (50%)	49,491	778,454 (71%)	322,538 (29%)	1,100,992
Total	81,612 (33%)	162,439 (67%)	244,051	2,205,633 (58%)	1,605,554 (42%)	3,811,187

Source: Authors based on Anup Karan (personal communication 16/07/2019), drawing from data used for a recent publication (2019)
[a]Includes allopathic doctors, dentists, and AYUSH
[b]Includes health assistants, sanitarians, dietitians and nutritionist, optometrists and opticians, dental assistants, physiotherapy associates, and pharmacist assistants

overall, notes the phenomenon of "pipeline leakage" from junior to middle management positions such that even as the number of working women in Indian corporations (including corporate hospitals) is on the rise, where 12.5% of management roles are occupied by women, executive leadership of women drops to 5%. This is something that must be explored further with an emphasis on the health sector and also in the Kerala context, as the state has already shown itself to diverge from national trends. For now, based on available information, we seek to contextualise the role women play in leadership from summary data, as above, and historical data, as follows.

Historical Context

In colonial India, women doctors began graduating as early as 1886, but the obstetric nurses in Kerala were first hired by the Travancore Medical Department as early as 1868 (Jeffrey, 2004). The first Kerala woman medical graduate, Mary Poonen Lukose, held the unique distinction of also being the first woman Surgeon General (to the Kingdom of Travancore) (Jeffrey, 1992a).[2] A closer look at her experience also typifies the aforementioned tension between respectability and resistance, as Jeffrey explains:

> From childhood, she [Mary] wanted to be a doctor, at a time when there were no women nurses or doctors in Kerala. Through her father's influence, and over the opposition of a conservative Scots mathematics professor, she entered the Maharaja's College, Trivandrum, to study for a BA. She was the first woman to attend classes and, for three weeks, the only female student in the college….in 1909, after becoming the first Kerala woman to take a BA degree, she began seven years in London and Dublin studying medicine, including the first 18 months of the First World War when women – especially skilled medical women – were increasingly called on to do jobs hitherto closed to them. In 1915 she became the first Kerala woman to graduate in medicine.
>   Amid this apparently 'westernised' way of life lay some of the tensions of a dying Kerala. Her lawyer uncle, for example, chose to marry off one of his daughters at the age of only 13, thus following a common Syrian Christian practice of early marriage. Attitudes that favoured the education and salaried employment of young women, which allowed Mary Poonen to become the most important female official of her generation, represented innovations. They resulted from some Syrian Christians drawing close to European missionaries, adopting some European Christian practices and profiting from the resulting opportunities. Just as matriliny had provided models of behaviour for those who wished to demonstrate their respectability in old Kerala, British practices, often mediated through Syrian Christians like the Poonens, provided models for the new Kerala. But under both old and new codes, women had room for manoeuvre that was unique in India and most parts of the world at the time. (Jeffrey, 1992a, p. 93)

This room for "manoeuvre" is a critical source of agency used by women leaders over time. The practice of matriliny—a kinship practice where ancestral descent

---

[2] The Travancore region also boasted the first woman judicial officer "in the entire Anglo Saxon world" (Pillai, 2016, p. 704).

was traced through maternal instead of paternal lines in certain influential Kerala communities, like the Nairs—dates back to the eleventh century and was legally dismantled in 1976 through the promulgation of the Kerala Joint Hindu Family System (Abolition) Act (Jeffrey, 2004). In Kerala, it is argued that "matriliny helped to create conditions in which salaried work for women became a desirable and respectable goal for all classes by the 1920s—which is when a woman first headed the Travancore Medical Department [Mary Poonen Lukose], the first woman to head a department in India" (Jeffrey, 2004, p. 656).

The precolonial legacy of matriliny is an important context that has shaped the trajectories not just of women in the castes like the Nairs but also other caste-religion groupings that emulated them, seeking salaried work in the fields of health and education, with a preference for the public sector (Jeffrey, 2004). Matriliny also cohered well with the push, in the early twentieth century through to the post-independence period, for women's workforce participation in the fields of education and health (Devika, 2012; Jeffrey, 2004). Additionally, education, particularly of women, was fostered in Kerala and other parts of colonial and postcolonial India by Christian missionaries and had an adjuvant effect on this push (Lankina & Getachew, 2013). In opening up new spaces for women, the changes were vexed by debates about the loyalties of married women and by their limits (for instance in rejecting women's participation in "unfeminine" work like policing or selling liquor) (Devika & Thampi, 2011). The compromise at the time was that married women's work was necessarily a fulfilment of her duties towards the home and, as such, a form of respectable femininity.

Thus, it would be premature to interpret female workforce participation per se as a fully liberating process for women. This, as J. Devika points out, "did not mean the undoing of patriarchy, but its re-doing, in ways that were complex and perhaps more difficult to resist" (2006, p. 46). For instance, "inborn capacities" of women in the domestic sphere were lauded, and in the nineteenth century, an argument was made that the modern home and the modern hospital were mirrors of each other. At the inauguration of the new Civil Hospital in Thiruvananthapuram in 1865, for example, the Maharajah of Travancore noted that the institution "will always be distinguished for its sanitary arrangements, for the attention and tender care of the sick and the suffering" (Devika, 2006, p. 49). The properties of tender care and sanitation were ascribed to women in popular discourse at this time. On the other hand, women's participation in politics required a rejection of a family life in pursuit of power or as having a lack of morality, in effect, an "un-gendering" to claim a kind of "honorary masculinity" (Devika & Thampi, 2011). An example of this is Gouri Amma, a leader in the communist movement of the state who in the 1950s "publicly proclaimed that women did not really need 4 months of maternity leave, and that women should be appointed as bus-conductors, an exclusively male job" (Devika & Thampi, 2011, p. 58).

In the 1990s, the 73rd and 74th of India's constitutional amendments advocated 33% representation of women in local self-government institutions under the larger rubric of political decentralisation. In Kerala, the waning legacy of health, education, and land reforms was giving way to privatisation in line with economic liberalisation occurring at a global scale. Decentralisation reforms seemed to embrace women's participation, seeking the betterment of Kerala's poor in "intimate" and everyday matters, such that the local self-governance institution, the *panchayat*, was "perceived as a non-political space, the space of development altruism—and therefore, by definition, demanding of 'feminine capacities' and thus to women as leaders/managers" (Devika & Thampi, 2011, p. 1168). In later work, this is described as the "gentle power" that women exercise in this role (Devika, 2012).

A study of panchayat women in leadership carried out about a decade ago pointed to three themes characterising these women's political mobility (Devika & Thampi, 2011). First, People's Planning Campaigns set in motion in the mid-1990s created pathways by which developmental activism could lead to positions of political leadership for women. This was very much an echo of the welfarism of the nineteenth century. Second, a majority of women in panchayat leadership came from families with at least two or three generations of allegiance/involvement with political parties. Third, pecuniary stability and access as well as spousal support gave these women leaders adequate "respectability" in their communities that enabled their fulfilment of their roles as leaders. The study, relying on life histories of 45 leaders, also found tighter controls and resistance exercised over interactions of senior party politicians, with those in more decentralised positions given greater "freedom" to act locally. The authors conclude that "unlike earlier times when politics was indeed a space in which 'un-gendered' women could occasionally seize power reserved for men, the new spaces, which held out the promise of political empowerment for women, seem to be reinforcing dominant gender norms" (Devika & Thampi, 2011, p. 1174).

Women's Voices

We were curious to see if these trends held for women working in the heath sector, one that is very squarely in the welfarist domain. As part of a larger study on health equity in Kerala, we have been identifying, through public record as well as peer nomination, women who occupy positions of leadership in the health sector in Kerala. The initial emphasis is on the public sector, specifically the Department of Health and Family Welfare, which was extended to include leaders in panchayats, prominent civil society activists working in the health sector, as well as a woman healer who has received public acclaim. Following institutional ethics committee-approved procedures, participants were apprised of our study, gave written informed consent, and were interviewed in Malayalam and/or English; summaries of interviews as well as transcripts were created and grounded coding methods (Glaser & Strauss, 2009) were used to analyse findings. Our fieldwork is ongoing; the findings presented here are drawn from interviews with 15 individuals aged 48 years and older, who occupy senior managerial positions at the state and district level in the state or who have founded and run women's health-related organisations, with 19–41 years of experience, and had served at least a decade in their current capacity.

A Career in Health and Progressing to Leadership Roles

A majority of the women interviewed reported receiving natal and marital family support throughout their careers in health/medicine, whether they chose this path or were led to it by circumstance. For some, family members—grandparents, parents, uncles, and aunts—were the inspiration that drove them to have ambitions of taking up leadership positions. Moreover, some of the women leaders expressed that earlier in their careers they had either chosen or been deputed into roles that involved "social commitment" like work in palliation, with the mentally ill or with communities that are underserved by the health system, like tribal and minority populations. These experiences, and in some cases strong mentorship from peers and seniors, played a formative role for them. On the other hand, some reported facing challenges with male superiors, especially when seeking leave for childcare.

The administrative cadre in the Kerala health service was introduced in 2010, and at this time, the option of entering this cadre was made available to many of our participants. A number of them noted that this is a gendered choice (men prefer to stay on in clinical work, while women like the stability of administration), while others chose this path specifically because they saw it as challenging. Some did note that administrative and managerial roles are more predictable, do not involve night duty strictly speaking, and can allow greater work-life balance. That said, most women said that their administrative and managerial tasks often extended into their family time including evenings and weekends. A senior state-level official noted that the more prestigious leadership positions, in multilateral organisations and abroad, would usually be taken up by males who would be more likely to be in a position to leave family to pursue such opportunities. It was also noted that the push into senior positions would typically begin once children were old enough to be fairly independent and did not require as much care and time from their mothers, as has been seen in South Africa as well (Semenya & Potgieter, 2014). Further, the ambition of leadership per se was not something that they had specifically envisioned as young mothers or at junior levels in their career. Yet without exception, every single woman leader we spoke to in Kerala underscored for us the importance of family support in making the transition to leadership. This was reflected upon not in terms of respectability in the community (as discussed earlier for panchayat leadership) (Devika & Thampi, 2011) but pragmatic support in terms of sharing childcare duties, picking them up from late-night travel, handling family chores while they were busy with work, etc. As one district-level leader noted, "There is no need for compromise, when everyone in the family co-operates".

Leadership Styles and Experiences

We noted that the majority of the women we spoke to did not have a single leadership style. They felt that a combination would be required, with adaptation to circumstance. Emphasis was placed on motivation and coalition building. Women crafted their roles and contributions as leaders through self-awareness, especially of their own limitations. Another strategy was close connection to and understanding of communities served by the health sector. Finally, a skill that many women leaders ascribed to themselves, as they saw as uniquely gendered, was the ability to multitask. Many said that they were simply better at this than their husbands and most men they knew. As one state-level official explained:

> First thing is multitasking. That is definitely there. ... I think most of the ladies have this capability. That is why, yeah definitely it is there. Because it is naturally there. By birth, traditionally we have it. Being caretaker of the baby, doing cooking at kitchen, men do not know that. So they do only one at a time. Just browse and that's it. I write this with hand, I talk in the phone with the other hand, and take decisions at the same time. That is actually unique in women. So now, the advantage of being multitasking person, is they can do time management well. If the working time is 10 am – 5 pm, some people do only one thing during that. And when we do things, simultaneously multiple work will be done and we can complete tasks quickly.

This was a source of power that allowed them to negotiate and balance their lives and roles within the times allocated to each. These types of responses seemed to echo the properties of "gentle power" which is highly reflexive, not imposing or assertive, but rather collaborative and community based. At the same time, women leaders noted that they had experiences of uncomfortable or confrontational interactions with peers and colleagues like disagreements with male colleagues about gender norms, backlash or disapproval when they raised issues of their concern (e.g. sex worker rights), and resistance to suggestions that gender be included as a theme in the medical curriculum.

On Recognition and Career Progression: Wanted and Unwanted Attention

As a result of a "gentle power" leadership style, almost every single woman leader we spoke to had experienced rejection or challenges to their pursuit of leadership and decisions made as a leader. One leader, a member of a political family, faced legal intimidation when she sought to achieve a senior position in the department, one that she felt she had earned even if out of turn in terms of seniority. On the other hand, we noted another senior state-level official using the seniority norm to assure her position in the department—so as not to be passed over by a man. She received a great deal of negative attention for this as well. In both cases, doubts were cast on the professional morality and competence of these individuals. There is definitely a gender norm dimension to this—that was acknowledged by another state-level leader: "Kerala is patriarchal: patriarchy operates very deeply and in subtle ways. So a woman, when [it] comes to leadership, has to struggle a lot for acceptance…men at times have resistance to women's leadership".

The following mantra, described by one district-level official, resonated with many others in other kinds of positions as well: "Do work whether you receive appreciation or not. If you look for recognition you will be disappointed". We noted in some cases experiences of direct discrimination across intersections of women's identities. Being a religious minority, one woman leader noted that she had faced discrimination because of her gender, her religion, as well as the region that she was from—being told upfront that "we cannot trust [people from your religious community], or women [from this community]". She was also told she had the wrong last name to work in the state capital.

Decentralisation Reforms and Primary Healthcare: Working for Communities

Many of the women leaders we spoke to made explicit reference to reforms of local governance institutions or panchayats. They reflected on how these reforms opened up possibilities for their contributions as women leaders. The reference here was not to women's representation per se, but the flexibilities introduced in panchayat functioning as part of reforms. For instance, one state-level leader mentioned that sensitisation and training related to children's welfare were able to be introduced in villages because of decentralisation. Another leader at the district level noted that gradually in her area the use of public institutions increased because the receptivity to their feedback and sensitivity to their needs was increasing. In her particular case, communities were affected by endosulfan (pesticide) poisoning: investments in sanitation, water, and health, including a high-functioning primary facility, were priorities. One panchayat leader noted that

"after the People's Plan Campaign came into existence, the local institutions were transferred to the local panchayats and [things] then changed. Hospitals started becoming popular and people started using them. The discussions about its facility provisions were then discussed in *Gram Sabhas* [village assemblies]. When people go there, we will be getting complaints from them. People depend on the private hospital when they think that the doctor is not available at PHCs [Primary Health Centres]. …When people go there only we will get to know about the limitations there, and if we know only, this can be demanded from the government".

Sometimes change was implemented even in cases where communities did not see them as priorities. Another district-level leader explained that

"we used the board meetings of panchayat and demanded help for these households without even letting the households know. Because most of them were economically stable before and weakened due to the out-of-pocket expenditure incurred during cancer treatment. The people here are very proud; they would not like such a help from external source, yet they need it the most"

Here we see echoes of local leadership being effective because of attention to local, intimate matters through exercises of developmental altruism. There is no doubt that this has had effects, particularly in the domain of health, which all women leaders see as important.

Many of the women doctors we spoke to noted that they had served in Primary Health Centres and that this had a very strong effect on their working style. For many of our women leaders, working closely with communities and balancing their expectations and concerns with the requirements and routines of the health department exposed them to a lot of the skills and sensibilities that they continue to draw upon. Many leaders talked about how this exposed them also to various additional health issues that they began to care about, like palliation, and sensitised them to the perceptions people had of the health system, which they also found they could change. As one state-level leader mentioned "[Rural district and PHC] It's a very different place. So it was big eye opener for me. To me, I always used to think, why do these doctors have to be so rude always? What stops you from being a little pleasant? Why don't you smile? …Even when I worked in a very busy outpatient department, I did not find it so difficult to be polite". This leader then talked about the degree of support she was able to get from the community to move ahead with some key community health projects and how this in turn gave her confidence to take on more such responsibilities and even greater ones.

Of Grey Areas (and Blind Spots)?

We found ourselves questioning our positionality in relation to comments from many women leaders regarding sexual harassment. There were no reports of this across the interviews we conducted. As one local leader put it, "Sexual exploitation is not happening that often because not all men on the street are bad. Women should be aware of what the[se men] are, where they are from". In a sense, then the onus for protecting oneself was on women—to stay aware and to not take those kinds of "risks". Another leader at the state level noted the irony:

> While travelling late nights, my husband used to come and pick me from bus stand or railway station, but people used make fun of me, [saying] 'You are a feminist and you cannot go by yourself at 10 and 12 o'clock!' I said 'No, I also have to take safety into consideration'.

They did note that female colleagues would, in their view, feel more comfortable speaking to females about such problems, but also indicated that this was less likely in part because of the growing representation of women in health. The logic here is that women do not harass other women, and the more women there are, the safer a space or sector can become. We were not in a position to interpret or take a broader view on this, yet this area did feel like something of a blind spot to us especially in light of the fact that in the course of doing this fieldwork one of us experienced sexual harassment in a public place in broad daylight. This is perhaps an area that is hard to broach in the first place through in-person interviews with fairly high-profile women leaders. We intend to explore and probe this further.

Bringing It Together

The legacy of women's leadership in Kerala, as in India (as perhaps in the world), is vexed. Women are the majority (especially in Kerala) but have achieved positions of leadership not necessarily through struggles in women's movements or claims to solidarity, but by campaigns and agendas that were external, paternalistic, and in many cases, patriarchal. However, women are well aware of this, and further, this does not wholly preclude them from finding their own ways of exercising agency. Whether in relation to their numerical majority, to the legacy that Kerala has of women exercising "gentle power", or the way Kerala women leaders in health have negotiated their paths, leadership styles, recognition and attention, contribution to communities, and gender norms, we see structural constraints, but we also see power. It is not the type of power asserted in patriarchy. Rather, these are individual, everyday acts of resistance, or what scholars have called "pragmatic agency", in describing women's responses to biomedicine and technology (Desai, 2016; Lock et al., 1998). These forms of agency are asserted at the individual level, negotiating the Foucauldian "micro-physics" of power (Oksala, 2016), i.e. in interactions between women and men, as well as women and other men. It comprises acts of defying expected "respectable behaviour": being disagreeable, "disobedient", asserting and advancing one's own claims and ways of being (sometimes with subterfuge), and simply persisting in the face of disapproval or disruption by others. Nair observes this of feminist historiography in India, as we do of contemporary women leaders:

> The question of female agency …whether that agency takes the form of consent, transgression or subversion, can neither be wholly contained within a delineation of structures of oppression nor exhausted by accounts of female presence in history, but must be posed within specific contexts and placed along a continuum where various forms of agency may coexist. (Nair, 1994, p. 83)

Pragmatic agency and everyday resistance are riddled with tension, a kind of bargain struck with patriarchy of "playing by the rules" in ways that fall short of a radical restructuring of power that may arise from a formal, organised, solidarity-based, feminist praxis exercised by women leaders in health. And yet, in these acts of resistance and perseverance, we see that the typical forms of power are not fully reproduced: we cannot ignore that bargaining with the powerful is undeniably agentive (Scott, 1989). Further exploration and critical, reflexive questioning around the terms of bargaining—i.e. where and how women leaders in health navigate their resistance and respectability—we hope, may afford lessons and insights on how women may share and sometimes change the nature of power. As young women and men in this sector looking for leadership and a way forward, we are counting on it!

Acknowledgements We are grateful for the support and inputs of Dr. Sreejini N (formerly Public Health Foundation of India) and Dr. Anup Karan (Indian Institute of Public Health-Delhi). This work was supported by the Wellcome Trust/DBT India Alliance Fellowship (grant number IA/CPHI/16/1/502653) awarded to Dr. Devaki Nambiar as well as the Global Women's Health Program of the George Institute for Global Health. We are grateful for the support of the Kerala Department of Health and Family Welfare as well as the State Health Systems Resource Centre, Kerala. Most of all, we are deeply grateful for the time and thoughtful reflections given to us by interview participants: women leaders who are extremely busy and made time for this exercise.

References

Ameerudheen, T. A. (2017). *Women have a large presence in Kerala's local government bodies, but it's often men who run the show [Text]*. Retrieved January 6, 2020, from Scroll.in website: https://scroll.in/article/837459/women-have-a-large-presence-in-keralas-local-government-bodies-but-its-often-men-who-run-the-show

Anand, S., & Fan, V. (2016). *The Health Workforce in India* (No. No. 16). World Health Organization. Retrieved from https://www.who.int/hrh/resources/16058health_workforce_India.pdf

Chadha, A. (2014). *Political participation of women: A case study in India* (SSRN Scholarly Paper No. ID 2441693). Social Science Research Network. Retrieved from https://papers.ssrn.com/abstract=2441693

Desai, S. (2016). Pragmatic prevention, permanent solution: Women's experiences with hysterectomy in rural India. *Social Science & Medicine (1982), 151*, 11–18. https://doi.org/10.1016/j.socscimed.2015.12.046

Devika, J. (2006). Negotiating women's social space: Public debates on gender in early modern Kerala, India. *Inter-Asia Cultural Studies, 7*(1), 43–61.

Devika, J. (2012). Rockets with fire in their tails? Women leaders in Kerala's panchayats. *India International Centre Quarterly, 39*(3/4), 42–53. Retrieved from JSTOR.

Devika, J., & Thampi, B. V. (2011). Mobility towards work and politics for women in Kerala State, India: A view from the histories of gender and space. *Modern Asian Studies, 45*(5), 1147–1175. Retrieved from JSTOR.

Dhatt, R., Theobald, S., Buzuzi, S., Ros, B., Vong, S., Muraya, K., … Jackson, C. (2017). The role of women's leadership and gender equity in leadership and health system strengthening. *Global Health, Epidemiology and Genomics, 2*, e8. https://doi.org/10.1017/gheg.2016.22

Glaser, B. G., & Strauss, A. L. (2009). *The discovery of grounded theory: Strategies for qualitative research* (7th ed.). Transaction Publishers.

Jain, D. (2012). UNDERSTANDING LEADERSHIP: Lessons from the women's movement. *India International Centre Quarterly, 39*(3/4), 1–12. Retrieved from JSTOR.

Jeffrey, R. (1992a). Mary Poonen Lukose (1886–1976). In R. Jeffrey (Ed.), *Politics, women and well-being: How Kerala became 'a Model'* (pp. 92–95). https://doi.org/10.1007/978-1-349-12252-3_7

Jeffrey, R. (1992b). *Politics, women and well-being—How Kerala became a "model".* Macmillan Press.

Jeffrey, R. (2004). Legacies of matriliny: The place of women and the "Kerala Model". *Pacific Affairs, 77*(4), 647–664, 622.

Karan, A., Negandhi, H., Nair, R., Sharma, A., Tiwari, R., & Zodpey, S. (2019). Size, composition and distribution of human resource for health in India: New estimates using National Sample Survey and Registry data. *BMJ Open, 9*(4), e025979. https://doi.org/10.1136/bmjopen-2018-025979

Kodoth, P., & Jacob, T. K. (2013). *International Mobility of Nurses from Kerala (India) to the EU: Prospects and Challenges with special reference to the Netherlands and Denmark* (p. 53). CARIM-India RR 2013/19, Robert Schuman Centre for Advanced Studies, San Domenico di Fiesole (FI): European University Institute. Retrieved from https://www.mea.gov.in/images/pdf/InternationalMobilityofNursesfromIndia.pdf

Lankina, T., & Getachew, L. (2013). Competitive religious entrepreneurs: Christian missionaries and female education in colonial and post-colonial India. *British Journal of Political Science, 43*(1), 103–131. https://doi.org/10.1017/S0007123412000178

Lock, M., Kaufert, P. A., & Harwood, A. (1998). *Pragmatic women and body politics*. Cambridge University Press.

Nair, J. (1994). On the question of agency in Indian feminist historiography. *Gender and History, 6*(1), 82–100.

Nandraj, S., & Nambiar, D. (2018). Kerala's early experience: Moving towards universal health coverage. In P. Prasad & A. Jesani (Eds.), *Equity and access: Health care studies in India*. Oxford University Press.

Oksala, J. (2016). Microphysics of power. In *The Oxford handbook of feminist theory*. https://doi.org/10.1093/oxfordhb/9780199328581.013.24

Pillai, M. S. (2016). *The ivory throne: Chronicles of the house of Travancore*. Retrieved from http://search.proquest.com/docview/1790311637/abstract/39A8F34376A447DCPQ/1

Rao, K. D., Bhatnagar, A., & Berman, P. (2012). So many, yet few: Human resources for health in India. *Human Resources for Health, 10*(1), 19. https://doi.org/10.1186/1478-4491-10-19

Scott, J. C. (1989). Everyday forms of resistance. *The Copenhagen Journal of Asian Studies, 4*, 33. https://doi.org/10.22439/cjas.v4i1.1765

Semenya, S. S., & Potgieter, M. J. (2014). Bapedi traditional healers in the Limpopo Province, South Africa: Their socio-cultural profile and traditional healing practice. *Journal of Ethnobiology and Ethnomedicine, 10*(1), 4. https://doi.org/10.1186/1746-4269-10-4

Sundar, P. (2012). Czarinas or girl Fridays? Women in the corporate sector. *India International Centre Quarterly, 39*(3/4), 69–80. Retrieved from JSTOR.

Thresia, C. (2018). Health inequalities in South Asia at the launch of sustainable development goals: Exclusions in health in Kerala, India need political interventions. *International Journal of Health Services, 48*(1), 57–80. https://doi.org/10.1177/0020731417738222

Interview with Sabina Faiz Rashid, Dean and Professor at the James P. Grant School of Public Health at BRAC University

Mehr Manzoor and Kate Hawkins

"Leaders need to create spaces for people to excel. I truly believe in capacity building and nurturing and encouraging leadership among mid-level and junior professionals".

Sabina Faiz Rashid, PhD, is Dean and Professor at the James P. Grant School of Public Health at BRAC University. A medical anthropologist by training, Dr Rashid has more than 25 years of work experience in Bangladesh. Her areas of expertise are ethnographic and qualitative research, with a focus on urban populations, adolescents, and marginalised groups. She is particularly interested in examining the impact of structural and intersectional factors on the ability of these populations to realise their health and rights.

How Did Your Career in Health Begin?

I was born in Bangladesh but my formative years were spent abroad, growing up in different countries, attending school in diverse places. My late father, a self-made man, began his career as a barrister and later joined the Foreign Service. This led to us leaving Bangladesh when I was 9, and I eventually ended up in Australia for my university studies. After completing my bachelor's degree in anthropology, my dear friend Kate and I decided to travel the world and we took off for Bangkok and then onto Dhaka, where we were meant to spend 1 week. During that "short" week my uncle said, "Since you are back in Bangladesh after such a long time, why don't you take some time to work here. There's an organisation called BRAC; maybe you can do some work there". I was open to the idea and was fortunate enough to receive an appointment with founder Sir Fazle Hasan Abed, who knew my father from their time in the UK. I was able to convince him to give me an opportunity and I joined

M. Manzoor (✉)
Department of Health Policy and Management, Tulane University, New Orleans, LA, USA
e-mail: mmanzoor@tulane.edu

K. Hawkins
Pamoja Communications Ltd., Research in Gender and Ethics (RinGs), Brighton, East Sussex, UK
e-mail: kate@pamoja.uk.com

© Springer Nature Switzerland AG 2022
R. Morgan et al. (eds.), *Women and Global Health Leadership*,
https://doi.org/10.1007/978-3-030-84498-1_11

the NGO BRAC's research and evaluation division around October 1993. So began my unplanned journey in the world of health research and the development world

For my first assignment I was sent to a village to explore the reasons for school dropouts in BRAC programmes. The experience of spending time in the village changed my life. It was the first time that I had visited a rural village. I learnt more about anthropology, health, and development in those 6 months than I did in 4 years of undergraduate studies. Not to undervalue the degree, but the experience of visiting communities and meeting strong and capable women and resilient community members transformed my life.

I was always interested in young women's lives and was irked at certain mainstream ideas about women in the Global South all being oppressed, and that only women in the North were somehow liberated. All these notions and assumptions were being proven wrong before my very eyes by rural women, many of whom were actively trying to transform their lives for the better, despite the challenges they faced. Having spent time in rural areas, I wanted to continue trying to better understand my own country and my space as a woman living in Bangladesh. Working with BRAC gave me that opportunity, and in the early 1990s I was able to conduct research focusing on women and adolescent girls in informal slums and rural areas.

My early learning continued with my master's thesis study on the use of Norplant and family planning among poorer women. From a personal standpoint, it shed light on the complexities of reproductive health rights, agency, and bodily integrity, and who can speak for whom in these contexts.

For my PhD I looked at the lived realities of impoverished adolescent girls in a Dhaka slum, and on my return to Dhaka in 2004, I joined the James P Grant School of Public Health at BRAC University as a senior lecturer. The School had just been established and I had to convince them to hire me as I wanted to expand my critical thinking around issues of development, and health and rights of vulnerable populations. I was excited at being able to continue doing research and teaching, with mentoring support from a faculty member from Columbia University at the time.

In 2013, the founder of the school, the late Sir Fazle Hasan Abed, asked me to consider taking over as dean. In all honesty, I was fearful of taking on the role and stated, "No, I don't think I can do this job…and I am not ready". I was fortunate that the founder persuaded me otherwise. He encouraged me to take on the position and stated that I was doing an excellent job as the associate dean, and becoming dean was the natural and logical progression. He insisted that I needed to take on the leadership mantle. I will forever be grateful to Sir Abed for this support and recognition. I was BRAC University's first woman dean at the time, and the youngest at 44.

What Challenges Have You Faced?

There were times when I just wanted to walk away because of the sexism. I remember participating at a meeting when I was an assistant professor and a senior manager of Bangladesh origin was visiting from North America. There were about ten of us in attendance, including a lecturer and an assistant professor. At one point, he looked at me and asked, "Do you know when the coffee is coming?" I said, "No. Am I meant to know when the coffee is coming?" As the only female in the meeting, it was assumed that I was responsible for organising the coffee and snacks, despite there being junior male colleagues present.

Such attitudes and biases unfortunately permeate many workspaces. It is not easily spoken about even though it is visible. At other times the discrimination is very subtle, and one can feel like one is over-reacting or imagining the bias, and so it can be confusing. In such instances, I usually reflect and check myself an have turned to trusted friends and my husband for advice and objective feedback.

Organisations like BRAC are committed to gender equality, but to change the kind of structural sexism and discrimination that persists in workspaces and in society takes time, patience, greater awareness, and sustained commitment for change. Often it is unintentional and so ingrained in our consciousness that in many conversations and discussions, slights and undermining of female colleagues is not even noticed. Gender equality and equity is not just about how many heads or leaders are women in that particular organisation, but also involves more subtle indicators, such as salary structures, respect, promotions, due recognition, and the manner in which women's and men's opinions are valued in the workspace in general. This is a challenge not only in Bangladesh but globally.

It is also important to acknowledge that the level of agency and support a woman receives in the workspace can also be influenced by her class, position, and location in the social hierarchy, and with the "right" family "name" and connections to the "right" people (i.e. people in powerful positions or well respected in the social milieu). These factors can and do play a role in reducing the level of gender discrimination compared to others. It is critical to understand that in this context, class and privilege automatically ease the path and allow both men and women to bypass varying levels of discrimination. But overall, I would argue that gender biases do persist for most women regardless of their competence, class, and backgrounds.

Boys' clubs are pervasive and exist all over the world, even in the best of institutions possessing the right intentions. Sometimes women, too, join that club. How one reacts to this is critical as one should try not to get demoralised but rather remain professional and focus on ensuring the work being undertaken meets the highest quality and standards. I have always been forthright about my views in my personal life, my social circle, and in the workplace. For that, I credit my parents for the manner in which they brought us up. We are three siblings and I am in between two brothers. I never experienced any discrimination in the way I was treated, be it in terms of schooling, personal and professional interests, or otherwise. Our parents urged us to speak up and nurtured us to be open about our feelings and experiences. All three of us were encouraged to aspire to a career and understand the value of hard work. Furthermore, I never faced the pressure of getting married in my 20s even when others pressured my father to find a "suitable boy" for me to settle down with. My father always told me, "You should aspire to work hard, be financially independent, and live a life of integrity. Don't work in a job for the money, rather do it because it is what you love to do". I consider myself fortunate to have had the right messages of work ethics, values, and honesty from a very young age.

It is important to recognise that becoming dean did not mean that suddenly everything had changed. What did shift, however, was the power, authority, and opportunities I now had within my grasp to create change within the school with the support of my colleagues. Our associate dean is also a woman, and we are close and have immense mutual professional respect for each other. We have wonderful mid-level and junior colleagues, who are extremely invested in the school—with 60% being women. Mid-level colleagues are encouraged to write and bring in small research grants, are involved in teaching, and many are publishing as first authors in peer-reviewed journals. I feel fortunate that we have set up policies at the school that allow for flexibility; that is particularly appreciated by women as they have to juggle many more demands on their time, from their husbands, children, in-laws, and parents. I personally do not face these pressures. My husband and I are child-free and my immediate family has been very supportive. My husband is a feminist just like my father and has always supported me in my career.

But even with all this support, there have still been times when I felt frustrated and defeated. Leading an institution entails a lot of pressure and stress as one is ultimately responsible for all staff, finances, audits, evaluations, and the quality of the research and education programmes. Unlike many other institutes and schools, we are a self-financed institution, meaning that we raise all of our own funds for running the school. While this keeps all of us excited at bringing in new grants and research collaborations, it also means that we have limited time to breathe!

What Are Your Thoughts on Leadership?

Hierarchy is prevalent in all societies—some more, some less—and Bangladesh is no different. I view leadership as being aware of the hierarchy that has enabled one to reach the level one is at, while at the same time speaking up and ensuring that people who face greater disadvantages because of this hierarchy have access to appropriate opportunities.

Leaders need to create spaces for people to excel. I truly believe in capacity building and nurturing and encouraging leadership among mid-level and junior professionals. We thus created an organogram to support this in a more systematic manner given our country context. If we simply borrowed from the North American system where you can only be an assistant professor if you have a PhD, then we are going to stifle growth and opportunities for many dynamic colleagues in the school. In our system if instead of a PhD you have many years of experience, that's just as relevant and one can avail of leadership roles in management, and in research, etc. This allows mid-level staff to take on the role of coordinators of research/capacity building projects, and they are closely mentored by senior professors and a team. We encourage junior and mid-level colleagues to be lead authors on publications, as this will establish their confidence in their own capacities. We encourage our colleagues to lead smaller research grants, or co-lead on large grants, depending on their capabilities. We have created mentorship within the school with opportunities to attend scientific writing courses, journal clubs, and a seminar series where colleagues can meet, discuss, critically review each other's work, and learn. We have a separate fund set aside for capacity building grants to allow for junior colleagues, when possible, to attend conferences. This allows for exposure and the opportunity to network and learn. Some of my female colleagues may not necessarily view research as a long-term career goal; however, in the last 6 or 7 years, more and more young women are being attracted to our institution, wanting to take on leadership roles. This makes me very proud.

I have experienced and continue to see the manner in which heads of organisations and institutions, irrespective of competency, overshadow opportunities for the next generation of young leaders, particularly for women. This can be very demotivating for very smart and dynamic junior and mid-level colleagues. If we don't address these systemic inequalities and cultural biases in our traditionally "deferential pro-ageist" system, then we will be unable to hold on to dynamic, capable colleagues who need to be encouraged to take on leadership roles, particularly women.

The workplace should be compassionate, open, and safe. We have policies on gender harassment, sexual harassment, religious tolerance, and sexual diversity, as well maternity and paternity leave policies. No one is allowed to comment on appearances, personal beliefs, or marital status or one's orientation. We also try to be mindful of personal challenges. When a colleague was going through an extremely difficult divorce from an abusive husband, we found her temporary safe housing, transport, and a lawyer. Being mindful of the personal challenges that people face ensures a safe and secure space for everyone, not only women but also those who are marginalised because of existing societal prejudices.

What Advice Do You Have for Younger Women?

First and foremost, it is important to believe in yourself. It is also important to remember that as one moves further up the work hierarchy, the competition becomes fiercer. To prevail in such an environment, you need to be sincere, hard-working, open to learning, and willing to contribute. It is important to maintain your integrity and share your views. You need to have the courage to stand your ground. Seek out where possible nurturing and encouraging peers who you can rely on and they on you. Work as a team. Learn negotiation skills to get your point of view across. It is also important to be reflective and to learn from failure. The challenges one faces along one's life journey will help to transform you into a stronger person.

I also believe very strongly that one must have tolerance, respect, and empathy, irrespective of a person's gender, age, faith, class, skin colour, language, cultural differences, disabilities, sexual orientation, or socioeconomic background. I had to relocate every few years to a different country and thus I was invariably an outsider in many of these new places. However, I did learn to adapt, and what I took away from meeting people of diverse backgrounds is that we are not all that different, but have similar fears, hopes, and dreams. Having empathy will enable us to set aside the labels and accept people without judgement and create better personal and work relationships. Not only would we then be far more productive, our societies would also be more fulfilled and just. I feel it is important to have gratitude and to not feel entitled. Stay the course, particularly if the work feels purposeful and meaningful. There are now many more women in positions of power who are great role models and are a source of inspiration for all of us.

Leading from the Front: Transforming Policy in Crisis for School-Based Sex Education in Ireland

Ann Nolan

Constance Markievicz, a suffragette and nationalist who won a seat at Westminster in the General Election of 1918, was the first woman to be elected to the UK parliament. When she was appointed Minister for Labour in the revolutionary Dáil Éireann (Irish Parliament) in early 1919, Markievicz became the first European woman to hold a cabinet position. A further 13 women were elected to Dáil Éireann during the 1920s and 1930s, numbers that in relative terms exceeded those to be found in other European states such as Norway and Denmark (Gardiner, 1993) more generally associated with gender equality. However, by the 1940s women's participation in national politics in Ireland had gone into significant decline, with just two women politicians routinely holding seats in parliament, and it was to be a further 40 years before there would be another female minister in an Irish government (Galligan, 2018).

This chapter will showcase the impact of one woman's leadership as Minister for Education (1987–1991) in introducing a sex education programme into the Irish school curriculum—a development that had effectively been thwarted by Roman Catholic Church authorities since the foundation of the State. It will explore the sociopolitical context in which she worked and her own personal challenges with motherhood and the demands of family life. Mary O'Rourke was an unlikely figure in the context of a liberal platform for sexual health, being a member of the conservative Fianna Fáil party[1] and a self-proclaimed practising Catholic, wife, and mother of two small boys who would not generally have been credited with strong feminist credentials. There are obvious dangers in attributing too much credit to one individual in shaping the course of historical events, but at the same time, the policy

---

[1] National centrist party descended from the republican (anti-treaty) side of Ireland's Civil War (28 June 1922–24 May 1923) that followed the War of Independence from Britain.

A. Nolan (✉)
Trinity Centre for Global Health, Trinity College, Dublin, Ireland
e-mail: NOLANA13@tcd.ie

literature emphasises the importance of key actors as agents of change, particularly in areas of policy-making that are highly contested (Kingdon, 2003; MacGregor, 2013; Oliver, 2006). O'Rourke's introduction of sex education into the Irish school system will be considered here in light of the unique circumstances surrounding the crisis posed by HIV/AIDS when she held the cabinet positions for health and education.

The content of this chapter is based upon: (1) research interviews conducted by this author—including a lengthy interview with Mary O'Rourke for a PhD study on the transformative impact of HIV/AIDS on Irish sexual health policy; (2) academic studies, by historians and social scientists; (3) O'Rourke's (2013) autobiography; and (4) Irish print and broadcast media coverage of the topics dealt with here.

"Mná na hÉireann" (English: The Women of Ireland)

The marginalisation of women within electoral politics in Ireland is best explained in the context of broader social and cultural developments in independent Ireland, and specifically in the context of the influence wielded by the Roman Catholic Church on popular culture and public policy. The Catholic Church had achieved considerable influence and power in nineteenth-century Ireland when the country as a whole was part of the then United Kingdom of Great Britain and Ireland. After independence from Britain, Catholic Church influence on successive Irish governments became more marked (Whyte, 1980). As Inglis (1998) put it, the Catholic Church in Ireland enjoyed a "moral monopoly": that is, it claimed for itself and was popularly granted a unique status in defining the morality in relation to a very wide range of individual, familial, and communal activities. On a day-to-day basis, Church influence was particularly notable in the spheres of education and healthcare, with many healthcare facilities and practically all schools being run by religious orders—despite the fact that health services and schools were primarily funded from the public purse—within the Catholic ethos (Whyte, 1980).

The idealisation of motherhood and the role of women in the home became central to the rhetoric of the new State in 1921 (Luddy, 2007). This contested ideal was and remains enshrined in Article 41 of *Bunreacht na hÉireann*, the Constitution of Ireland:

> In particular, the State recognizes that by her life within the home, woman gives to the State a support without which the common good cannot be achieved. (Bunreacht na hÉireann, 41.2.1)

Professor Yvonne Scannell has described the all-male drafting of this Article in the 1937 Constitution as "the grossest form of sexual stereotyping" that "fails to recognise that a woman's place is a woman's choice" (Scannell, 1988, p. 125). Even so, the idea of women as predominantly mothers and homemakers maintained ideological dominance in Irish society for much of the twentieth century and was reinforced by a "marriage bar" which prohibited women from remaining in the public service on marriage up until 1973 (Maguire, 2008). Consequently, Irish women were subject to a kind of "double jeopardy" in that they were obliged to live under a social policy regime that some, at least, found oppressive, while simultaneously experiencing difficulties in challenging this regime through participation in political processes.

Women's Leadership in the Context of the AIDS Crisis

As international momentum unified around a response to AIDS that was characterised by value-neutral public health principles, the Irish State, and particularly the statutory health sector, was compelled to balance the views of a conservative voting majority at home (95% of whom were Roman Catholic in 1982) with the liberal consensus that was defining the response at European Union (EU) and global levels. When the first cases of AIDS were diagnosed in 1982, homosexual acts were criminalised; Ireland had no genitourinary consultancy posts and poorly developed diagnostic and treatment services for sexually transmitted infections (STIs). There was no mandatory sex education in schools, and contraceptives were restricted to married couples on prescription. Although a liberal platform had begun to emerge in relation to sexual and reproductive health and rights in Ireland during the pre-HIV/AIDS era, this was a marginal movement, representing a minority view. Consequently, the AIDS crisis presented an opportunity for liberal reform among those who had been dissatisfied with Ireland's conservative approach to sexuality and sexual health.

The AIDS pandemic was preceded by a second wave of the women's rights movement in the 1970s, and in Ireland, women's rights gained traction through membership of the European Economic Community (EEC now EU) in 1973. This ideological shift appears to have prompted a 260% increase in the number of women elected to parliament between the 1970s and 1980s, among them a secondary school teacher and member of the Athlone[2] Urban District Council, Mary O'Rourke. O'Rourke was first elected to parliament in 1982. While she did not run for election on a platform of sexual and reproductive health reform, as Minister for Education she took advantage of the global momentum in response to the AIDS crisis to introduce a highly contested programme of school-based sex education. The *AIDS Education Resource* that was introduced in schools nationwide in 1990 was effectively sex education by stealth. The programme embodied liberal public health principles that ran contrary to the prevailing value system in Ireland and largely reflected global policy for HIV and sexual health that was ascendant at the time.

When compared with the AIDS history literature in other Western contexts including the United States and the United Kingdom (Berridge, 1996; Berridge & Strong, 1993; Harden, 2012), the Irish context points to significant leadership from

---

[2] Athlone is a small town in central Ireland with a population of 21,351 (2016).

women, not least among them Professor Fiona Mulcahy, Ireland's first genitourinary consultant who transformed sexual health treatment services, and Justice Gillian Hussey who chaired the first national AIDS policy response, the church-led National Task Force on AIDS (Nolan & Butler, 2018). From a political perspective, however, Mary O'Rourke is notable because she used the AIDS crisis to liberalise policy for school-based sex education notwithstanding a sustained campaign of bitter opposition from well-placed and influential conservative Catholic groups. In a subsequent role as Minister for Health and Children (1991–1992), she was also instrumental in establishing a uniquely multisectoral and diverse task force of stakeholders to take forward a progressive multisectoral and participatory response to sexual health and drug use through the development of a national AIDS strategy.

A number of studies have stressed the ways in which crisis can work to promote opportunities for mobilisation by women and sexual minorities (Bedford, 2009; Borland & Sutton, 2007; Lopreite, 2008). It is also well recognised that AIDS had a transformative impact on rights across the world (Altman, 1995; Berridge & Strong, 1993; Harden, 2012; Nathanson et al., 2007; Northern Ireland Assembly, 2020). In documenting female leadership for sexual health policy in Argentina, however, Jennifer Piscopo emphasises that evaluation of the success of female leadership for health cannot be divorced from the sociopolitical context (Piscopo, 2014). The same caveat must also apply to an assessment of O'Rourke's impact on the highly contested domain of school-based sex education: while O'Rourke's personal agency and pragmatic, no-nonsense leadership style were important factors in her success, any assessment of her role cannot be divorced from the fact that AIDS generated a climate of fear to present what might be described as a "window of opportunity through crisis" (MacGregor, 2013, p. 232). In Argentina, reform of the laws governing access to contraception coincided with an increase in female leadership in parliament but also increasing civil society activism. Similarly, Mary O'Rourke's political career was ascendant at a time of sociopolitical transformation in Ireland following membership of the EU, with an increasingly visible minority platform for gender equality coupled with the looming threat of the AIDS pandemic.

Such qualifications are not intended to downplay O'Rourke's role in driving an agenda for change, but in our efforts to understand the ways in which women leaders for health progress the concerns of women, it is imperative that we don't lose sight of structural and institutional movements that may occur simultaneously to ease the pathway for change. While women leaders for health may be more responsive to the needs of the whole population, particularly minority groups (Dhatt et al., 2017), this is not exclusively so. There are men and women leaders in Ireland's political context who have been advocates for women's health and those who have actively obstructed progress.

Women's priorities for sexual and reproductive health can also depend on their own personal priorities and life experiences (Kohen, 2009). O'Rourke's determination to promote a liberal programme of sex education notwithstanding fierce opposition from colleagues and highly vocal conservative Catholic interest groups was, in part, inspired by her own personal experiences (O'Rourke, 2011). As a town counsellor she had met young mothers whose fertility was controlled by their husbands, and her constituency had witnessed the tragic death of a young 15-year-old girl who was found at a grotto of the Blessed Virgin by three schoolboys in late January 1984. Ann Lovett's dead infant son lay close beside her and her short life made her town "the whipping boy for the guilt of a whole nation" (2008). It also provided a catalyst for a public debate on sex education and O'Rourke with a bold agenda for change.

"I Don't Want to Be Put in a Cupboard with 'Women's Affairs' on a Label"[3]: Mary O'Rourke, Minister for Education (1987–1991)

O'Rourke's first demonstration of her political independence as a woman politician occurred in January 1983 when she rejected then-leader of the Fianna Fáil party, Charles Haughey's offer of Shadow Minister for Women's Affairs. At what she described as this "defining moment in my career", O'Rourke told Haughey (O'Rourke, 2013, p. 38):

> I don't want to be put in a cupboard with "Women's Affairs" on a label on the door and to only get out whenever there are women's affairs to be discussed. I will always be discussing women's affairs because I am interested in them and I am a woman – but I don't want to be pigeon-holed like that. (O'Rourke, 2013, p. 39)

This was a bold but potentially impolitic move since "Mr Haughey", as O'Rourke habitually referred to him, was a domineering political figure who was unaccustomed to being gainsaid. She reflected in later years that she didn't know where her "audacity" had come from, but this determination to speak her mind and take bold decisions was to become a defining feature of O'Rourke's political career. She was subsequently offered and accepted the position of Shadow Minister of Education, becoming Minister when Fianna Fáil took power after the general election in February 1987 at the height of the AIDS pandemic.

O'Rourke had been the opposition party spokeswoman on education when Ann Lovett died and the story was brought to national attention by Emily O'Reilly, one of a number of recently appointed female journalists who wrote for the first time about the darker realities of women's lives in Ireland. The story sparked a national debate about clandestine pregnancies and the need for sex education such as had never previously occurred in Ireland. Then-Minister for Education Gemma Hussey—who championed initiatives to combat sexism and sex stereotyping in textbooks while also establishing a working party to examine the position of women in Irish higher education during her tenure as Minister (Mooney, 2017)—announced that the Department was "taking steps" to develop a programme of sex education appropriate to Irish schools. She referred to "the terribly tragic case this year which concentrated all our minds on the necessity to develop programmes of sex and

---

[3] Source: O'Rourke, M. (2013). *Just Mary: A memoir*. Dublin: Gill and Macmillan, p. 39.

human relationships education" (Murphy, 1984). O'Rourke, in political opposition, supported Hussey's proposal and successfully urged her party to reject a motion that objected to Government's efforts to introduce sex education in schools (Coghlan, 1985).

Notwithstanding all-party support in the wake of Ann Lovett's death, there was substantially more opposition. Highly vocal and well-organised lay Catholic groupings that had formed in defence of traditional family values over the course of the abortion referendum in 1983 mounted sustained opposition to the introduction of sex education in schools. While constituting a small if highly visible and vocal minority, these conservative lobbyists were supported by the Catholic Archbishop of Dublin and other influential Bishops throughout the state (Kevin McNamara Archbishop of Dublin, 1987). Government plans to introduce school-based sex education were abandoned in the face of such sustained and powerful opposition.

O'Rourke was appointed Minister for Education when Fianna Fáil came to power in 1987. She reflected that the Assistant Secretaries of the Department who came to advise her were all men and at her first Cabinet meeting that she felt "…so junior, so untried, so green-horned, so naïve…it didn't seem like the time to put my usual rule of speaking up into practice" (O'Rourke, 2013, p. 43). Once she found her feet, she was not afraid to be controversial. One of her first objectives as Minister for Education was to champion the deeply unpopular spread of multidimensional education, which marked her out as a politician who had no intention of maintaining the status quo. Frank and pragmatic, O'Rourke was not afraid to talk about sex and was forthright and direct in her approach:

> Well I do think issues like that [i.e., sexual] you have to lead from the front. You just have to lead from the front. If you wait until 95% of the population are in agreement with you, you'd be long dead. I think if you feel strongly about a thing yourself, but you must have your own belief in it and you must have your own belief in yourself. That's hugely important. And once you'd have that, well then you should fire off. (O'Rourke, 2011)

The policy literature generally concludes that controversial issues are particularly unattractive to policy-makers. Political theorist, John Kingdon, highlighted a tendency by politicians to "duck hot issues" and pass them to administrative agencies, but O'Rourke demonstrated quite the opposite tendency throughout her tenure as Minister in that she confronted controversial issues (2013, p. 38).

By early 1988, it was announced in the Seanad that the Ministers for Education and Health were discussing plans for the provision of an AIDS education programme in schools to ensure that "no child should leave school without being aware of the facts about AIDS" (Seanad Eireann Debate, 1988). In the climate of fear generated by HIV/AIDS in the 1980s, there was significant but not unanimous political support for the introduction of an explicit programme in schools. Some politicians remained hostile to the idea and conservative Catholic lay groups protested outside the Department of Education on a daily basis (Nolan, 2018).

At that time over 95% of schools were owned and run by the Catholic Church in Ireland, and as such, the Bishops had a right to be consulted about the proposed programme. O'Rourke recalled that they were "…a bit alarmed and they wondered if it could be done without the word sex in it…I said, well it's about sexuality" (O'Rourke, 2011). She reflected that her status as a woman, a mother, and a Fianna Fáil T.D. may have wrong-footed them:

> I think they were a bit surprised: I was late forties, married, two little boys at home and kind of the paragon of all that is great and good. Suddenly here I was talking about these matters, as well as talking about educational matters. So I think that sort of frightened off people, you know, or frightened off a certain section of the Catholic hierarchy who would be in constant interaction with the Department of Education…. (O'Rourke, 2011)

It is significant that some of the Catholic hierarchy were "frightened off" by what O'Rourke claimed was her representation of "all that is great and good". She emphasised, however, that they didn't hold up any barriers to the introduction of the programme which suggests a level of acceptance among the Bishops that the state had a role to play in sex education in light of the threat posed by AIDS (A. Nolan, 2018). She would not be drawn into open controversy with the Bishops at the time stating firmly to media sources, "they [the Bishops] have their bailiwick[4] and I have mine" (Walsh, 1990).

The more significant opposition to the proposed introduction of an AIDS education resource, which was school-based sex education by another name, came from conservative Catholic lay groups:

> … they [Catholic lay groups] came up to lobby me that I shouldn't be doing this and I shouldn't be doing that and all that. It was amazing, they had a great hold: they had a great foothold at that time … I said of course, the parents are the first educators, according to our Constitution. So I would be all for parents being the ones to convey all that information. But in many, many, many cases, parents didn't do it … I don't like to be always down on right-wing Catholics, but certainly they were wrong on these issues, certainly wrong because if they weren't going to convey the news to their children, the State had a duty to do it. (O'Rourke, 2011)

Using the AIDS crisis as an entry point, Mary O'Rourke stood firm against all opposition and oversaw the development of a programme of school-based sex education that was, by the standards of the time, quite explicit, marking a turning point in Ireland's relationship with sexuality. The AIDS Education Resource was officially rolled out in schools throughout the country on 2 October 1990. It retained controversial elements which the Bishops had objected to including references to anal sex, oral sex, condom use, and masturbation (Department of Education & Department of Health, 1990). This programme became the basis upon which a mandatory programme of school-based sex education was introduced in Irish schools in 1997 by another female Minister for Education, Niamh Breathnach.

---

[4] One's sphere of operations or area of interest (Oxford English Dictionary).

Discussion and Conclusion

What does this case study tell us, if anything, about women's leadership in areas of contested health policy like sex education in schools? It would be both naïve and indeed incorrect to suggest that only women champion such issues in Ireland: a number of male doctors had long made the case for sex education in Ireland supported by some Ministers for Health (Desmond, 2000; Freedman, 1984; Thornton et al., 1979). The international literature appears to suggest that gender differences in attitudes to various sexual and reproductive health and rights are not particularly marked and, if anything, women can demonstrate more conservative attitudes to abortion, for example (Barkan, 2014; Shapiro & Mahajan, 1986). However, AIDS, more than appears to have been the case for crisis pregnancy or the death of Ann Lovett, opened a "window of opportunity" for women in Ireland to progress sexual health and sexual rights along liberal lines.

The reasons for this are not clear but in this case study it is notable that the ministerial champions of school-based sex education in the Department of Education were all women. Building on the groundswell of support for the introduction of school-based sex education in the wake of Ann Lovett's death, Gemma Hussey was the first Minister of Education to develop a policy response, but her efforts were stymied by fierce opposition mounted by conservative right-wing groups. The AIDS crisis provided her successor, Mary O'Rourke, with an opportunity to prioritise a policy she had championed in opposition. As one contemporary commentator called it, the AIDS Education Resource was "…sex education by stealth" (Dublin AIDS Alliance Archive, 1988). O'Rourke was ultimately the right person, in the right place, at the right time. Was her gender significant and pivotal to her success?

There is no doubt that as leader of the government, Charles Haughey was committed to Ireland's membership of the European Union where gender equality and modernisation of Ireland's political and administrative culture were made a condition of membership under various European directives. It was also the case that the European Court of Human Rights (ECHR) had in 1988 found Ireland to be in breach of Article 8 of the European Convention on Human Rights in respect of Ireland's criminalisation of homosexual acts. Homosexual acts were not decriminalised in Ireland until a female Minister for Justice, Máire Geoghegan-Quinn, brought forward legislation in 1993. Ireland's laws regulating access to contraception and the provision of sexual health treatment services were also in the spotlight with criticism coming from the World Health Organization and other regional health bodies (Nolan, 2014). While change was afoot, Ireland was at the time out-of-step with more liberal countries in Europe and that was a source of embarrassment to the political establishment at home. Furthermore, the "national mood" was changing in the context of other modernising forces, increasing access to education, and, of course, the crisis presented by AIDS guaranteed majority support from O'Rourke's parliamentary colleagues. As such, while O'Rourke's personal determination and tendency to "lead from the front" on controversial issues were important factors in her success, they cannot be divorced from the sociopolitical context.

As highlighted in the Introduction, Mary O'Rourke's political career was ascendant at a time of transformation following Ireland's membership of the EU. A new, young, and dynamic generation of journalists brought issues of concern to women to the fore in broadcast and print media; there was an increasing focus on gender equality and the rights of women, while the 1980s was the decade in which the dominance of Catholic morality in Irish life began to be challenged, if, as historian Diarmaid Ferriter claims, "not always confronted successfully" (Ferriter, 2004, pp. 8–9). Add into that mix the fear generated by the AIDS pandemic and the appointment of Dr. Fiona Mulcahy, Ireland's first genitourinary consultant, leading the AIDS response at a clinical level. The "window of opportunity through crisis" presented itself, and O'Rourke was the right person, in the right place, at the right time to seize the opportunity for change.

Mary O'Rourke has left a detailed account of her experiences as a woman, a mother, a parliamentarian, and Minister for Education and Health. She is honest about feeling at times overwhelmed and concerned for the welfare of her two boys. As a woman working outside the home, she was in the minority at a time when traditional family values prevailed. In assessing O'Rourke's contribution, it is important to take account of the ways in which gender intersects with socioeconomic status and other markers of privilege and oppression. Intersectional approaches demonstrate the convergence of gender with health systems to promote a deeper understanding of health outcomes (Zeinali et al., 2019). O'Rourke was a well-educated, middle-class woman whose family had been embedded in Ireland's political establishment. This is what she meant when she reflected that her status as a woman, a mother, and a Fianna Fáil T.D. may have wrong-footed the Bishops in their opposition to her plans. She was aware that her status in Irish society and in the eyes of the Bishops gave her leverage.

By the early 1990s as sexual abuse scandals made headlines, the moral authority of the Catholic Church in Ireland went into decline. Simultaneously, economic growth and increasing prosperity gave new impetus to the liberal platform. While Niamh Breathnach encountered some opposition when she introduced sex education as a mandatory component of the second-level curriculum in 1997, it was nothing like the kind of resistance experienced by Hussey or O'Rourke. Ireland was by that time in transition from a society in which Roman Catholic morality defined the regulation of sexual and reproductive health and rights to one in which a secular liberal agenda was ascendant.

In 2015, Ireland became as the first country in the world to approve same-sex marriage by popular vote, and in 2018, an overwhelming majority voted to remove the constitutional ban on abortion. The sociopolitical and economic landscape of Ireland has been transformed, and yet those development gains are fragile and vulnerable to the global retreat of sexual and reproductive health and rights. There is a prevailing sense that Mná na hÉireann have overthrown the Ancient Régime, and yet in the centenary since 1918 when women won the right to vote and Constance Markievicz was the first woman elected to the British House of Commons, only 9% of elected members to Dáil Eireann (lower house) have been women with 11% in the Seanad (upper house) (Oireachas Library & Research Service (b), 2018). Of the

200 senior ministers in Irish governments from 1919 to 2019, only 19 (9.5%) have been women. Some of those have been changemakers in Irish life, and it must be acknowledged that O'Rourke demonstrated significant courage in refusing to evade what she saw as her responsibility to create a sex education programme that matched the needs of the time: a time when AIDS was still an acute, fatal condition commonly transmitted through sexual contact. Whether a male politician could have or would have achieved what O'Rourke achieved is a moot point. It is difficult, however, to resist the conclusion that this was an example of a woman politician who dealt with primarily male and patriarchal opposition with significant skill and whose achievements could not easily be matched by a male politician of this period.

References

Altman, D. (1995). Political sexualities: Meanings and identities in the time of aids. In R. Parker & J. Gagnon (Eds.), *Conceiving sexuality: Approaches to sex research in a postmodern world*. Routledge.

Barkan, S. E. (2014). Gender and abortion attitudes. *Public Opinion Quarterly, 78*(4), 940–950. https://doi.org/10.1093/poq/nfu047

Bedford, K. (2009). Gender and institutional strengthening: The World Bank's policy record in Latin America. *Contemporary Politics, 15*(2), 197–214.

Berridge, V. (1996). *AIDS in the UK: The making of policy, 1981-1994*. Oxford University Press.

Berridge, V., & Strong, P. (Eds.). (1993). *AIDS and contemporary history*. Cambridge Cambridge University Press.

Borland, E., & Sutton, B. (2007). Quotidian disruption and women's activism in times of crisis, Argentina 2002–3. *Gender and Society, 21*(5), 700–722.

Coghlan, D. (1985, April 1). *Another setback for lobby opposing sex education*. The Irish Times.

Department of Education, & Department of Health. (1990). *AIDS education resource*. Stationary Office.

Desmond, B. (2000). *Finally and in conclusion*. Dublin New Island Books.

Dhatt, R., Theobald, S., Buzuzi, S., Ros, B., Vong, S., Muraya, K., et al. (2017). The role of women's leadership and gender equity in leadership and health system strengthening. *Global Health, Epidemiology and Genomics, 2*, e8. https://doi.org/10.1017/gheg.2016.22

Dublin AIDS Alliance Archive. (1988, December). Interview with Dr James Walsh, National AIDS Co-ordinator. *AIDS Resources Newsletter*.

Ferriter, D. (2004). *The transformation of Ireland: 1900-2000*. Profile Books Ltd..

Freedman, D. (1984, February 15). *Sexually transmitted diseases: The Irish problem*. Paper presented at the Federated Dublin Voluntary Hospitals and St. James's Hospital Annual Conference, Dublin.

Galligan, Y. (2018, August 31). *Women and politics in Ireland since 1918*. Lecture to O'Connell Summer School, Co. Kerry, Ireland.

Gardiner, F. (1993). 'How women voted in the election'. In Gallagher, M., Laver, M. (Eds), *'How Ireland Voted 1992'*. Folens PSAI Press. Dublin.

Harden, V. A. (2012). *AIDS at 30*. Potomac Books.

Inglis, T. (1998). *Moral monopoly: The rise and fall of the catholic church in modern Ireland*. University College Dublin Press.

Kevin McNamara Archbishop of Dublin. (1987). *Curriculum and values in education*. Veritas Publications.

Kingdon, J. W. (2003). *Agendas, alternatives, and public policies* (2nd ed.). Longman.

Kohen, B. (2009). The effectiveness of legal strategies in Argentina. In J. Jaquette (Ed.), *Feminist agendas and democracy in Latin America*. Duke University Press.

Lopreite, D. (2008). *Challenging the Argentina gender regime? The politics of reproductive rights after democratization*. Paper presented at the Annual Meeting of the American Political Science Association, Boston.

Luddy, M. (2007). Sex and the single girl in 1920s and 1930s Ireland. *The Irish Review, 35*, 79.

MacGregor, S. (2013). Barriers to the influence of evidence on policy: Are politicians the problem? Drugs: Education. *Prevention and Policy, 20*(3), 232.

Maguire, M. (2008). *The civil service and the revolution in Ireland, 1912-38*. Manchester University Press.

Mooney, B. (2017). Thirty years of Education Matters: An absorbing journey. *Education matters yearbook 2017-2018*.

Murphy, C. (1984). *Hussey urges sex education*. The Irish Times.

Nathanson, C. A., Sember, R., & Parker, R. (2007). Contested bodies: The local and global politics of sex and reproduction. In R. Parker, R. Petchesky, & R. Sember (Eds.), *Sex politics: Reports from the front lines*. Sexuality Policy Watch.

Nolan, A. (2014). *'Marriage is not an anti-viral agent': The transformation of sexual health policy in the initial decade of AIDS in Ireland*. (PhD). Trinity College Dublin, the University of Dublin, Unpublished.

Nolan, A. (2018). The transformation of school-based sex education policy in the context of AIDS in Ireland. *Irish Educational Studies, 37*(3), 295–309.

Nolan, A., & Butler, S. (2018). AIDS, sexual health, and the catholic church in 1980s Ireland: A public health paradox? *American Journal of Public Health, 108*(7), 908–913.

Northern Ireland Assembly. (2020, June 23). *Official Report (Hansard)*. Belfast.

O'Rourke, M. (2011, March, 18) *Author's interview with former Minister for Education, Mary O'Rourke (1987-1991)/Interviewer: A. Nolan*.

O'Rourke, M. (2013). *Just mary: A memoir*. Gill and Macmillan.

Oireachas Library & Research Service (b). (2018). *Women in parliament: Percentage of women and men elected to Dáil Éireann (1918-2018)*. Houses of the Oireachtas.

Oliver, T. R. (2006). The politics of public health policy. *Annual Review of Public Health, 27*, 195–233.

Piscopo, J. M. (2014). Female leadership and sexual health policy in Argentina. *Latin American Research Review, 40*(1), 104–127. https://doi.org/10.1353/lar.2014.0013

Ruane, M. (2008, August 20). *Action group to exploit Granard's historical link with Michael Collins*. The Irish Times.

Scannell, Y. (1988). The constitution and the role of women. In B. Farrell (Ed.), *De Valera's constitution and ours* (pp. 123–136). Gill and Macmillan.

Seanad Eireann Debate. (1988, February 25). *Information and Education Programme on AIDS: Motion*. Dublin.

Shapiro, R. Y., & Mahajan, H. (1986). Gender differences in policy preferences: A summary of trends from the 1960s to the 1980s. *Public Opinion Quarterly, 50*(1), 42–61. https://doi.org/10.1086/268958

Thornton, C., Brennan, R., Denham, P., & Browne, A. (1979, February). Sex education by the gynaecologist: Analysis of a school programme in Ireland. *Irish Medical Journal*.

Walsh, J. (1990, October 2). *Bishops likely to accept new aids plan for schools*. The Irish Times.

Whyte, J. H. (1980). *Church and state in modern Ireland*. Gill and Macmillan Ltd..

Zeinali, Z., Muraya, K., Govender, V., Molyneux, S., & Morgan, R. (2019). Intersectionality and global health leadership: Parity is not enough. *Human Resources for Health, 17*(1), 29. https://doi.org/10.1186/s12960-019-0367-3

Interview with Ilona Kickbusch, Independent Global Health Consultant, Former Director of the Global Health Centre at the Graduate Institute of International and Development Studies, Geneva

Sulzhan Bali and Roopa Dhatt

"Lead with an exclamation mark!"

Ilona Kickbusch is a German political scientist best known for her contribution to health promotion and global health. Ilona has had a distinguished career with the World Health Organization (WHO), at both regional and global levels, where she led the Global Health Promotion Programme and initiated the Ottawa Charter for Health Promotion and a range of projects including Healthy Cities and Women's Health Counts. Previously, Ilona served as the Director of the Global Health Centre at the Graduate Institute of International and Development Studies, Geneva, and also led Yale University's Global Health Program (1998–2003). She is a member of WHO's Independent High-Level Commission on Non-Communicable Diseases and is the co-chair of the Universal Health Coverage 2030 Steering Committee, Council Chair for the World Health Summit, and a member of the Global Preparedness and Monitoring Board, and several other advisory boards in the health policy arena. She has been an advisor to a number of organizations, government agencies (including the German Federal Ministry of Health), and the private sector on health policies. Further, she launched the think-tank initiative Global Health Europe: A Platform for European Engagement in Global Health and the Consortium for Global Health Diplomacy. During her career, Ilona has received several awards, including the Adelaide Thinker in Residence Award and the Cross of the Order of Merit of the Federal Republic of Germany, in recognition of her invaluable contributions to global health governance and global health diplomacy.

S. Bali (✉) · R. Dhatt
Women in Global Health, Washington, DC, USA
e-mail: sulzhan@gmail.com; roopa.dhatt@womeningh.org

© Springer Nature Switzerland AG 2022
R. Morgan et al. (eds.), *Women and Global Health Leadership*,
https://doi.org/10.1007/978-3-030-84498-1_13

133

Why Is Gender Equity at the Senior Leadership Level Important for Global Health Governance?

I could answer like Mr. [Justin] Trudeau [Prime Minister of Canada] and say because it is 2019! It is just the principle of equity. I belong to the generation of women where our starting point was that we have two genders and they are equal and should have equal participation in everything we do in society. This is, of course, more complex today as we must recognize a much wider range of gender identities. There is also the principle of diversity in decision making and governance—men and women have different approaches to problem solving, how they see the world, what they consider important. Research highlights that diversity in decision making brings better results.

So, Not Just Gender Equity, but Diversity Makes for Better Leadership?

Yes! Unfortunately, traditionally leadership in global health governance has been a lot of "white men with white hair." The field is not only male dominated but also dominated by academics and experts from one part of the world. They are very committed. However, in an international organization, all parts of the world need to be reflected in senior leadership. So, you can't only look at gender alone. You really need diversity to be able to create a global culture and have representation of a diversity of voices. While gender is incredibly important, you also have to make sure that you are bringing in women who bring in different types of cultural experiences and different styles. And today, of course, we need to think beyond the women's issue only. My comments relate to the changes my generation sought to bring about.

Do Men and Women Differ in Leadership Capability or Styles?

Women can lead just as well as men. There is no difference in capability, but they can lead differently. You have examples such as Angela Merkel who is a very different type of leader, but then you also have leaders like Indira Gandhi whose leadership style was no different from her male peers. Unlike men, women negotiate more, create consensus, and are less status focused. So, there is a lot of difference in leadership styles, and that is influenced by cultural leadership styles. You have a different notion of what constitutes a leader in the United States than in an Asian country or an African country.

Is the Perception of Leadership and Failures Different Because of Their Gender?

Many people are of the opinion women are not on the top of the totem pole because they are not made for leadership. Even women who've made it to the top of the totem pole have difficulties in being accepted as leaders. So, when a woman fails, there would always be that gender component. It's rarely said the other way 'round', or that success of women leaders is attributed to gender. Just look at the strong response to the COVID-19 pandemic in countries with strong women leaders.

As the male form of leadership is the type of leadership one tends to often see and expect, women who don't lead like that are seen as weak and therefore they are sometimes also not supported by other men and even women. There are many examples, Angela Merkel being one, of journalistic pieces on why she isn't considered as insistent, definitive, like some of the male chancellors before her. Another example would be Margaret Chan. In many cases, if people are not satisfied with the form of leadership and that leader tends to be a woman, they will tend more to put it down to the gender issue than just say, "this person is a crappy leader." They will say, "well, what can you expect, this is a woman leader." Women leaders always have that extra problem if they don't do things as expected, and if they are not as successful for any reason.

There is often a tendency to consider gender a significant component in "leadership weakness." Frequently if something goes wrong, and it goes wrong for men as well as for women, the tendency will be to say, "well, we're not surprised, she's a woman, she tried this strange leadership style and no wonder nothing came out of it," kind of thing. Around a woman the failure is often put down to gender or criticism gets personalized, whereas a man won't be criticized because he's a man and sort of, well it's just "normal" that a man is there. Of course, they'll be criticized about other things, but it's, there is always that additional component of criticism for women, at least that's been my experience.

Do People Respond to Male and Female Leaders Differently?

People can often feel at unease in responding to some female leadership styles, which are more cooperative and collaborative. I partly experienced this in my work when I was heading large divisions in WHO, where the majority of my staff were men and most of them were older than I was. They were all medics. Even when I got my first position as a director, the people that were most opposed to me as a director were my secretary and my administrative assistant because they wanted to work for a man and not for a woman. It took them time to get used to my style of leadership. A participatory approach, collaborative approach, was actually interpreted as a weakness until they found out that I could take some really tough decisions.

As a Woman Leader, What Other Obstacles Did You Face?

It was difficult at times and people were unfair or criticized me when I came into the WHO, because I brought three criteria that weren't usual. First of all, I was a woman. Second, I was much younger than most other WHO professionals. And third, I was a social scientist. All that sort of bundled together. When I became a director, I was younger than all the program managers in my staff. Most of them were medics. So you've got that mix. So, they got a boss who was female, who was younger than them, who sort of came from a different area of expertise—a social scientist. They considered it reasonably unfair and it took quite some time for them to appreciate that there was a reason why I was given that job, and as it turned out, I was quite good at it. So, there were structural barriers as well and attitudes such as medics don't report to social scientists.

How Did You Address the Obstacles in the Perception and Acceptance of You as a Leader?

Well, I worked through it. I confronted them with it. First of all, you need to get yourself what I've always called the duck's skin or feathers. You can't let yourself be victimized. I've always opposed being a victim. So, it became important to me to move forward, to convince people, and to remember that they weren't criticizing me as Ilona. They couldn't deal with a woman in the job. They couldn't deal with a social scientist or a person younger to them. It wasn't necessarily Ilona the person. It definitely helped not taking it personally. That was the characterization of my generation of feminists. We built a movement; we came out of a movement. So, we had a very strong focus on the structural and understanding that personal was actually political.

Mentorship helped of course, it is important to have trusted people with whom you can talk and ask, "do you really think I did the right thing here and should I have approached it differently?" So, it's very, very important to really be in constant dialogue. You've got to have a certain amount of integrity and continuity and an understanding that this is what I want to achieve, and this is how I should go about doing it. I found it very important to listen to people and also do things that others didn't do. Sometimes it's incredibly small things. When I became the director in headquarters, I shocked people by actually walking into their offices. Nobody had ever done a walk about.

The other thing is, that if you have a more flat and cooperative leadership style, people who adhere to the other styles, they interpret you as weak and try to push things around you or past you. Then they get a surprise when they see that this is not weakness, but a way of doing things and that they are found out and that certain things are not accepted.

Did You Have to Change the Way You Dressed or Spoke Because of Your Gender?

I dress more formally if I go to a conference or I have a speaking role or whatever. I did try to change early on though. Joining WHO, I tried to dress down or wear those pantsuits in blue. As I grew older, the more I dressed for myself than on the basis of what others thought I should wear. So yes, women change the way they dress or speak because women are also judged by how they look. Men can come along with any old suit but if a woman comes in looking crinkly, then it can distract people from what you're doing. So, there's more push toward women to dress a certain way. How we dress, how long our skirts should be, should we wear pants, suits, or bright colors, or whatever. So, yeah, it remains a problem because you are judged on appearances and that is not good.

Are There Any Mentors That You Credit for Your Success?

Oh yes, of course. Most of them were men, but interestingly, nearly all of them were Scandinavian men. When I was still a researcher, I had a strong mentor who was a woman Italian professor who later became a politician; she helped me talk things through. I also had a very supportive male professor at the university. At the WHO, there was the regional director who hired me, he was Finnish. There was Halfdan Mahler, who supported me and selected me to do a very challenging job. He was Danish. I had the director in the regional office of the division who was Swedish, from whom I learned a tremendous amount. And then there was Joshua Cohen—an advisor to the director general—who really took me by the hand and taught me a lot of things about leadership and how to move forward. So, I had incredible support.

How Do You Deal with Rumors at the Workplace?

On the other hand, because all these mentors were powerful in a sense, and here I was, this young, 30-ish person and female. So, of course the room abounded with rumors, with whom I was sleeping or not. One just had to disregard them and get on with the business. I don't think you can do anything else. You can do a good job. You can be as open and transparent as possible. Many people were just envious. I mean, aside from the regional director, I was the only one in the office who could pick up the phone and call DG Mahler directly. So, people were very, very jealous. They just couldn't understand what is so special about this kid that she can get this project, that she has this access. The only way to respond was to do a good job. If I hadn't done a good job, it would have seemed like favoritism or seemingly confirmed rumors that there were sexual favors involved. There's very little you can do against these things except just ignore and do your job well.

What Measures Can Institutions Take to Inculcate Greater Representation of Women in Leadership Positions?

First of all, they have to be committed to mentoring everyone in the organization—women *and* men. So there has to be a basic principle of a learning organization, which is committed to diversity, providing access to leadership and power through formal mentorship. I benefited from both. I benefited from supervisors who supported me. It is important that organizations really look carefully at their senior staff. Are they supporting the people that they are responsible for?

I also benefited from people who had no hierarchical relationship to me directly. Part of this is also that you have to be willing to seek out mentorship and to ask "Will you help me? Will you support me?" It is not a weakness to do so. It can be challenging, especially for women who might think, "I won't ask for this because then people will think I'm not up to the job."

When I was cast in the leadership position as the first woman director, I got coaching support from a consulting agency. There was a fantastic person there with whom I met around every 2 weeks or so to just talk things through with them. So, organizations must have a willingness to financially invest in mentorship and coaching because in some cases, external coaching is more helpful. When I was appointed in headquarters, I called the personnel office and I said, "Ok, now I'm responsible for this enormous bunch of people and budget, so who's going to coach me now?" And they said, "there is no program." And so, I said, "that's a problem." So, they said, "Let's go and find yourself one, we'll pay for it." It was a bad sign for the organization that they were not prepared but good that they were willing to pay for it and I sought out the help. It needed a proactive approach. Making financial and time resources available helps. It is a mix of things and needs a high awareness in the human resources team, and willingness at the top leadership of the organization.

Are There Any Organizations That Are Changing This?

Not fully yet. The awareness is more now, particularly in the UN organizations. Representation of women is also being measured numerically and that's a good step forward. When Dr. Tedros [Adhanom Ghebreyesus] hired all these women in senior leadership roles, some with no prior WHO experience, he inculcated an induction program to help them understand the organization, its culture and rules. It is very important to set a goal (say 50% of women in leadership) and push toward it. However, you also have to complement it with internal support, particularly when women are hired from the outside as leaders because the people within the organization who might have hoped for moving up might see these positions going to "outsiders." Frequently, when you set yourself a gender goal, you won't have enough women in the organization in leadership positions, so you have to bring in people from outside but you also have to pave the road by complementing it with a culture change by helping people within the organization accept women (especially outside talent) as leaders.

How Important Are the Peer Networks for Inculcating Leadership?

You definitely need a peer support network. So, all the stuff we said about mentors applies, but also to have support of a partner, family, or close friends. You need a work-life balance too. I've seen too many women who have then only worked and had no real personal life. That's not good.

What Advice Would You Give to Young Women Who Are Aspiring to Be Global Health Leaders?

Well in a sense, all of the above. Don't take it personally, be professional, be yourself, show integrity and coherence, show how goal oriented you are, be persistent in fighting for your rights and making sure you get paid as much as your male colleagues do.

Never take no for an answer. When I was appointed at WHO, the position had been advertised as a P5 and then I saw my contract, which said P4. So, I didn't sign it. I insisted on a meeting with the Regional Director, and I said, "this is advertised as P5, I want to be paid as a P5." We agreed that after appraisal of my first year's performance, I would get P5. Always be professional about it though. It is always good to say, "this is what I expect, and this is the respect that I want." One needs a view beyond the organization for this. You can develop this with a good support network. One also needs the courage to leave if one is in the wrong place. You have to take risks and develop courage, that's where the support network becomes even more important. Never think you can do it alone. Find friends, ask questions, ask for support, and never, ever think that asking for support is a sense of weakness.

If You Could Have a Billboard for Other Women Leaders, What Would It Say?

"Lead with an exclamation mark!"

Levelling the Terrain for Women in Global Health Leadership: A Case Study of Sub-Saharan Africa

Stella Bakibinga, Elizabeth Bakibinga, John Daniel Ibembe, and Pauline Bakibinga

Introduction

Sub-Saharan Africa (SSA) is among the world's most gender-unequal regions and the lack of parity extends to all components of society, including health leadership in the region. With an average gender gap of 33.7%, sub-Saharan Africa records the third-largest gender gap among the eight regions in the World Economic Forum (WEF) Gender Parity Index. The WEF report covers 33 of 46 countries in SSA (WEF, 2018a). The women of Africa make a sizeable contribution to the continent's economy: they are more economically active as farmers and entrepreneurs than women elsewhere worldwide, grow most of Africa's food, and own one-third of all businesses. However, numerous constraints such as the time lost doing unproductive domestic chores, prevailing restrictive cultural norms, alcohol abuse, and poverty, which promote early/teenage pregnancies and school dropout, hold back women in SSA from fulfilling their potential, whether as leaders in public life, in the boardroom, or in growing their businesses (African Development Bank Group, 2015).

SSA has high female labour force participation, the majority of whom are nurses, but this does not reflect a complementary number of women in positions of leadership in the health sector (Munjanja et al., 2005). Since 1990, SSA has witnessed greater democratisation, which has increased women's participation in politics and

S. Bakibinga
Örebro University, Örebro, Sweden

E. Bakibinga (✉)
Commonwealth Secretariat, London, UK

J. D. Ibembe
Department of Anthropology, Washington University in St Louis, St. Louis, MO, USA

P. Bakibinga
Health and Systems for Health Research Unit, African Population and Health Research Center, Nairobi, Kenya

© Springer Nature Switzerland AG 2022
R. Morgan et al. (eds.), *Women and Global Health Leadership*,
https://doi.org/10.1007/978-3-030-84498-1_14

141

led to improvements in gender equality with the aim of levelling the field for everyone (Blankenship & Kubicek, 2018). Emphasis has been placed on achieving gender parity, increasing women's access to positions of leadership in elective politics, and access to education, but not on increasing the number of women in positions of leadership across the different sectors of the economy, including the health sector. Globally, the UN Economic and Social Council's resolution 2011/17 on science and technology aims at providing support for women seeking entry into science careers. Regionally, the East African Community (EAC), Southern Africa Development Community (SADC), and Economic Community of West African States (ECOWAS) have in place the gender and science, technology, and innovations (STI) frameworks, gender policy, and the African Union Kwame Nkrumah Regional Award for Women Scientists, respectively. In spite of these global, regional, and national commitments to narrowing the gender employment gaps, the gender disparity persists as the discussion below reveals. Of the science professionals in SSA, women make up 30.4% of the total (UNESCO, 2017).

Despite these initiatives and the progress noted in improving gender equality in science and in the workplace in the region, the status of women and girls in SSA is still a cause for concern. The political promises to make it mandatory for workplaces to create women- and career-friendly workplaces, and to provide funding for quality education for disadvantaged girls, among others, do not appear to have generated great impact. Some SSA countries have put in place policies and initiatives which promote women in science, but their implementation is weak or non-existent; thus, there is underrepresentation in leadership positions (Prozesky & Mouton, 2019; Gregorio, 2019). Gender-based affirmative initiatives were instituted in different countries. In Uganda, Kenya, and Tanzania, the affirmative action on education, interpreted and implemented in different ways, saw an increase in the numbers of girls enrolling in institutions of higher learning (Onsongo, 2009). However, cultural norms, patriarchal attitudes and practices, stereotypes Pappas (2016) and discrimination in the workplace, and poor funding and planning for education and science initiatives served to limit the growth of women in science leadership positions. There are women who have made it to senior management positions, but men's dominance as key decision-makers prevails. This is partially because there are generally fewer women in the sciences, something that affects their employability in health. In 2013, women constituted only 30% of workers in research and development in SSA with gender disparities manifesting at all levels (Muthumbi & Sommerfeld, 2015).

The conflicting choice between career and family imposed on women by societal customs affects their progress into senior health leadership, compared to men (OECD, 2018). Additionally, the scarcity of local female role models in SSA affects career choices (Qureshi, 2016; Mcunu, 2018).

Globally, a number of outstanding women have struggled to overcome gender barriers and achieved considerable success as a result of national policies on education for all and extended maternity cover, amongst other enablers. Yet in SSA, young women have to create paths to their successful science careers without benefitting from mentors or enabling environments (Roca et al., 2018).

Background

Despite political commitments, legislative amendments, and positive change registered in certain areas in the years following the Beijing Plan of Action, SSA is still one of the poorer performers globally as reported in the 2014 edition of the Social Institutions and Gender Index (SIGI) synthesis report (OECD, 2014). There are high to very high levels of discrimination in more than half of the countries across the SIGI and most SIGI sub-indices (see Fig. 1). It is critical to note that the high numbers of parity targets in some African countries like Ethiopia and Rwanda are skewed by the scores from the political arena, and do not necessarily reflect the increased participation of women in civil society, business, and other sectors of the economy. The situation is not much better in the private sector, where women globally occupy less than a third of senior and middle management positions (UN, 2017).

The World Health Organization (WHO) reports that one in every three women has suffered violence, which manifests in many forms including economic abuse, sexual harassment, and exposure to harmful traditional practices which hamper women's meaningful engagement in the economy. The World Bank's 10-year report on Women, Business, and the Law reveals that there has been great progress towards legal gender equality over the past decade but that a typical economy only gives women three-quarters the rights of men in the measured areas (World Bank, 2019). Many laws and regulations deter women from entering the workforce or starting a business, discrimination that can have lasting effects on women's economic inclusion and labour force participation (World Bank, 2019).

The mixed picture showcases the need to continuously make long-term investments in gender equality that not only ensure the introduction of necessary law, but that the law is implemented or enforced to give results right from the grassroots.

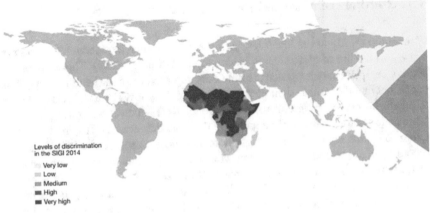

Levels of discrimination
in the SIGI 2014

　Very low
　Low
　Medium
　High
　Very high

Fig. 1 Levels of discrimination in the SIGI
Source: OECD (2014), "Social Institutions & Gender Index (SIGI) 2014 Synthesis Report: Sub-Saharan Africa", https://www.oecd.org/dev/development-gender/BrochureSIGI2015-web.pdf

This should notably be through engaging men and boys to inspire social norm change and holding law enforcement agencies accountable.

According to the United Nations Development Programme (UNDP), perceptions, attitudes, and historic gender roles limit women's access to health care and education and lead to disproportionate levels of family responsibility, job segregation, and sexual violence (WEF, 2018b). The evidence based on the representation of women in global health leadership shows that women remain largely under-represented in the upper echelons of health leadership in SSA as in other parts of the world (Dhatt et al., 2017). This low representation is also attributed to their role as primary caregivers to their families, as combining both family and career responsibilities is very challenging (Fenny, 2018).

The SSA region has one of the highest percentages of women representatives in parliament worldwide, yet this is not reflected at the policy change level. Women still face challenges in property ownership, gender-based violence, culturally driven harmful practices, and early marriages (OECD, 2014).

More than a century will be needed to close the equality gap between women and men in SSA, and yet the ratios of women's participation in four thematic areas, including economic participation and opportunity, educational attainment, health and survival, and political empowerment, are worsening (WEF, 2018a; Chutel, 2018). It is therefore important to expose the underbelly of the monster of inequality in SSA in order to reach gender parity in less time. Women in SSA do not have adequate access to the labour market and to productive assets due to continued legal discrimination, negative gender norms and stereotypes, and women's disproportionate care burden (Lusigi, 2018). Additionally, negative perceptions, attitudes, and historic gender roles transmitted as lower education opportunities limit the choice of jobs or professions for women (Lusigi, 2018).

The Numbers of Women in Health Leadership in SSA

Women are mostly at the lower levels of the decision-making hierarchy and rarely make it to the top of global health leadership (Dhatt et al., 2017). This emphasises another perspective that women are not under-represented in the health occupations per se, but that the issue is their distribution along the salary scale and various levels of organisations' organograms that raises concerns (Fielden et al., 2001). There are more male doctors than female doctors. In the United States, in 2015, the Bureau of Labor Statistics reported that though more and more women are entering medical school, men are still more likely than women to be physicians or surgeons (63.7% men), while women continue to be much more likely than men to become nurses (90% women) (Stephens et al., 2016). There is a gender seniority gap in the health sectors as in other areas, where fewer women hold higher paying positions and positions of seniority in organisations (Daly et al., 2018). In Economic Community of West African States (ECOWAS)' West African Health Organization (WAHO), the Director General and his three predecessors are male (WAHO, 2019). The lack of women researchers limits the nature of the evidence generated, as female perspectives are largely absent in the health agendas. Within the healthcare provision sector, women mostly take on nursing and/or midwifery professions, careers that rarely benefit from leadership opportunities due to the gender dynamics in the health sector identified above and the privileges and vulnerabilities that come with. The society is stratified and privilege follows accordingly. There is unequal bargaining power in terms of influence, access to resources, etc. A look at the leading health research institutions, selected based on the authors' knowledge and availability of information on their respective websites, reveals that most of the executive directors are male (Table 1). Women tend to occupy junior positions in the organisations. In the absence of data, factual/anecdotal evidence shows that doctors lead or dominate the leadership of medical and health professional associations. Nurses lead in nurses' associations and as more men enter the nursing field, women are edged out. This goes back to issues of gender and participation mentioned earlier.

Women scientists, such as the heads of ICIPE and APHRC (Table 1), having weathered many storms in their career paths, are inspiring examples for other women. These and a few others are beneficiaries of generous maternity leave policies and flexible working hours, amongst other opportunities that provide women with work-life balance (Sipalla, 2019).

In other regional organisations, the numbers show a limited representation of women. A man heads the African Medical and Research Foundation (AMREF) International's board, which has 3 female directors out of 11 board members. The man-led executive committee has 12 female members out of 16 committee members. AMREF's senior management team is led by a man and has 16 female members out of 27 members. On the other hand, men head 3 of 27 National Committees of the Inter-African Committee on Traditional Practices (IAC). IAC is an international and African regional body that works to eliminate practices that are harmful to particularly women and children such as female genital mutilation (IAC, n.d.).

Table 1 Selected leading health research institutions in SSA

Institution	Head/executive director
African Academy of Sciences https://aasciences.ac.ke/secretariat	Male (M)
African Population and Health Research Center (APHRC) https://aphrc.org/	Female (F)
African Institute for Development Policy https://www.afidep.org/	M
International Centre of Insect Physiology and Ecology (ICIPE) http://www.icipe.org/about/senior_management	F
Ifakara Health Institute http://ihi.or.tz/about/	M
KEMRI-Wellcome Trust https://kemri-wellcome.org/	M
East, Central and Southern Africa Health Community https://ecsahc.org/	M

The executive director and principal health officers of the East African Health Research Commission (EAHRC), which handles health matters and research and provides advisory services to the EAC, are male and of the 16 commissioners, only 1 is female (EAHRC, n.d.).

Having established the status quo of women's participation in health leadership in SSA, it is critical to survey the legal and policy environment with a view to making recommendations on how these laws and policy mechanisms can be harnessed to boost women's participation in global health leadership.

Legal and Policy Mechanisms

SSA has demonstrated its commitment to promoting gender equality, specifically increasing women's participation in development processes, through the African Union (AU) and other regional blocs including the East African Community (EAC), the Economic Community of West African States (ECOWAS), the Economic Community of Central African States (ECCAS), and the Southern Africa Development Community (SADC). Many individual SSA states have committed to ensuring gender parity as attested to by the legislative instruments they accede and ratify. Regional bodies like the ECOWAS, the EAC, the ECCAS, and the SADC have set up initiatives aimed at gender parity. Leaders have committed to empower women, eliminate harmful traditional and cultural practices, and ensure gender equality through the AU's Agenda 2063. ECOWAS' Gender Policy sets to gender mainstream all its activities (OECD, 2004). In 2016 in Kenya President Uhuru Kenyatta launched the Africa Regional Human Development Report 2016 on Accelerating Gender Equality and Women's Empowerment in Africa (Lusigi, 2018). In 2018, the EAC Secretariat adopted a gender policy to ensure equal rights and opportunities to address the disparities in employment, inter alia (EAC, 2018). SADC's Protocol on Gender Equality seeks to boost women and girls' participation in science (SADC, 2012). African governments have committed to promote women's participation in science under the joint strategic priority area "Investing in people—education, science, technology and skills development", in which Africa and the European Union (EU) acknowledge the importance of youth, especially girls and young women, and those living in disadvantaged or vulnerable environments (African Union, n.d.).

Most countries in SSA have signed up to or acceded to the Convention on the Elimination of All Forms of Discrimination Against Women (CEDAW), the International Labour Organization's international labour standards relevant to women workers' rights and the promotion of gender equality in the world of work (ILO, 2017), and the Maputo Protocol to the African Charter on Human and People's Rights. Many are parties to regional and international legislative instruments that call for equal participation of men and women in society. The Maputo Protocol remains one of the most relevant instruments applicable in SSA for it provides a legal framework for women's rights and requires states to develop laws that prohibit discrimination.

International organisations have also worked in concert with governments and regional bodies to bridge the gap. The United Nations Educational, Scientific and Cultural Organization (UNESCO) is involved in implementing some of the continent's aspirations, particularly the AU's Agenda 2063 which aims at having a gender-inclusive Africa (UN, 2015a, 2015b).

Research by the World Bank as reported above shows that gender discriminatory legislation remains on the statute books of a number of several SSA countries. Where no lacunae exist in the law, poor implementation of legislative commitments works against women (Hughes, 2017). According to the World Bank, despite daunting challenges, several economies in SSA are making progress in enacting laws that promote equality between men and women (World Bank, 2018a). However, women encounter widespread legal barriers in SSA and other parts of the world that keep them out of jobs and prevent them from owning a business, says the biennial report, which now monitors 189 economies globally, including 47 in sub-Saharan Africa (World Bank, 2018a). Kenya, the Democratic Republic of Congo, Tanzania, and Zambia collectively carried out 13 reforms among 34 reforms to remove legal barriers to women's economic inclusion carried out throughout SSA (World Bank, 2018b). However, protecting women against violence, including that which denies them access to economic resources, jobs, physical security, and safety from sexual violence outside the home, remains a challenge for the region, despite recent progress. Of the world's 45 economies with no laws against domestic violence, 19 are in SSA, earning the region an average score of 46 on this indicator. Nine of the region's 47 economies score 0 on this indicator. The World Bank has observed that achieving gender equality requires more than just changes to laws and that the laws need to be meaningfully implemented—and this requires sustained political will, leadership from women and men across societies, and changes to ingrained cultural norms and attitudes (World Bank, 2019).

The Role of Civil Society in Promoting Gender Parity

Professional bodies, civil society, and non-governmental organisations (NGOs) have always been at the forefront of promoting new ideas and in encouraging governments to implement them. They often represent the voice of the people with roles of advocacy, education, and training and are active in monitoring what has, or has not, been achieved (Haslegrave, n.d.). Under the Commonwealth Principles on the Three Branches of Government, generally known as the Latimer House Principles, governments are encouraged to work with civil society organisations, including professional societies, to encourage gender balance and diversity at all levels (Commonwealth Secretariat, 2004). The SSA region has a number of professional bodies that bring together women health professionals. The Medical Women Association of South Africa (MWASA), Kenya Medical Women's Association

(KMWA), Medical Women's Association of Nigeria, and the Association of Uganda Women Medical Doctors are examples of women's medical associations in SSA that unite medical workers and dental practitioners. Uganda's association includes all medical students. These associations promote the interests of their members and provide mentorship, networking, Ludwig et al. (2018) and training for career development, roles that are seen as providing a boost for females choosing to join and remain within the health workforce. With longer work experience and further career development, women's chances of climbing the ladder to positions of leadership in health are higher.

The Impact of Social, Cultural Norms, and Stereotypes

Failure to consider power asymmetries in Africa, especially those facilitated by norms and stereotypes, hampers the quest for gender parity. The primary development policies in many countries still do not take into account the differences in income and power between men and women, hampering efforts to finance programmes that reduce inequality (Mutume, 2005). In addition, Mutume (2005) observed that the majority of African women face major challenges and obstacles including denial of education and employment and have limited opportunities in trade, industry, and government. Illiteracy, limited land ownership, and restrictions on agency and mobility all are some of the barriers that have had a dramatic impact on social and economic progress which thereafter kick-starts conditions that lead to keeping girls out of school and exposing them to harmful traditional practices like child, early, and forced marriages. Young women raised in societies in which they are the primary caregivers for both children and elderly family members typically regard a successful career and raising a family as mutually exclusive. Additionally, society perceives girls as intellectually weaker and discourages them from pursuing science subjects, which explains their under-representation in the higher level of health sector management. In some instances, male juniors do not listen to women in senior leadership due to the subordinate role culture assigns females (Fielden et al., 2001).

Access to education for girls has increased in SSA compared to that of the boys; however, completion rates show that social norms and cultural practices make girls drop out earlier resulting in fewer girls enrolling and graduating from universities and colleges (UNESCO, 2014; World Bank, 2018c). Although the number of women entering higher education in SSA has increased, gender disparity remains, and only 30% of science professionals are women. As a result, women are under-represented in the professions, most especially in science, technology, engineering, and mathematics (STEM) and research, management, and corporate governance, all of which are areas critical to women vying for and getting positions in global health leadership (Roca et al., 2018). The summation of the effect of negative norms and stereotypes leads to a reduction of women available to participate in global health leadership.

Factors Promoting High Attrition Rates

Health worker performance, including retention, is a complex issue to address, as a variety of determinants influence staff behaviour at different levels, namely, health worker characteristics (individual level), health system and facility characteristics (macro and micro levels), characteristics of the wider political and socioeconomic environment (contextual factors), and community/population characteristics (contextual factors) (Dieleman & Harnmeijer, 2006). Having made it to the health profession and into positions of management, evidence shows that more women leave the workforce before reaching the apex positions of leadership. Lack of access to child-friendly workplaces, flexible working hours, generous maternity policies, and quality childcare hinder the integration of women into the workplace. Sexual harassment and bullying do not make it easier for women professionals in a male-dominated work environment. A toxic work environment results in high attrition rates, which hampers women professionals from acquiring the seniority that is required for global health leadership (Newman et al., 2017). Outside the organisations, there exist societal gender norms that converge to diminish the presence of women in the top echelon of leadership (OECD, 2018).

Levelling the Terrain: The Way Forward

After considering the barriers to women's participation in global health leadership, we make recommendations on ensuring adequate recruitment, retention, and motivation of women to sustain them at upper echelons of global health leadership. Overall, gender-sensitive interventions, remedial mechanisms, processes, and outcomes are required.

Four interconnected pathways would achieve more equal human development outcomes but also enhance women's participation in leadership, including in global health. The pathways include completion of existing legal and policy reforms for more gender equality; engagement of women in decision-making at all levels through elimination of discriminatory social institutions that block women's health and education; provision of equitable access to economic, financial, and natural resources; and keeping track of progress through data collection and measurement.

Legal and Policy Interventions

Legal and policy frameworks and partnerships that support equality, enhanced education for girls, continuous professional development, and positive work environments will go a long way in providing the foundation required for more women participation in health leadership. It is common knowledge that legislation that guarantees equal pay encourages women to compete for top positions. This coupled with re-emphasis on gender mainstreaming in health institutions and policies, and establishment of gender units within the health sector are progressive interventions. These interventions are costly and may not fit in with development planning, thus the need for partnerships.

Employers will have to address sexual harassment in the workplace. Governments will have to ensure that social movements like *#MeToo* and *#TimesUp* have an impact on the enactment and enforcement of legislation on sexual harassment and codes of conduct.

Stakeholders need to focus on the partnerships in finance, technology, capacity building, and systemic issues promoted in SDG 17 of Agenda 2030, a blueprint adopted by all UN member states to ensure prosperity and peace in the world (UN, n.d.). The AU's Agenda 2063 aims at promoting girls' involvement in the science, technology, and innovations frameworks through provision of career guidance and in partnership with several UN agencies. It has undertaken projects to increase women's employment and leadership in science (Muthumbi & Sommerfeld, 2015). UNESCO, in partnership with the Korea International Cooperation Agency (KOICA), between 2014 and 2017 provided mentorship to girls in Kenya, which focused on helping them make informed career choices in STEM (Development Education Research Centre, 2018). Measures that equalise the gender balance among teachers improve girls' education, boost numbers and quality, and widen the pool of available leadership candidates at all levels in health.

Stakeholders should replicate UNDP's partnership with public, private, and multilateral institutions at national, regional, and global levels to implement an action plan that sees private companies step up to promote gender equality in the workplace through a Gender Equality Seal Certification on standards that foster equality of opportunities. The quest to have this certification will motivate establishments in health to put in place systems that allow women to fairly compete for leadership roles.

Civil society plays the role of advocate and can get involved in the policy and strategy development that advances the agenda of promoting women to senior positions in health. Enactment of such gender equality policies and laws, which level the employment field, requires a lot of political commitment and will. In SSA today, gender equality activism has been de-politicised. Most activists in civil society groups refrain from delving into the politics involved. NGOs and professional bodies should continue to advocate for more women representation in management and leadership at all levels in health.

Mentorship, Financing, and Cultural Shifts

Successful achievement of Agenda 2030 and the AU's Agenda 2063 will strongly rely on addressing discriminatory social institutions, including those in the health sector. Putting social norm change at the core of future actions could be one of the most effective means to guarantee that the region will be on track to fulfil its promises on gender equality and women's empowerment. The SIGI Regional Report offers new analysis and good practices to support countries in tackling these key areas and moving from commitment to progress on the ground, and policy leaders should embrace what it offers. Change of social norms and practices is a complex and iterative transaction, which requires a lot of awareness raising, training, negotiations with power holders, as well as financial investment. To achieve this paradigm shift, civil society needs to have close and cordial working relations with the legislative and cultural leadership and for all stakeholders to recognise and have a complete understanding of the politics involved, and address issues.

Mentoring programs can provide career support and networking among women working in health. The small number of female role models in global health leadership will have to mentor girls and young women into STEM and beyond. Through mentorship programmes, women who currently hold leadership positions need to share their experiences through visits, talks, and workplace shadowing. Where there is a complete lack of interdisciplinary role models, women leaders in other science fields can fill this gap (Fielden et al., 2001). Men in health can mentor girls (Vogel, 2017). Mentorship initiatives such as Project Girls for Girls, which empowers girls to lead (Project Girls for Girls, n.d.), and the International Science Programme Gender Equality Activity which promotes the activities of female physicists and mathematicians (ISP/UU Alumni Network, n.d.) are commendable. UNESCO should make young girls and women aware of role models through its strategy that highlights Africa's great women in history and their contribution to development. The development and maintenance of a talent pool of women leaders is another way of giving visibility to outstanding women in global health.

Strategies that prioritise the integration of women in African public and private research sectors and encourage women's participation in regional and global conferences are encouraged. One such example is the Women Leaders in Global Health Conference (RBM Partnership, 2019).

Gender budgeting that favours STEM education for girls and women will provide the requisite finances.

Measurement, Monitoring, and Evaluation

In the absence of a monitoring and evaluation framework, there is need to examine the impact of recommended and other equality initiatives on women in global health leadership. The examined impact could specifically include the four pathways identified earlier on in levelling the terrain. There is need to conduct more research on employment in the health sector in the region, and statistics on the matter will show the gaps which need to be filled. The definition of female leaders in health should include women employed in the field such as economists and managers (Vogel, 2017).

There is need to look beyond parity. Besides gender, there are other dimensions of equality such as race and social class, which affect the numbers of women in leadership (Zeinali et al., 2019). In South Africa, the Medical Research Council which offers grants to health professions, decided to overhaul its application review process upon realisation that it mainly benefited men. Today, the competition for grants is distributed to different career levels and ages considering that some women re-join or join health research when they have completed childbearing (Vogel, 2017). Unfortunately, most of the global focus on gender to date has been on women in the West or those living in urban areas. Rural women, and particularly poor female farmers in SSA, have not yet benefited from the recent focus on gender equality. The unique obstacles that African women confront must become part of the global dialogue to attain gender parity. The World Bank should be invited through Africa Region's Gender Innovation Lab (GIL), to assess and evaluate the role of women in global health leadership so as to better inform new interventions to generate knowledge on which policies work (or not) to close gender gaps in earnings, productivity, and agency (World Bank, 2014). It is important for stakeholders to work with the African Development Bank in its endeavours to involve policymakers, civil society, and governments at major regional gatherings to enrich the Gender Equality Index to ensure that it takes participation of women in health leadership into account.

Conclusion

Levelling the terrain for women in global health means that ultimately the evidence will show more women in positions of leadership. Countries will have to benchmark and develop a clear pathway galvanised by legislative and policy interventions, backed by political will and action and informed by existing national, regional, and global commitments.

References

African Development Bank Group. (2015). *Gender equality index*. Retrieved September 1, 2019, from https://www.afdb.org/en/topics-and-sectors/topics/quality-assurance-results/gender-equality-index

African Union (n.d.), *Investing in people—education, science, technology and skills development*. Retrieved September 20, 2019, from https://www.africa-eu-partnership.org/en/strategic-priority-areas/investing-people-education-science-technology-and-skills-development

Blankenship, J., & Kubicek, P. (2018). Democratization and gender equality in sub-Saharan Africa. *The Journal of the Middle East and Africa, 9*(1), 27–50. https://doi.org/10.1080/2152084 4.2018.1449458

Chutel, L. (2018) *It will take 135 years to close the gender gap in sub-Saharan Africa*. Retrieved July 1, 2019, from https://qz.com/africa/1503278/global-gender-gap-index-africas-gap-widens/

Commonwealth Secretariat. (2004). *Commonwealth principles on the three branches of government*, https://thecommonwealth.org/history-of-the-commonwealth/latimer-principles

Daly, A., Liou, Y.-H., & Bjorklund, P. (2018). Pay, position, and partnership: Exploring capital resources among a school district leadership team. *Transformational Approaches in Teaching and Learning*. https://doi.org/10.1007/978-3-319-77237-0_8

DERC. (2018). *Global education digest 2015–2017*. Retrieved June 16, 2019, from https://angel-network.net/sites/default/files/Digest%202015%20-%2017%20online.pdf

Dhatt, R., Theobald, S., Buzuzi, S., Ros, B., Vong, S., Muraya, K., & Jackson, C. (2017). The role of women's leadership and gender equity in leadership and health system strengthening. *Global Health, Epidemiology and Genomics, 2*, e8. https://doi.org/10.1017/gheg.2016.22

Dieleman, M., & Harnmeijer, J. W. (2006). *Improving health worker performance: in search of promising practices*. Retrieved July 1, 2019, from https://www.who.int/hrh/resources/improving_hw_performance.pdf

EAC. (2018). *EAC launches gender policy*. Retrieved September 1, 2019, from https://www.eac.int/press-releases/146-gender,-community-development-civil-society/1217-eac-launches-gender-policy

EAHRC. (n.d.). *About EAHRC our team*. Retrieved July 1, 2019, from https://www.eahealth.org/about-eahrc/our-team

Fenny, A. (2018). Raising African women leaders in global health. *The Lancet, 392*, 2662–2663. https://doi.org/10.1016/S0140-6736(18)32841-1

Fielden, S., Davidson, M., Gale, A., & Davey, C. (2001). Women, equality and construction. *Journal of Management Development, 20*(4), 293–305.

Gregorio, M. D. 2019. *3 challenges faced by female researchers in the developing world*. Women in STEM talk about how international foundations and editorial boards can support gender equality. Retrieved from https://www.elsevier.com/connect/3-challenges-faced-by-female-researchers-in-the-developing-world

Haslegrave, M. (n.d.). *The role of NGOs in promoting a gender approach to health care*. Retrieved July 1, 2019, from https://www.un.org/womenwatch/daw/csw/role_ngo.htm

Hughes, C. (2017). *Legislative wins, broken promises: Gaps in the implementation of laws on violence against women and girls*. Retrieved September 1, 2019, from https://www-cdn.oxfam.org/s3fspublic/file_attachments/rr-legislative-wins-broken-promises-vawg-080317-summ-en.pdf

IAC. (n.d.). *About IAC*. Retrieved July 1, 2019, from https://iac-ciaf.net/about-iac/

ILO. (2017). *ABC of women workers' rights and gender equality*. Retrieved July 1, 2019, from https://www.ilo.org/wcmsp5/groups/public/%2D%2D-dgreports/%2D%2D-gender/documents/publication/wcms_087314.pdf

International Science Programme. (n.d.). *Gender equality activity*. Retrieved July 1, 2019, from http://www.isp.uu.se/isp-alumni-network/

Ludwig, S., Dhatt, R., & Kickbusch, I. (2018). Women leaders in global health—The importance of gender equality in global health. *European Journal of Public Health, 28*(4). https://doi.org/10.1093/eurpub/cky218.020

Lusigi, A. (2018). *Gender equality as the organizing lens for development planning*. Retrieved July 1, 2019 from http://www.africa.undp.org/content/rba/en/home/blog/2018/gender-equality-is-so-much-more-than-a-goal-.html

Mcunu, N. (2018). *Tradition and few chances are keeping black South African women out of science*. Retrieved from https://qz.com/africa/1202388/tradition-and-few-chances-are-keeping-black-south-african-women-out-of-science/

Munjanja, O. K., Kibuka, S., & Dovlo, D. (2005). *The nursing workforce in sub Saharan Africa*. Geneva. Retrieved March 23, 2009, from http://www.icn.ch/global/Issue7SSA.pdf

Muthumbi, J., & Sommerfeld, J. (2015). *Africa's women in science*. Retrieved June 09, 2019, from https://www.who.int/tdr/research/gender/Women_overview_piece.pdf

Mutume, G. (2005). *African women battle for equality*. Retrieved July 1, 2019, from https://www.un.org/africarenewal/magazine/july-2005/african-women-battle-equality

Newman, C., Chama, P. K., Mugisha, M., Matsiko, C. W., & Oketcho, V. (2017). Reasons behind current gender imbalances in senior global health roles and the practice and policy changes that can catalyze organizational change. *Global Health, Epidemiology and Genomics, 2*, e19. https://doi.org/10.1017/gheg.2017.11

OECD. (2004). *Gender equality in West Africa*. Retrieved September 1, 2019, from http://www.oecd.org/swac/topics/gender.htm

OECD. (2014). *Social institutions & gender index 2014 synthesis report*. Retrieved June 21, 2021, from https://www.oecd.org/dev/development-gender/BrochureSIGI2015-web.pdf

OECD. (2018). *Gender equality in West Africa? The role of social norms*. Retrieved June 16, 2019, from https://oecd-development-matters.org/2018/03/08/gender-equality-in-west-africa-the-key-role-of-social-norms/

Onsongo, J. (2009). Affirmative action, gender equity and university admissions—Kenya, Uganda and Tanzania. *London Review of Education, 7*(1), 71–81.

Pappas, S. (2016). Male doctors, female nurses: Subconscious stereotypes hard to budge -06-20T21:56:51Z *Human Nature*. Also available at https://www.livescience.com/55134-subconcious-stereotypes-hard-to-budge

Project Girls for Girls. (n.d.). *Project Girls for Girls-Empowering Women to Lead*. https://www.projectg4g.org

Prozesky, H., & Mouton, J. (2019). A gender perspective on career challenges experienced by African scientists. *South African Journal of Science, 115*(3–4), 1–5. https://doi.org/10.17159/sajs.2019/5515

Qureshi, M. W. (2016). Women in science: Africa needs more role models. Retrieved from https://blogs.worldbank.org/education/women-science-africa-needs-more-role-models

RBM Partnership. (2019). *Women leaders in global health conference 2019*. Retrieved September 1, 2019, from https://endmalaria.org/events/women-leaders-global-health-conference-2019

Roca, A., et al. (2018). Retrieved from https://www.thelancet.com/journals/langlo/article/PIIS2214-109X(18)30063-9/fulltext) .

SADC. (2012). *SADC protocol on gender and development*. Retrieved September 1, 2019 from https://www.sadc.int/issues/gender/

Sipalla, F. (2019). *Workplace support for breastfeeding mothers at APHRC*. Retrieved September 3, 2019, from https://aphrc.org/?p=10743).

Stephens, T., Spevak, R., Rogalin, C. L., & Hirshfield, L. E. (2016). Drawing doctors vs. nurses: Gendered perceptions of health professionals. *Journal of the Indiana Academy of the Social Sciences, 19*(1), 6. Retrieved from http://digitalcommons.butler.edu/jiass/vol19/iss1/6

UN. (2015a). *Transforming our world: Agenda 2030 for sustainable development*. Retrieved June 16, 2019, from https://sustainabledevelopment.un.org/post2015/transformingourworld

UN. (2015b). *Sustainable development goals*. Retrieved September 1, 2019, from https://sustainabledevelopment.un.org/?menu=1300

UN Economic and Social Council. (2017). *Progress towards the sustainable development goals: Report of the secretary-general (E/2017/66)*.

UNESCO. (2014). *UNESCO priority gender equality action plan: 2014–2021*. Retrieved June 20, 2019, from https://unesdoc.unesco.org/ark:/48223/pf0000227222

Vogel, L. (2017). Celebrating more women leaders in global health. *CMAJ: Canadian Medical Association Journal = Journal De L'Association Medicale Canadienne, 189*(46), E1433–E1434.

WAHO. (2019). *Director general*. Retrieved June 16, 2019, from https://www.wahooas.org/web-ooas/en/a-propos/directeurs-generaux

WEF. (2018a). *Global gender gap report 2018 sub-Saharan Africa*. Retrieved July 1, 2019, from http://reports.weforum.org/global-gender-gap-report-2018/, http://www3.weforum.org/docs/WEF_GGGR_2018.pdf

WEF. 2018b). *Financial inclusion is key to tackling Africa's gender inequality*. Retrieved July 1, 2019, from https://www.weforum.org/agenda/2018/07/financial-equality-for-africa-s-women-farmers

World Bank Group. (2014). *Improving gender equality in Africa*. Retrieved July 3, 2019, from https://www.worldbank.org/en/region/afr/brief/improving-gender-equality-in-africa

World Bank Group. (2018a). *Women, business and the law 2018*. World Bank. © World Bank. Retrieved from https://openknowledge.worldbank.org/handle/10986/29498. License: CC BY 3.0 IGO.

World Bank Group. (2018b). *Four African economies among most improved in removing legal barriers against women, says WBG report*. Retrieved July 1, 2019, from https://www.worldbank.org/en/news/press-release/2018/03/29/four-african-economies-among-most-improved-in-removing-legal-barriers-against-women-says-wbg-report

World Bank Group. (2018c). *World development report (WDR) 2018—Learning to realise education's promise*. Retrieved July 1, 2019, from www.worldbank.org

World Bank Group. Women, Business and The Law. (2019). A decade of reform. Retrieved from http://pubdocs.worldbank.org/en/702301554216687135/WBL-DECADE-OF-REFORM-2019-WEB-04-01.pdf

Zeinali, Z., Muraya, K., Govender, V., Molyneux, S., & Morgan, R. (2019). Intersectionality and global health leadership: Parity is not enough. *Human Resources for Health, 17*(1), 1–3.

Interview with Sameera Al Tuwaijri, Global Lead on Population and Development at the Health, Nutrition and Population Global Practice of the World Bank

Sulzhan Bali

"Be true to your loved ones. Be true to everything you cherish. Most of all, be true to yourself."

Sameera Al Tuwaijri is the global lead on population and development at the health, nutrition, and population global practice of the World Bank. She is a board-certified OB/GYN who had over 10 years of experience in clinical practice before she embarked on studying public health. She earned a master's in public health from Harvard University and a doctorate in health policy and completed a post-doctoral fellowship at Johns Hopkins University. Prior to joining the World Bank in 2010, she was the Regional Adviser, Reproductive Health Policy for the United Nations Population Fund, Arab States, and the Director of the International Labour Organization's programme on public health and safety and served as the first Regional Director, Arab States, UN Women.

Do You Credit Any Mentors or Influential People Along Your Career Path Who Have Helped You Succeed as a Leader?

Absolutely. My father. There is no question about it. I am so much like him. We would always say the same thing at the same time. We challenged each other. He was my backbone. He was the man that I would have done everything that he asked me not to do. Just to show him that I could. The flame of passion comes from him as well. I always aspired to impress him and to actually have that wow look in his eyes. Also, in my career I came across wonderful people who influenced me positively. Some are famous, some are not, but all these people recognized the potential in me and challenged me to push the boundaries. That's exactly what I've been doing.

S. Bali (✉)
Women in Global Health, Washington, DC, USA

© Springer Nature Switzerland AG 2022
R. Morgan et al. (eds.), *Women and Global Health Leadership*,
https://doi.org/10.1007/978-3-030-84498-1_15

At the Bank, I cherish my colleague David Wilson, who is brilliant but so low key, so good with advice, I always say, "Oh my God, that was so valuable. I could not have come up with it myself." He's been there for me since day zero. I also take special pride in being friends and colleagues with Fadia Saadah. She is so generous with her support, and she will take the initiative and ask you "Why are you doing this?" I have had long talks with her about women from Middle Eastern countries being under-represented in global health and how can we change that.

I worked with a very nice adviser at Harvard, Ian Atkin, who was also there for me. In fact, when I just prepared to graduate from the Master of Public Health program at Harvard, I competed to deliver the commencement speech, and I put it together, and it was so personal. I was hesitant to share it though, but he really encouraged me. He said, this needs to have like 3,000 pairs of ears to listen to.

Why Is Representation of Women (Especially Women of Color) Important?

Representation is important because it's an equality issue. Women are disconnected across the globe. The long hour yardstick should not be used to measure success. I think that women have many responsibilities, among which, and only among which, is 9 to 5, or 9 to 6, or 9 to 9 is the work we do, while men don't have to do the same. By design, we are under-privileged and discriminated against. Unless you don't want the family, you don't want children. Even then, if you are passionate, you're emotional. If you are driven, you're abusive, while those very same characteristics, those very same personality traits, are transferred into something else for men. The fact that I am Arab, the fact that I am not white, the fact that I come from a society that does not recognize women's work as valuable, the fact that I actually had to scratch nail and teeth into something for it to come to me. You find yourself swimming upstream, and guess what, it's exhausting, and you look at yourself at one point in time and say, "Why am I doing this?"

How Did You Address Conflicts as You Progressed in Your Career?

In the beginning it was tough, especially in certain parts of the world where I worked. People look for the man in the team. I have learned how to assert myself from the very beginning. Sometimes it's a body language thing that "I am the team leader here. All of these people you see around me, men and women, small and big, and young and old, are my team, so I am here." I think there's an art to it.

Being a young physician in hospitals, people never took me seriously, because I looked 10 years younger than my 23 years. I was a woman, and I am a small person.

People asked if there was an older doctor after they recognized the fact that I was actually a doctor.

As you mature, and as you assume your position as a policy dialogue member of the team, expect the treatment to become a bit better. It doesn't always unfortunately, unless you foresee it. I learned how to sometimes even be aggressive. It needed to be very tactful because you cannot be aggressive all the time. Sometimes, unfortunately though, we need to assert ourselves in ways that we don't like, but it's just nature of the game.

Do You Change the Way You Speak or Dress When You Attend High-Profile Meetings?

I am always careful with what I wear. Because I come from a conservative cultural background. I cover my head, and I cover myself when I go home. It would be hypocritical not to respect other people's culture. I always research where I am going, and I always dress according to the occasion.

I do change my attitude sometimes, sometimes by being assertive, knowing when to speak, and other times by listening and restraining myself, and letting the course of the confrontation run its normal mandate. When people disagree with me, I unpack everything that was said, and refute what needs to be refuted and agree with what needs to be agreed with. As a member of an international organization, I also realize that it is our responsibility to learn from countries, work with them, and ensure we are at their service, basically.

How Did Marriage Influence Your Career Choices and Trajectory/Journey?

I had a bad marriage experience. I sometimes feel that marriage was designed to enslave women. In all walks of life, and in all societies, to different degrees, from 10% to almost 70%. I wanted to marry somebody who takes me as I am, not try to change me, accepts my beautiful things, as well as my not so beautiful things, and I do the same. I remember meeting my future husband, and I introduced him to my adviser at Hopkins, and he had one piece of advice for both of us. We were just about to get married. He said each one of you should get this marriage at 80%. I didn't get even 10% at the end.

I also paid a high social price because my marriage didn't fulfill the expectations of my family. He wasn't from Saudi Arabia. I took a chance on something that I thought was my right. I don't regret making that choice because I feel it's a human right to choose who you want to spend the rest of your life with. In a difficult relationship like mine though, for example, there was little encouragement or support, only a lot of hurdles and a lot of heartache. To the point that, I was about to give up on my career completely at one point, because it was just difficult to fight all of these fights at the same time.

How Did You Address Obstacles in Your Journey, Especially Juggling Multiple Roles?

I think this happens to women in all walks of life, even with willing partners. Because if you just take the issue of childcare, even if you have someone living with you, having to leave young kids frequently, and having to move frequently, it has its benefits, there's no question about it. It was also challenging.

At the beginning, it was denial. No, no, no, this is not happening to me. After the denial came the realization that you know what, this is as good as it gets. I invested in my resilience. I woke up every morning and counted my blessings rather than my problems, and I persisted. I tried to line up my trips in the calendar to try to be with my daughter. I am happy to say that I have not missed a birthday ever in the 18 years. I had my siblings, but I was on my own most of the time because of the choices I made. What really helped was that I had a social network that was very solid, I reached out and supported my fellow women, and they supported me. I babysat kids. It was almost like a fraternity club. We supported one another.

Importance of Social Network and Peer Support

I have a lot of women friends that I chose all over the world. We support each other. One of us was involved in domestic violence. Without any coordination, we all said the same thing in the same breath: "Leave him and come stay with me." So we all created a box where we would have keys to our homes, with the address and the phone number for emergencies. We called it the salvage box. We just put together some framework, like, do not call, do not send that text message, because you have a home wherever we are. I still have one of those boxes. It has grossed 73 keys now. I have never, luckily, had to use it. In the time it was created, I think it was 17 years ago, I had somebody knocking on my door. The idea that you have 73 choices if something goes wrong in your life, that is powerful.

Have You Experienced Failure or Made a Mistake?

Well, I obviously have some low points in my career, some very low points, but I don't think it was gender-related. I think it was circumstantial more than anything else. I recall once that I was pushed into something that I didn't want to get involved in. I had a lot of pressure from my superiors, and I had to, at the end and it didn't work out, and I was very upset because obviously, I am not someone who takes failure easily. I do, I mean I fail, of course like everybody else, but I try not to most of the time.

Did You Ever Feel Discriminated or Overlooked Because of Your Gender?

I've had moments in my life where being a woman was a major factor into pushing me to the forefront. However, being a Saudi woman works against me much more than being a woman alone. We are not valued for who we are. The unspoken statement I come across often is "you could stay home and work, and there's plenty of money". You have to be gainfully employed. I am not underestimating the value of making money, but at the same time some of us are not in Saudi Arabia, not because we cannot find employment but because we have different aspirations.

How Did You Address Discrimination or Being Overlooked?

I just let my work speak for me. I really cherish what I do. I mean, I always liked what I did. I cannot be a mediocre bureaucrat who's pushing papers. I need that excitement and challenge. Because what I pay against it is a very high price. I am away from my family, I am away from my roots, I am away from everything that's safe, secure, content, and comfortable. Not to push limits but realize a dream that's only in my head.

How Can Organizations Improve Representation of Women in Senior Management and Also of Women of Color?

By walking the talk. Because the idea of diversity and inclusion, it's not just the check the box mentality. We don't just need to break barriers at the top of the leadership but all across the organization. All the way from the leadership to the security guards, to the cleaning crew, because that is not something you do. It needs to be systematic. It needs to be sustainable, and it needs to be merit-based.

Also, we cannot possibly continue only hiring the Harvards and the Browns and the Stanfords of the world, while the University of Kenya, or the University of Johannesburg, or King Saud University have equally talented pool of students but may be overlooked. This is the biggest inequality. The inequality of privilege, especially as tuition is a huge obstacle. To improve representation, we need to look into hiring beyond the Ivies.

Because if you are the PhD from Harvard, jobs are going to be thrown at you. You don't need to go around and look for something. But if you are a graduate of Cairo University, you'd have to dig your way. I am not advocating for less-quality individuals. Of course not. We need to have the top notch, the top one percent. But the top one percent reservoir is not just limited to the Ivies. That's how organizations can break barriers, by targeting full packages and talent irrespective of Ivy degrees.

What Advice Would You Give to Young Women Who Are Aspiring to Be Global Health Leaders?

First, weigh in your priorities. If you want to have a family, you should have every opportunity. If you want to be a mother; you should do that. But weigh in your priorities. Plan your life in a way that it gives you a maximum opportunity. Be cognizant of the fact that you cannot have everything at the same time. We are all driven and ambitious, so if something fails, it's not a disaster. Guess what, it's okay. It happens! The second thing is give yourself credit. For even the menial tasks. You deserve the credit for a job well done. The third thing is persistence. There are going to be so many factors and so many people to put you down. Small minds, small people. Stay focused.

If You Could Have a Billboard for Other Women Leaders, What Would It Say?

"Be true to your loved ones. Be true to everything you cherish. Most of all, be true to yourself."

Responses to Sexual Abuse and Exploitation in the Wake of the Oxfam Sex Scandal and Their Implications for Women's Leadership

Cheryl Overs and Kate Hawkins

International development and overseas aid are significant drivers of the global health sector—mobilising financial and human resources to support the cause of better health in low- and middle-income countries and contributing to the development of policy frameworks and norms. Much of this assistance is channelled through the non-governmental sector. In recent years, issues of sexual abuse and exploitation in the development and humanitarian sectors have come to the fore. This dovetails with an increased interest in sexual harassment—within the health sector, health research, programming, and health governance architecture—and its deleterious effect on the ability of women to work and lead with ease.

The sexual abuse and exploitation of women by staff of United Kingdom (UK) international aid agencies working in the Global South came into sharp focus in 2018 as a result of revelations involving Oxfam staff that were exposed in the media (O'Neill, 2018; Ratcliffe & Quinn, 2018; Ratcliffe, 2018a, 2018b; Press Association, 2018; Aitkenhead & Beaumont, 2018; Beaumont, 2018; Elgot & McVeigh, 2018; Rawlinson, 2018). Against the background of #MeToo, complex conversations about sexual abuse and exploitation, and how to respond to it, took place. The government embarked upon information gathering and subsequent policy change which has ramifications for global health and development beyond UK-financed projects and programmes.

The introductory section of this chapter makes the link between gender-based violence and women's leadership in global health. It then explores the incidents that sparked a renewed interest among the British establishment in safeguarding women in humanitarian and development settings. It outlines the norms and narratives that

C. Overs
Michael Kirby Centre for Public Health and Human Rights, Monash University, Clayton, VIC, Australia

K. Hawkins (✉)
Pamoja Communications Ltd., Research in Gender and Ethics (RinGs), Brighton, East Sussex, UK
e-mail: kate@pamoja.uk.com

underpin new policies and guidelines to address sexual exploitation and abuse. It considers the potential impact of these new policies on women in the Global South, focusing on sex workers as a way of exploring the impact on the most marginalised women and who benefits from reform.

Measures developed in the Global North to address sexual exploitation and abuse focus primarily on better training, enforcement of strengthened workplace policies, and better use of the national laws that should, but frequently do not, act as a system of protection, prevention, and punishment. There is potential for these approaches, which together are called safeguarding, to fizzle out and become a box-ticking exercise and to have negative unintended consequences for women whose sexual safety the policies aim to protect. This will impact upon women's progression within the development and humanitarian sector and their ability to lead, including on global health.

Sexual Exploitation and Abuse and Women's Leadership in Global Health

In their 2018 statement, the Global Health Fieldwork Ethics Workshop noted the irony that while gender-based violence has become an increased focus of the global health world,

> [T]he women who participate in global health—the program managers, fieldworkers, researchers, local promoters, and community members—have not been appropriately acknowledged as susceptible to gender-based violence, potentially made more so through their global health engagement. (Global Health Fieldwork Ethics Workshop, 2018, p.134)

Despite evidence gaps it appears that gender-based violence, whether often framed as harassment or abuse, is prevalent in the academic, medical, political, and civil society spaces that make up the global health world (Ridde et al., 2018). In academic medicine, studies have demonstrated that sexual harassment can have a direct impact upon women's leadership potential by affecting their productivity, funding, earnings, and likelihood of continuing in the field (Fairchild et al., 2018).

Within the global health workforce, the WHO's research demonstrates that sexual harassment from co-workers, patients, and the community is a barrier to leadership and that, "Female health workers face the burden of sexual harassment causing harm, ill health, attrition, loss of morale, stress" (WHO, 2019, p. 2). This harassment starts early on within professional careers. A meta-analysis of harassment in medical training concluded that 59.4% of medical trainees had experienced harassment (Fnais et al., 2014).

The international political architecture of global health, through the United Nations (UN) organisations that set norms and programmatic priorities, has also been found to be blighted by sexual harassment. A 2018 independent evaluation of UNAIDS suggested that there were a "vacuum of accountability" and "a broken organisational culture" in relation to harassment (UNAIDS, 2018). UNICEF brought in new guidelines on sexual harassment in 2018 when their Deputy Executive Director was found to have behaved inappropriately in a previous position (Crossette, 2018).

A survey of 1005 women from more than 70 organisations in the humanitarian sphere found that nearly 50% of women respondents report having been "touched in an unwanted way by a male colleague in the workplace and even more are subject to persistent sexual advances from their colleagues" (Humanitarian Women's Network, 2016). The staff of civil society organisations, particularly those that take a more activist or campaigning approach to health, may face backlash from communities who are concerned about changes in power relations.

Sexual harassment has even been of issue at the People's Health Movement Assembly (a global network bringing together grassroots health activists in a social justice movement). Their statement on the matter explained, "There is often an assumption that spaces populated by progressive movements, networks and organisations are free of incidents of sexual harassment but clearly that is not the case" (PHM, 2018).

Sexual harassment is a serious problem within global health. This harassment not only violates the rights and dignity of the individual, but it erodes women's participation and as a result excludes their skills and knowledge from the field.

Data on gender-based violence within global health is hard to come by—perhaps because of low reporting rates and the stigma that prevents the victims from sharing their stories. There is some research that looks at both race/ethnicity and gendered discrimination in the health sector (although it is lacking). It is hard to find data that is from low- and middle-income settings or that is disaggregated in terms of social position, class, and/or place in occupational hierarchies. As a result, it is difficult to understand whether there are other intersecting aspects of inequity which might amplify or compound gender-based violence and how this plays out in a range of geographical settings.

It is widely acknowledged that the bulk of health promotion and care is provided by local women, offering leadership within their own communities. Yet these women are less prominent in the literature on sexual harassment in global health. When local women are considered in the sexual harassment discourse, it tends to be as beneficiaries of health programmes and research rather than as workers and active participants in the global health process.

A Scandal That Rocked the Aid World

On 9 February 2018, *The Times* newspaper published a story on accusations that had been made and investigated in 2011 about parties allegedly attended by sex workers in an Oxfam employee residence in Port-au-Prince, Haiti. According to a whistle-blower, at least five undressed women were in attendance at the gathering which they referred to as an orgy. Two of the women, who were alleged to be sex workers, wore Oxfam T-shirts.

Reports that emerged in the wake of the newspaper article showed that the then Oxfam country director in Haiti, Roland van Hauwermeiren, a Belgian, had been questioned by Oxfam investigators about those parties and about paying for sex himself. As well as parties at staff residences occurring while he was director, Van Hauwermeiren admitted to being visited at his residence by sex workers and to having a non-paying sexual relationship with a Haitian woman who he described as neither a sex worker nor a victim but rather an older woman with honour. He was allowed to resign and given one month's notice.

In the wake of this incident, two male Oxfam staff, who were accused of "using prostitutes", bullying, and CV (curriculum vitae) fraud left, and others were dismissed for buying sex, accessing pornography, and "failing to protect staff". Further allegations emerged soon after, that male employees paid for sex in Chad in 2006, when Van Hauwermeiren was running operations there, and that he and others had gone on to new posts within Oxfam and to posts in other organisations supported by references from Oxfam (Ratcliffe & Quinn, 2018). At the same time, claims emerged that Van Hauwermeiren had been forced out of another British charity seven years earlier after an investigation into paid sex (Ratcliffe, 2018a, 2018b). Oxfam was accused of further failures in Haiti by keeping a senior aid worker there for more than a year despite reported sexual harassment claims (Press Association, 2018). As with sexual abuse cases in the Catholic Church, this heralds an emerging pattern of two tiers of offending—the unacceptable behaviours and the covering up of such behaviours.

After investigators reported to Oxfam trustees, UK International Development Secretary Penny Mordaunt MP threatened to cut Oxfam's funding unless all information on its workers' use of sex workers in Haiti was handed to the Charity Commission to enable it to launch a statutory inquiry into Oxfam workers and sexual exploitation (Booth, 2018). Mark Goldring, the chief executive of Oxfam Great Britain (GB), quickly claimed that attacks were out of proportion and accused critics of an anti-aid agenda (Aitkenhead & Beaumont, 2018). However, Oxfam International published the 2011 inquiry into the Haiti sex abuse, revealing that three staff who were under investigation had physically threatened a colleague to ensure that person's silence (Beaumont, 2018). "Humblest apologies" were offered to the Haitian government amid resignations of celebrity patrons such as Minnie Driver and Desmond Tutu and reduced donations. The charity is reported to have lost 7,000 regular donors since the scandal emerged (Elgot & McVeigh, 2018). In May 2018 Goldring announced he was to stand down as chief executive insisting that the organisation was taking steps towards recovery (Rawlinson, 2018).

A Renewed Focus on Sexual Exploitation and Abuse

The cascade of accusations against Oxfam shook the UK aid sector. In July 2018 the UK Government International Development Select Committee published a report which outlined evidence of widespread sexual exploitation and abuse by aid personnel concluding that the aid sector had failed to give it due attention which was a display of "complacency verging on complicity" (International Development Committee, 2018, p.29). The report described detailed response strategies and recommended specific policies to curb sexual exploitation and abuse in aid settings including beneficiary education in relation to their rights, the creation of standardised reporting on safeguarding from the UK Department for International Development (DFID) grantees, a victim- and survivor-focused approach, the creation of whistle-blowing systems, a culture of transparency in relation to sexual exploitation and abuse, and independent oversight and UN leadership in this area.

The report frames sexual abuse as including non-consensual sex of any kind. Sexual exploitation is sexual behaviours and interactions which are forbidden despite being consensual. There is universal support for criminal law and all other measures that address rape and other sexual assault and sex with children, and for policy that addresses unwanted sexual advances and harassment in workplaces as discrimination. Unsurprisingly, conversations about preventing and responding to clear-cut cases of sexual abuse are less contentious than conversations about sexual exploitation, which is a shifting and often ill-defined concept.

The Oxfam matter, and subsequent governmental attention, turned out to be just one of several stories unfolding in global aid and development programmes around the world. It would bring the architecture of international aid into question, and ultimately policy was rushed through that set up an official atmosphere of zero tolerance for sexual exploitation and abuse. However, in that rush to protect programmes and reputations, there has been little discussion of the implications and meanings that underpin safeguarding efforts.

If we are interested in women's leadership, we should be wary of the idea that women in communities where aid agencies work are too powerless to consent to sex, in contrast to the women who live near the head offices of those agencies. It has ramifications for the way that vulnerability and agency are conceptualised among local women, those who are the beneficiaries of aid programmes and staff and volunteers who are implementing programmes that may undermine empowerment efforts.

Tackling Sexual Exploitation and Abuse in Practice

Despite an atmosphere of general and often vigorous agreement that abusive and exploitative practices in aid settings should end, and general support for the UK government's sexual exploitation and abuse recommendations, a larger conversation about safeguarding has begun in mainstream and social media. Questions about the ethics and gender dimensions of aid and the problematic aspects of relationships between institutional and individual aid providers from the Global North and aid recipients in the Global South are emerging.

The question of how such a widespread issue could have escaped attention for so long has been raised by almost everyone. The clearest answer is that the #MeToo movement finally provided a context in which sexual exploitation and abuse were being recognised and that women working in the aid and development sector who spoke out were joining their counterparts in every other industry.

Abuse in international aid settings is perpetrated by individuals and organisations whose role is to offer help and to alleviate human suffering, not inflict it. In most cases, international humanitarian and aid agencies are charities as well as registered not-for-profit companies. Unlike private commercial enterprises beholden only to law and shareholders, the voluntary or third sector is accountable to donors and government and relies on philanthropic reputations to attract donations, volunteers, and other resources. Although the charitable role and human rights-based ethos may protect the aid agencies, some have suggested that it may also contribute to staff developing an inflated sense of power—sometimes referred to as the white saviour or hero complex—which justifies bad behaviour by people who are working for a good cause.

In the light of this, there is a perception that different standards of behaviour apply where people are operating in difficult environments and away from home for long periods of time. That men in difficult circumstances are entitled to sexual hijinks and subject to lower ethical standards than when they are at home is universally accepted thanks to military traditions. It is neither surprising nor debatable that these values extend to aid agencies. The evidence is in the very language they use to describe the "missions" by their "officers" to "the field". Like warzones the geographical sites of aid are represented as "hearts of darkness", or less poetically, as US President Trump has put it, as "shitholes" (Gopal, 2018). One of the main characteristics of these settings is the (perceived) lack of the rule of law which removes the state from its role as enforcer of fair rules against sexual misconduct.

A common justification for bad sex in bad places is that the bodies that occupy those sites, including those of aid workers, lack the social and economic context and cohesion that are necessary to follow civilised sexual mores. British University of Cambridge academic Mary Beard (2018) articulated this on Twitter: "Of course one can't condone the (alleged) behaviour of Oxfam staff in Haiti and elsewhere. But I do wonder how hard it must be to sustain 'civilised' values in a disaster zone".

Beard was criticised by her Cambridge University colleague, Priyamvada Gopal, for characterising Western aid workers as resistance fighters. "Black agency, Haitian agency", she said, "figures nowhere in your vision, however much on the side of the anticolonial you might consider yourself to be … Still more troubling is your notion that moral bearings ('civilised values'!) understandably disappear in spaces where people struggle with the worst things that can happen to human beings" (Gopal, 2018).

Gopal is right to identify black agency as missing and to draw attention to the racist implications of assuming that bad sex happens in bad places. This view echoes assumptions made in the popular novel *Emergency Sex (And Other Desperate Measures): True Stories from a War Zone,* a book widely read by aid workers (Cain et al., 2006). The book is a first-hand account, and to some extent a celebration, of hyper-sexual culture among aid workers (both men and women) set in Cambodia in the 1980s when that country was emerging from the genocide. It illustrates the perceived value of sexual freedom in difficult situations which provides a clue as to the difficulty of enforcing rules to ensure that if young aid workers can't access "good sex" they need to accept its less popular cousin, abstinence.

What is absent from the novel is recognition of who has sexual freedom and the power of aid workers to obtain "bad sex" unethically. In her seminal work, "Thinking Sex: Notes for a Radical Theory of the Politics of Sexuality", Gayle Rubin (2012) articulates the sexual hierarchy which organises sexual practices:

According to this system, sexuality that is 'good,' 'normal,' and 'natural' should ideally be heterosexual, marital, monogamous, reproductive, and non-commercial. It should be coupled, relational, within the same generation, and occur at home. It should not involve pornography, fetish objects, sex toys of any sort, or roles other than male and female. Any sex that violates these rules is 'bad,' 'abnormal,' or 'unnatural.' Bad sex may be homosexual, unmarried, promiscuous, non-procreative, or commercial. (p. 152)

These notions about "good" and "bad" sex and a thoroughly heteronormative structural bias underpin development and humanitarian efforts (Lind, 2009; Jolly, 2011; Hawkins et al., 2014). It is important to consider what rules prohibiting consensual adult sex mean in theory and how that translates to enforcing them in places where aid workers have no access to the partners of similar racial and economic status other than work colleagues required for "good sex". Few commentators have tackled assumptions about the "good sex" that male aid workers might have at "home" with partners of the same colour, economic status, and age being replaced by bad sex that they deserve or need to cope with the horror of poverty and/or conflict.

Furthermore, the task of understanding and combatting sexual exploitation and abuse in the aid sector is confounded by key differences between domestic workplaces and overseas aid settings. Primary among these differences is that the women and girls of interest in relation to safeguarding measures don't have any formal or legal status in respect of the aid sector. Nor do they have any say in the policies and enforcement procedures that governments and aid agencies from the Global North put in place to protect them from sexual abuse and exploitation perpetuated by their staff in the Global South.

This voicelessness of female citizens of beneficiary countries was evident in the public conversation about sexual exploitation and abuse in the aid sector which seemed to have had something for everyone—from conservatives wanting to end all aid, feminists focusing on female victimhood, to those advocating radical decolonisation of aid. However, the only affected women in the conversation were agency staff from the Global North who had either experienced sexual harassment in the workplace or witnessed sexual behaviour of male staff and local women which they considered inappropriate. Above all, no sex workers' voices were raised in the conversation despite the fact that women selling sex was the main issue that sparked the conversation about sexual exploitation and abuse and that they were one of the main targets of the new safeguarding policies. This is also despite the many sex worker advocacy groups in developing countries, several of whom are sponsored and overseen by the main UK and United States (US) aid agencies.

Sex Work and Transactional Sex

Many feminists and the UK government define any sex between people between whom there is a power differential as exploitation, and thus sexual relations between aid agency staff and local people in recipient countries would be classed as exploitation. However, this notion does not fit easily with a belief in adult agency and the right of competent adults to refuse or consent to sex. This is particularly important, especially when we keep in mind that the women involved in the events that sparked the "Oxfam scandal" in Haiti were in fact consenting adults. Sex work is central to this issue because events of 2018 were set in motion by accusations of paid sex and because new rules about sexual behaviour in aid settings will affect sex workers, particularly those whose livelihoods depend on foreign clients.

Where sex with all local women is banned, transactional sex, the name given to relationships that are driven by financial incentives, will also be assumed to be exploitative and prohibited. There are important ethical dimensions to the impact of aid workers in environments in which economic crisis enables commercial child sex abuse and drives women who don't want to sell sex to do so. However, defining consenting adult sex work as sexual exploitation is controversial. The UK Development Committee report said that the sector had been aware of sexual exploitation and abuse by its own personnel for years without giving it the attention it deserved. But while that's true of some forms of sexual exploitation and abuse—underage sex, rape, sex for aid—it is not true for buying sex, which has only recently been categorised as exploitation and prohibited. In 2018, Oxfam GB's Code of Conduct strictly prohibited staff, volunteers, and other representatives from buying sex:

> Oxfam does not make a judgement against individuals who participate in selling sex in exchange for money or something else such as gifts or material support ("transactional sex"). However, in line with the IASC Core Principles on PSEA, Oxfam has banned this activity in order to prevent sexual exploitation and abuse from occurring. (Oxfam GB, 2018, p.5)

The sex worker rights movement strongly protests against policy that forbids buying sex as a way of ending exploitation arguing that prohibitions on sex buying, like those on selling, violate the right to bodily autonomy and fail to recognise agency and competent adults' right to consent. Demanding that consensual adult sex work be differentiated from sexual exploitation, abuse, and trafficking, sex workers have argued that the measures needed to enforce a ban on paying for sex take attention and resources away from combatting actual sexual abuse.

The existence of black and brown women in poor countries who negotiate and make decisions about sex on a similar basis to white women in rich countries ill fits with this binary view of perpetrators and victims. This raises practical as well as ethical questions.

Penny Mordaunt MP said of the reforms that it was important that survivors' voices were heard and that the charitable sector needed to show that victims are a priority (Ratcliffe, 2018a, 2018b). But this rhetoric about listening to and believing "survivors" offers nothing to women who have sold sex or had foreign boyfriends in transactions they do not see as exploitative. Thus, defining consenting adults as victims of exploitation is incompatible with a "victim-centred approach".

The question of how to help people who do not share the helpers' vision of the problem is much discussed in respect of sex workers and trafficking victims. Although there is little research on the topic, a common response taken by anti-trafficking organisations globally is to isolate women and girls who have been selling sex and "educate" them until they agree that they are victims (Ramachandran, 2015; Thomas Reuters Foundation, 2019).

Like many who urge the criminalisation of buying and/or selling sex, Pauline Latham MP deals with this problem by denying the agency of such women by reclassifying them as victims. She rejected the notion that these women should be classed as "prostitutes" and instead characterised them as trafficked women and girls at the mercy of abusive men (Ratcliffe, 2018a, 2018b). This begs the question of who Latham thinks deserves to be "called a prostitute" and how prostitutes should be treated that differs from victims. The view that women in poor countries only sell sex out of desperation brought about by disaster is a fiction, even a whitewash. In reality, large numbers of women, men, and people of other genders sell and trade sex in all circumstances including the peaceful prosperity of Latham's own constituency.

Bans on sex as an expression of zero tolerance for sexual exploitation place sex workers, and women who *might* sell sex, out of bounds, not just for sexual transactions but also socially and professionally. They effectively declare them "persona non grata" in their own communities. This is clearly a violation of human rights and gender equality and flies in the face of the theories about community participation and leadership that aid agencies expound. It could be seen as particularly hypocritical on the part of agencies that are committed to equality and funded to operate programmes to improve sex workers' health, economic, and human rights status.

Placing certain women, and to a lesser extent men, outside of acceptable sexual and social activity is fraught with practical risks too. A recent study of garment workers in Sri Lanka illustrated the ways in which attempts to prevent sex being bought and sold as an exercise in safeguarding, underpinning the UK Modern Slavery Act, degenerated into a box-ticking exercise that discriminated against the garment workers it was intended to protect (Hewamanne, 2019). It also raised the possibility that, like many formal ethics procedures, the key purpose of the reporting and monitoring systems for safeguarding against sexual exploitation was not in fact protection of "vulnerable women" but protection of the industry in which it is applied. It is not unreasonable to suspect that sexual exploitation and abuse of safeguarding could be similarly driven in view of the seriousness of the fiscal and reputational losses experienced by British aid agencies.

Implications for Future Action

To some, reducing the rights of adult women to protect them from sexual exploitation unjustifiably limits the right to choose and to exercise agency. Although prohibiting sex between categories of consenting adults with different levels of power is a proven tool for reducing sexual abuse and exploitation in some settings, such as universities, where sex between staff and students is routinely forbidden, the implications of such bans to entire populations in aid settings are unknown.

What is known is that historically, prohibitions on adult consenting sex have been implicated in a range of unintended consequences including discrimination against women and sustaining sexual exploitation and abuse rather than reducing it. There is also evidence that enforcing bans on consensual sex erodes the goodwill necessary to make safeguarding work as well as wasting resources that could be better used ending the sexual abuse of children and adults.

Furthermore, essentialist, heteronormative, and conservative ideologies that recognise promiscuous, mercenary, or fleeting sex as exploitative by definition are associated with rules about sex that cast too wide a net. Moreover, rules that define all or almost all women as vulnerable and any sexual contact with them as exploitation almost invariably increase control over women's behaviour as much or even more than that of the male potential perpetrators.

Ultimately the success of efforts to safeguard local populations and aid agency staff against sexual exploitation and abuse by aid workers depends on the quality of safeguarding procedures. They will only work in situ and avoid further stigmatising and dividing good from bad women if they are grounded in sound understandings of human sexuality and behaviour and respect for human rights.

It is very difficult to imagine the secure, accessible, fair, and interlinked systems along with reliable reporting, training, documentation, and victim protection/support being achieved in most aid settings and it is impossible in some. Moreover, along with evidence that in-country exploitation and abuse is linked to non-sexual abuse, bullying, and financial corruption, it is clear sexual exploitation and abuse safeguarding could be a knee-jerk, isolated exercise in meaningless box-ticking without root and branch reform in the ways aid providers interact in aid settings at both institutional and personal levels.

Former aid worker Shaista Aziz has argued that racism, power, patriarchy, and neocolonialism within the aid system are the mechanisms through which sexual abuse is enabled and that the lenses of safeguarding and IT are insufficient (Aziz, 2018).

It is crucial to avoid the moral panic that characterises so much law and policy on sex and gender. Laws that address human sexuality work best when they place as few limits as necessary on consenting adults and when they focus intensely and realistically on abuse with the sharpest tools available. Organisational policy, expectations, and norms around sexual behaviour are therefore most workable where they recognise rather than deny the value of sex and sexual pleasure and the human right to bodily autonomy. Moreover, such recognition has an important role to play in ensuring that the tools are sharp—that resources are very carefully targeted, that rules are grounded in independent research and tied to a strong ethical framework. This means that reporting and evaluating the efficacy of sexual exploitation and abuse safeguarding must be independently monitored for real impact.

Beyond the practical aspects of new sexual exploitation and abuse policies for the aid sector, current reforms play an important role in conceptualising women politically which in turn has implications for women's participation in non-governmental organisation (NGO), government, and community, and for aid policy and programming. Research has shown that the sexual rights of adult women to exercise agency in relation to their choice of sexual partner have clear linkages to their ability to make claims in other areas of their lives and that supportive intimate relationships are often a prerequisite to women's ability to take up leadership positions (Hawkins et al., 2011). The new safeguarding rhetoric contains strong messages about women's power—how and when women may share power with men and which women are rendered powerless by vulnerability, what the limits of power are, and the place of sex and sexuality in geopolitical relationships. These need to be viewed with a critical eye.

As we seek to tackle sexual harassment, we must ensure that procedures to protect against, and respond to, abuse are fit for purpose. They must protect not only the few elite women who have reached leadership positions in global health in the Global North but to the millions of potential leaders in the Global South whose voices are seldom listened to. Attention should be paid to who is driving and shaping the response to gender-based violence in global health, who evaluates the appropriateness or success of these initiatives, and whose interests they serve.

References

Aitkenhead, D., & Beaumont, B. (2018). Oxfam chief accuses critics of 'gunning' for charity over Haiti sex scandal claims, *The Guardian*. Retrieved February 16, 2018, from https://www.theguardian.com/global-development/2018/feb/16/oxfam-chief-accuses-critics-of-gunning-for-charity-over-haiti-sex-scandal-claims

Aziz, S. (2018). We interrupted Penny Mordaunt to demand aid sector abuses end now, *The Guardian*. Retrieved October 18, 2018, from https://www.theguardian.com/commentisfree/2018/oct/18/aidtoo-sexual-abuse-charity-sector

Beard, M. (2018). *Twitter update*. Retrieved from https://twitter.com/wmarybeard/status/964613592833253376

Beaumont, P. (2018). Trio on Oxfam's Haiti team threatened key witness, report reveals, *The Guardian*. Retrieved February 19, 2018, from https://www.theguardian.com/world/2018/feb/19/trio-oxfam-haiti-team-threatened-key-witness-confidential-report

Booth, R. (2018). Oxfam warned it could lose European funding over scandal, *The Guardian*. Retrieved February 12, 2018, from https://www.theguardian.com/world/2018/feb/12/haiti-demands-oxfam-identify-workers-who-used-prostitutes

Cain, K., Postlewait, H., & Thomson, A. (2006). *Emergency sex (and other desperate measures): True stories from a war zone*. Ebury Press.

Crossette, B. (2018). With scandals rife across the UN, are managers at fault? *Passblue*. Retrieved from https://www.passblue.com/2019/04/24/with-scandals-rife-across-the-un-are-managers-at-fault/

Elgot, J., & McVeigh, K. (2018). Oxfam loses 7,000 donors since sexual exploitation scandal, *The Guardian*. Retrieved February 20, 2018, from https://www.theguardian.com/world/2018/feb/20/oxfam-boss-mark-goldring-apologises-over-abuse-of-haiti-quake-victims

Fairchild, A. L., Holyfield, L. J., & Byington, C. L. (2018). National Academies of Sciences, Engineering, and Medicine report on sexual harassment: making the case for fundamental institutional change. *JAMA, 320*.

Fnais, N., Soobiah, C., Chen, M. H., Lillie, E., Perrier, L., Tashkhandi, M., et al. (2014). Harassment and discrimination in medical training: A systematic review and meta-analysis. *Academic Medicine, 89*(5), 817–827. https://www.ncbi.nlm.nih.gov/pubmed/24667512

Global Health Fieldwork Ethics Workshop. (2018). #MeToo meets global health: A call to action. *Health and Human Rights, 21*(1), 133–139. https://www.ncbi.nlm.nih.gov/pmc/articles/PMC6586977/

Gopal, P. (2018). Response to Mary beard, medium. Retrieved February 18, 2018, from https://medium.com/@zen.catgirl/response-to-mary-beard-91a6cf2f53b6

Hawkins, K., Cornwall, A., & Lewin, T. (2011). *Sexuality and empowerment: An intimate connection, pathways policy paper, October 2011*. Pathways of Women's Empowerment RPC. Retrieved from https://opendocs.ids.ac.uk/opendocs/bitstream/handle/123456789/5846/Sexuality%20and%20Empowerment%20Policy%20paper.pdf?sequence=1

Hawkins, K., Wood, S., Charles, T., He, X., Li, Z., Lim, A., Mountian, I., & Sharma, J. (2014). *Sexuality and Poverty Synthesis Report*. IDS Evidence Report 53, IDS: Brighton.

Hewamanne, S. (2019) Modern Slavery Act is having unintended consequences for women's freedom in Sri Lanka, *The Conversation*, Retrieved July 11, 2019, from https://theconversation.com/modern-slavery-act-is-having-unintended-consequences-for-womens-freedom-in-sri-lanka-112258

Humanitarian Women's Network. (2016). *Discrimination, harassment and abuse of women aid workers: Survey results and way forward*. Retrieved from https://interagencystandingcommittee.org/system/files/hwn_background_paper.pdf

International Development Committee. (2018). *Sexual exploitation and abuse in the aid sector, Eighth Report of Session 2017–19*. Retrieved July 23, 2018, from https://publications.parliament.uk/pa/cm201719/cmselect/cmintdev/840/840.pdf

Jolly, S. (2011). Why is development work so straight? Heteronormativity in the international development industry. *Development in Practice, 21*(1), 18–28.

Lind, A. (2009). Governing Intimacy, Struggling for Sexual Rights: Challenging heteronormativity in the global development industry. *Development, 52*, 34–42. https://doi.org/10.1057/dev.2008.71

Ratcliffe, R. (2018a). Oxfam's disgraced Haiti official left earlier post over 'sex parties', *The Guardian*. Retrieved February 13, 2018, from https://www.theguardian.com/global-development/2018/feb/13/oxfam-disgraced-haiti-official-liberia-post-roland-van-hauwermeiren

Ratcliffe, R., & Quinn, B. (2018). Oxfam: fresh claims that staff used prostitutes in Chad, *The Guardian*. Retrieved February 11, 2018, from https://www.theguardian.com/world/2018/feb/10/oxfam-faces-allegations-staff-paid-prostitutes-in-chad

Ridde, V., Dagenais, C., & Daigneault, I. (2018). It's time to address sexual violence in academic global health, it's time to address sexual violence in academic global health. *BMJ Global Health, 4*, e001616. https://gh.bmj.com/content/4/2/e001616

Thomas Reuters Foundation. (2019). *Thai sex workers reject anti-trafficking raids and rescue*. Retrieved from https://www.freedomunited.org/news/thai-sex-workers-reject-anti-trafficking-raids-and-rescue/

O'Neill S (2018) Oxfam in Haiti: 'It was like a Caligula orgy with prostitutes in Oxfam T-shirts,' *The Times*. Retrieved from February 9, 2018, from https://www.thetimes.co.uk/article/oxfam-in-haiti-it-was-like-a-caligula-orgy-with-prostitutes-in-oxfam-t-shirts-p32wlk0rp

Oxfam GB. (2018) *Protection from sexual exploitation and abuse (PSEA) policy*. Retrieved from https://www.oxfam.org.uk/~/media/Files/OGB/What%20we%20do/About%20us/Plans%20reports%20and%20policies/Safeguarding/PSEA%20Policy%20approved%20May%202018.ashx

PHM. (2018). *Statement from the People's Health Movement (PHM) against sexual harassment*. Retrieved from https://phmovement.org/statement-from-the-peoples-health-movement-phm-against-sexual-harassment/

Press Association. (2018). Oxfam 'kept aid worker on in Haiti despite sex harassment claims,' *The Guardian*, Retrieved from March 17, 2018, from https://www.theguardian.com/world/2018/mar/17/oxfam-kept-aid-worker-on-in-haiti-despite-sex-harassment-claims

Ramachandran, V. (2015). Rescued but not released: the 'protective custody' of sex workers in India, *Open Democracy*. Retrieved from https://www.opendemocracy.net/en/beyond-trafficking-and-slavery/rescued-but-not-released-protective-custody-of-sex-workers-in-i/

Ratcliffe, R. (2018b). MPs accuse aid groups of 'abject failure' in tackling sexual abuse, *The Guardian*. Retrieved from July 31, 2018, from https://www.theguardian.com/global-development/2018/jul/31/mps-accuse-aid-groups-of-abject-failure-in-tackling-sexual-abuse

Rawlinson, K. (2018). Oxfam chief steps down after charity's sexual abuse scandal, *The Guardian*. Retrieved from May 16, 2018, from https://www.theguardian.com/world/2018/may/16/oxfam-head-mark-goldring-steps-down-sexual-abuse-scandal

Rubin, G. (2012). Thinking sex: Notes for a radical theory of the politics of sexuality, In *From gender to sexuality*, Duke University Press.

UNAIDS. (2018) *Report of the independent expert panel on prevention of and response to harassment, including sexual harassment, bullying and abuse of power at UNAIDS Secretariat Submitted to the UNAIDS Programme Coordination Board Bureau 19 November 2018.* Retrieved from https://www.unaids.org/sites/default/files/media_asset/report-iep_en.pdf

WHO. (2019). *Delivered by women, led by men: A gender and equity analysis of the global health and social workforce.* World Health Organization. (Human Resources for Health Observer Series No. 24) https://apps.who.int/iris/bitstream/handle/10665/311322/9789241515467-eng.pdf

Interview with Juno Roche, Trans Writer and Campaigner, Patron of cliniQ, and Author of Three Books: Queer Sex, Trans Power, and Gender Explorers

Cheryl Overs

"Community leadership isn't a career for me ... I prefer a much quieter form of leadership grounded in writing".

Juno Roche is an internationally recognised trans writer and campaigner, and founder of Trans Workers UK and the Trans Teachers Network. On the Independent's Rainbow List 2015 and 2016, she is Director of cliniQ, a queer-inclusive and non-judgemental holistic well-being and sexual health services for trans clients, members of the trans community, and their friends and families. She is a trustee of the Sophia Forum, which promotes and advocates for the rights, health, welfare, and dignity of women living with HIV through research, raising awareness, and influencing policy. In 2015, Juno received the Blair Peach Award for her campaign "Why Trans Teachers Matter". She regularly contributes to publications including Diva, The Guardian, *and* Vice *and is the author of two books:* Queer Sex *(longlisted for the Polari First Book Prize) and* Trans Power, *which was published in 2019.*

How Did You Get Involved in Health Activism?

My campaigning began in the 1980s as part of the group that set up the first LGBT housing co-op in London. We were very young and most had been more or less kicked out of home and ended up squatting in East London. We began working with social services and getting quite good funding from government to take over housing, do it up, and provide homes. It was very successful, and ever since I have always been annoyed by the deficiencies of the state on issues that are simple to solve. In the 1980s, HIV was a distant ghoulish thing on the horizon, and by the time

C. Overs (✉)
Michael Kirby Centre for Public Health and Human Rights, Monash University, Clayton, VIC, Australia

© Springer Nature Switzerland AG 2022
R. Morgan et al. (eds.), *Women and Global Health Leadership*,
https://doi.org/10.1007/978-3-030-84498-1_17

it fully descended on us I had already learnt a lot about problem solving from the housing work.

More recently I have been working on trans equality issues with unions and in education. I've been really lucky as a campaigner that most of my work in recent years has been pretty well supported. I have been working on a campaign "Finding our T-spot", which examines current research around the transgender community and sexual health care and asks the question "what research do we need to make viable structural changes to improve sexual healthcare for all the transgender community including non-binary people?"

It is about finding and creating safer spaces for people that don't identify as cis. It's driven by the idea that trans-friendly policies aren't enough. To make safe spaces we need education and structural change and that's what I'm interested in, not the well-meaning policy making. If there are 19 chairs and 20 students you need clearly need to bring in another chair, not a policy. It's the same with equalities. If every book in your library only talks about cis people having babies, I as a trans woman am forever going to feel at least slightly excluded.

I don't see myself as an activist, but a campaigner and I only get excited about it when I can see the creative challenges. My degree was in fine art and philosophy, and years ago I made art installations. I still aim to create installations around issues such as risk and stigma, which is fascinating. Who do I bring together and how? Do I hold a roundtable, make a film, write about it, speak at an event?

Some work I did within the Catholic Church is a good example. I was invited to help on issues affecting both trans students and teachers which involved thinking creatively about how to ground trans equality in Catholic scripture. We had a meeting of priests and teachers where we looked at the impact of stigma and the burden imposed on trans people for whom school is not a safe space. Rather than talk about toilet policy, we came up with the notion of kindness as primary in policy making and it went from there into making a big picture of what that looks like. It was phenomenal really. That diocese rolled out a programme called "Kindness" for trans kids in their schools. In fact, that began with a room full of men who just needed someone to hold their hand and tell them everything will be alright. So that's what I did. I'm very good at that.

What Challenges Have You Faced in Your Career?

One of the main drivers around HIV for me was my own diagnosis and subsequent experience of discrimination. I had been an addict in London, woke up one morning in the late 1980s, and decided to make a break from it and go to university on the Sussex Coast. It happened really quickly; the university, becoming drug-free, took a bit longer. When I tested positive for HIV in my first year the university told me to leave because their insurance did not cover having an HIV-positive student. I was on an art course and I made stuff, and they said I could cut myself and what would happen then? I had this stigma placed on me that I had "bad blood" and it was my legal and moral responsibility, and this would thwart my plans.

But more than that, I was the first of my extended East End working-class family to go to university and my attitude was fixed—if I was going to die, I was going to die with a degree. I grew up in a family with a lot of addiction and circumstances that meant that if I did get to university, I was not going to show up bright-eyed and bushy tailed. If I got there, I was going to be a mess. And I was, and I needed support. Amazingly, since I was still on drugs, I did get that degree, but with a 2.1, not a first which I think I would have got if I had the support I needed.

So, navigating, that was my first real fight. Stigma and discrimination fired me up then and it still does. The question becomes "what does it take to enable people like me to get an education?" I learnt from that experience that stigma goes far beyond name calling in the street. It is structural and has to be challenged on that basis to get thorough and systemic reform.

I have always been aware of limitations and strengths of organisations. I primarily work alone but I deal with all of the NGOs in the field—my company name is Just Juno. Someone commented that I am oppositional, but I don't think I am an inherently oppositional person. But the times we live in and the issues I am dealing with put me in that position. I am continually fighting my way in. That's not just about being trans, even my [working-class] accent marks me out as different. I realised I had to do work to be there. I had to learn a new language. We hugely underestimate the impact of class in our society which may be subsumed by race, gender, and otherness.

As a working-class trans woman, I can be the easiest person to shut down if I oppose the dominant narrative. I've become quite good at setting it out to organisations that invite me to their events that they know what I will say, they know exactly what dynamic I bring, and they are utilising that dynamic so they need to respect it. I won't be used to call out people or issues by organisations who want to tick boxes but then won't listen to the solutions I propose. I spoke at a union conference of 800 teachers after I had been doing a project on trans issues in schools. After a few minutes, people were stamping the floor because they wanted me to get off the stage which I refused to do. Sheer bloody mindedness overcomes me in such moments. I thought, I'm the only trans woman you are going to hear from probably all year so I'm not budging. I feel driven and I feel attached to my campaigns, I like public speaking, and it helps to know that what I was saying was right and to view it as a performance which takes you to a different space.

In terms of leadership, I don't see myself as a leader but as a creative person making just a bit more space for myself and others to breathe. Life as a person with HIV or an addict or trans or whatever can be very suffocating, and activism can be rushing towards a place that you may well emotively bounce off. I try to do it differently. I say things that other people find difficult to say.

In some sense I am happy to throw myself under the bus, perhaps because I am older now. I don't need other trans people, or sex workers, or addicts to believe in me to make changes that make life easier for us. Hopefully they will breathe easier, go off and get a job, be treated well in services, and have a good life without thinking about the politics of it all. For example, one of my campaigns was around trans students being sent to toilets in schools that were further away than the male and female toilets. It meant they spent 27% more time outside the classroom which is illegal discrimination. I threatened legal action and the problem was solved by some closer toilets being designated non-binary. Future users of that space can benefit without needing to know about me.

Lack of good research is an ongoing challenge. We need good research because it's how we quantify and qualify each other. I am very engaged by the question of what good research looks like, what do we get back from it, and how do we do it. For example, I questioned the sources of a man at the Trade Union Congress conference who said in his presentation that 40% of trans people attempt suicide and 80% [attempt] self-harm. He wasn't happy about being questioned, but I persisted because if you are going to present such a gloom and doom picture, it has consequences, and it has to be right if you are going to tell a trans kid they are more than likely to self-harm. On closer examination it turned out they were extrapolated from questionable data from lesbians in Holloway prison. There's a bit of a rush to research trans people in the UK at the moment so I am working to bring the right people together to think about that.

There are big gaps in the evidence. For example, there's no therapy available post-gender reassignment therapy. Ageing is a big issue for trans women. The average age of transition for trans women in the UK is 42 years old, in part because it's not until then women have economic stability. At 42 you are coming into the period where women are invisible and treated badly in the workplace anyway.

People are very keen to do qualitative research because it gives them the narrative they want—alienation, violence, suicide, HIV, depression, etc.—but less keen to do quantitative work. We need both. Next week I am making a film about research with the Terrence Higgins Trust, and I plan to grill researchers about why we should trust them. I think their answers will tell us more than the actual research results.

At the moment, I am talking a lot about the notion of HIV risk for trans men and trans women. The information is very poor. We can't go on talking about trans women as a "key population" for HIV in England. Maybe you can do that elsewhere but not England. Trans men's risk is not understood at all. Including trans women as a key population sets up a bunch of misconceptions, becomes very paternalistic, gives nothing back, and diverts attention from the real risks in places we are not looking. People in the HIV organisations think they know the agenda and the best way to deal with it. They will say to me "I've got your back" to which I reply, "No, the last thing I need is for anyone to have my back. I need you to get out of the way. I need you to give up your place at the table".

Where Are You Now and What Advice Do You Have for Young Women?

Results and sustainability are very important to me so I spend a lot of time thinking through how to achieve them. For example, I followed up that work I mentioned in the Catholic diocese by setting up the links to expand it to other areas via a head teacher network, which worked well.

I have a company and an agent and requests all go through those so I don't do anything unpaid. Trans women are in the top 10% for education and the bottom 10% for employment. So, if I'm going to be some kind of model and true to myself, I at least have to make sure that my own house is in order.

It was always important to me to make a public statement that community leadership isn't a career for me. I prefer a much quieter form of leadership grounded in writing. I live in the back of beyond in Spain now in a small village and that's where I write. It means I don't get caught up here in London. I come and go. I say what I want to say and go back there. I always think I could have done more.

Perhaps one of the beauties about getting to a certain age is you can say, "You know what, I'm alright. I'm not perfect but I'm alright and I'm kind of happy with myself". When people say things that make you feel less OK with yourself, about how you were too shouty or whatever, it goes in and stays for a second and goes out the other side. Don't let people push you into stuff. I resist being pushed into rubber-stamping research that I don't think will be helpful, for example.

I think the important thing is to know your position. Know what it you want to do, what has to be achieved. You don't necessarily know how to change it but that's where the creativity comes in. Do your homework. Don't try to think cleverly, think simply and practically and directly about good outcomes for people.

Women in Health Systems Leadership: Demystifying the Labyrinth

Zahra Zeinali

Health systems are defined as "consisting of all people, institutions, resources, and activities whose primary purpose is to promote, restore, and maintain health" (Global Health U, 2015). They are the vessel through which health is promoted and health care delivered. The health workforce are an essential building block of health systems (WHO, 2014a) enabling healthcare delivery, without which it is impossible to bridge the supply and demand sides of health care. Therefore, the World Health Organization (WHO) has declared "no health without a workforce" as a universal truth (WHO, 2014b).

According to the WHO, the proportion of women working in the health sector across the globe is on average higher than any other sector (High-Level Commission on Health Employment and Economic Growth, 2016); in many countries, close to 75% of people working in the health sector are women (Librarian, 2018). Despite women making up the majority of healthcare positions within the health workforce pipeline and training institutions, the top levels of leadership in the health sector remain dominated by men. This holds true about top global institutions in global policy and governance, decision-making structures, governments, and the public or private sector (Dhatt et al., 2017). For instance, in 2018 the percentage of countries with a woman Minister of Health, disaggregated by WHO region, is as follows: Africa 38%, Europe 36%, the Americas 31%, Eastern Mediterranean 24%, Western Pacific 19%, and Southeast Asia 18% (Women in Global Health, n.d.). None of these regions are near parity. This means globally, despite 70% of the health and social workforce and 90% of long-term care workforce being women, only an average of 31% of Ministers of Health are women (Women in Global Health, n.d.).

Leadership in health systems has a vague definition given the myriad types of health systems existing and operating around the world. Often, health leadership refers to individuals at the highest levels who are steering a health system, i.e.,

Z. Zeinali (✉)
Johns Hopkins Bloomberg School of Public Health, Baltimore, MD, USA
e-mail: zzeinal1@alumni.jh.edu

© Springer Nature Switzerland AG 2022
R. Morgan et al. (eds.), *Women and Global Health Leadership*,
https://doi.org/10.1007/978-3-030-84498-1_18

183

people working in health ministries and departments. But in the everyday function of health systems, leadership in health is distributed at various levels and dealt with by different actors. For the sake of having a unified understanding of health leadership throughout this chapter, the following broad three levels of leadership in health systems are considered (Chunharas & Davies, 2016): First is the national level where policy making and priority setting happen. Second is the subnational level where policy implementation happens; this is where policies from the national level are translated across the system. Third is the operational level (including community) where program managers, health workers, and providers implement policy and practices and deliver health care (Chunharas & Davies, 2016). At any of these levels, health systems leadership is considered to encompass both the hardware and software of health systems: the hardware being the structural aspects, such as different types and cadres of the health workforce as well as governance and institutional legislation. The software, however, includes the social aspects such as norms, values, trust, interests, affinities, and power that underpin the relationship of the actors and elements of the health systems and influence their actions (Gilson, 2017; Sheikh et al., 2011; Gilson et al., 2017).

Global data shows that about 75% of the health workforce in most countries is comprised of women (Librarian, 2018). However, moving up the hierarchy of health systems, at any of the three aforementioned levels, women take up only about 25% of leadership positions (Hawkes & Buse, 2019; World Health Organization, 2019). This underrepresentation at the leadership level is clearly not due to a shortage in the pipeline of health workers, rather a multitude of barriers and biases that hinder women's equal participation in leading health systems. Gender leadership gaps are due to stereotypes, power imbalances, privilege, and discrimination (World Health Organization, 2019). While most of these barriers are not specific to the health sector, and in fact obstruct women's presence in leadership in all sectors, we examine them in the health systems setting specifically. The underrepresentation of women in the leadership roles of health systems poses a major challenge as the women who run the health systems' operations do not have the same power in the design and delivery of health systems as the men do (World Health Organization, 2019). This disparity poses significant inefficiencies that contribute to imbalances in health worker training, recruitment, deployment, retention, and attrition in health systems (Newman, 2014).

The Third Global Human Resources for Health Forum's Political Declaration on Human Resources for Health committed to "promote equal opportunities in education, development, management and career advancement for all health workers, with no form of discrimination based on gender, race, ethnicity or any other basis" (GHWA, 2013). According to the WHO, gender biases in power, resources, entitlements, norms, and values are manifesting in the underrepresentation of women in leadership positions across health systems, the pay gap, and physical and sexual violence and harassment (High-Level Commission on Health Employment and Economic Growth, 2016; Commission on Social Determinants of Health, 2008). Closing the gender gap in health systems leadership is an important step in addressing women's health issues and outcomes (Hawkes & Buse, 2019).

The WHO Commission on Social Determinants of Health recommended the empowerment of women and marginalized groups at the micro-level of individual people, as well as ensuring their representation at the macro-level political economy and decision-making structures, including within the health system, to improve health outcomes that are a result of social inequities (Commission on Social Determinants of Health, 2008). Evidence from randomized trials has demonstrated that compared to men, women in leadership positions of governmental organizations implement policies that are more supportive of women and children (Downs et al., 2014).

Increasing women's leadership in health systems at the global, national, and subnational levels is a vital step toward addressing women's health challenges and empowering and recognizing the majority of the health sector's workforce. It is important, however, that diverse groups of women are included within health systems' distributed leadership. In aiming to achieve the ambitions of the Declaration on Human Resources for Health, approaches are needed which seek to understand and address different manifestations of discrimination and marginalization within human resources for health, including health systems leadership.

Policies thus far have tried to fit women into inequitable systems, but there is now a momentum to catalyze change and improve the systems and work environments to close the gender gap in leadership (World Health Organization, 2019) and give women who run the health systems an equal say in the design and delivery (World Health Organization, 2019). In this chapter we will explore some of the persisting issues women face in health systems which affect their leadership journeys.

Bias

Gender stereotypes and biases are the bedrock of gender inequities observed in leadership. Stereotypes are the "cognitive shortcuts" that allow classifying people based on identities and social locations such as gender, race, age, or migration status. A bias is a belief that forms after being exposed to stereotypes and is not easily changed (Project Implicit: Frequently Asked Questions, 2011; Northouse, 2015; The American Association of University Women, 2016). Gender is often subject to stereotyping and once a stereotype is adopted, it becomes the filter through which information is selectively used and recalled (The American Association of University Women, 2016). Stereotypically male characteristics have long correlated with expectations of leadership and its attributes (The American Association of University Women, 2016). This has led to both men and women demonstrating explicit and implicit bias toward women and their ability to fit leadership positions. Due to the feminized nature of health systems and health workforce, women are tangibly disadvantaged in this sector when it comes to career progression toward leadership positions.

Addressing the gendered nature of the health workforce requires investigating how health work is conceptualized, stratified, and valued (George, 2007). Health systems reflect the prevalent gender norms of the society, and hence, gender bias has often led to differentially valuing or undervaluing women's contributions to health, especially in the social care workforce or at the lower levels of the health workforce such as with community health workers. This under-recognition often leads to expectations of unpaid work (George, 2007; Gupta et al., 2019). Gender inequities and biases originating from society's restrictive gender norms can cripple or even incapacitate a health system's functions (Gilson, 2017).

While efforts to reduce gender imbalance in global health leadership are critical and gaining momentum, it is imperative that we look beyond gender parity and recognize that women are a heterogeneous group and that the privileges and disadvantages that hinder and enable women's career progression cannot be reduced to a shared universal experience, explained only by gender. Therefore, when addressing gender inequity, we must always adopt an intersectional framework to take into account the ways in which gender intersects with other social identities and stratifiers, such as age, socioeconomic status, race, ethnicity, nationality, religion, disability, and ability, to create unique experiences of marginalization and disadvantage (Zeinali et al., 2019).

Occupational Segregation

A WHO gender analysis of human resources for health notes that "gender, among other power relations, plays a critical role in determining the structural location of women and men in the health labor force and their subjective experience of that location" (George, 2007).

Gendered societal norms and expectations have a significant influence on women's ability and interest in health leadership. Equal opportunity and gender equality in the health sector can lead to several positive outcomes such as equal access to professional knowledge and education, an increased health worker pipeline, an equal chance of being hired, being fairly paid and enjoying advancement opportunities, better work-life balance, and improved health services (Newman, 2014). Improving women's representation within health system leadership is therefore beneficial to all (Gilson, 2003).

Moreover, gender equality in the workforce has been defined as "a condition where women and men can enter the health occupation of their choice, develop the requisite skills and knowledge, be fairly paid, enjoy fair and safe working conditions, and advance in a career, without reference to gender" (Newman, 2014; Williams, 2006). Gender essentialism, on the other hand, is the conviction of assuming men and women are different in multiple aspects including their skills and working styles, leading to assumptions that women have a natural tendency for choosing caring, nurturing jobs and men are more prone to managerial jobs (World Health Organization, 2019; Newman et al., 2011).

Gender bias stratifies the location of men and women in the health workforce (George, 2007). Occupations that require fewer years of education and training, earn lower salaries, and are more insecure during health systems' reforms are often highly feminized. In contrast men are occupying jobs that are generally more precisely defined, with better earnings and room for promotion (George, 2007). This phenomenon is called occupational gender segregation and is an enduring form of workforce inequality and discrimination. Occupational gender segregation is affected by both supply side factors such as personal choice (often heavily influenced by societal gender norms as well) and demand side factors such as bias and discrimination in the workplace (Reskin, 1993). Occupational segregation happens in two axes, vertical and horizontal segregation (Gender Equality Glossary and Thesaurus, n.d.). Vertical segregation, defined as a concentration of men or women in different positions, grades, or levels of responsibility (Gender Equality Glossary and Thesaurus, n.d.), is the more readily visible problem in the health sector. Horizontal segregation refers to the concentration of men and women in different sectors or jobs (Gender Equality Glossary and Thesaurus, n.d.). In the health sector, this is translated to a more prominent presence of women in jobs that have traditionally been attributed to women and "female traits" such as caring, for instance, nursing and midwifery. To this day, far fewer women are physicians (Librarian, 2018), a traditionally male occupation which is also considered more elite in leadership positions (Dhatt et al., 2017). These elite cadres are historically male-dominant, leading to cadre inequality which can be further exacerbated by gender inequity. This contributes to lack of motivation and low morale, disempowerment, and maldistribution of the workforce (Newman, 2014). The concept of occupational segregation is pervasive to all countries, whether they are classified as high- or low- and middle-income (Dr. Richard Anker MHMM, n.d.).

Occupational segregation affects all genders' work experience, presenting itself in various forms such as narrower set of choices and job opportunities for a specific gender (for instance, the limited participation of men in nursing, social care, or midwifery workforce) as well as the stereotypes that lead to the widening of the gender pay gap and the resulting unequal power structures in the health systems (World Health Organization, 2019).

Pay Gap

It is estimated that women, as the main healthcare providers, deliver health care to 5 billion people around the world and contribute US$3 trillion annually to global health, nearly half of which is in the form of unpaid care work (Langer et al., 2015). But inequalities persist even in the paid workforce. In fact, if the unpaid care and social work is taken into account for calculating the pay gap, the pay gap between men and women would increase considerably (World Health Organization, 2019). Employment sectors with a female majority workforce, such as health care, are usually attached to lower social value and pay (World Health Organization, 2019). Additionally, gender bias leads to women earning less than men even in the same occupational category (George, 2007; U.S. Bureau of Labor Statistics, 2018; Robinson, 1998; Rytina, 1982). A comparison of women's monthly wage against their male counterparts in 13 countries in different national income groups found a persistent gap in the following categories of the health workforce: 32% less for physicians, 28% less for dentists, 16% less for professional nurses, 8% less for auxiliary nurses, and 7% less for X-ray technicians (Robinson, 1998). According to the American Association of University Women, three of the top ten jobs with the highest gender pay gap in the United States in 2017 are in the healthcare market, including physicians and surgeons, registered nurses, and medical and health service managers (Advisory Board Daily Briefing, n.d.).

Factors leading to the pay gap are complicated and interlinked and include productivity-related indicators such as training and qualifications, work experience, hours worked per day, and career breaks. Other factors include the aforementioned underestimation of feminized markets such as health care, inflexibility of the market with regard to women who want to combine childcare with their career, and employment in public versus private sectors (Fitzgerald, n.d.). But studies show that these factors do not account for all of the discrepancy observed in the remuneration of men and women in the same occupations. For instance, in Australia, only 40% of the pay gap is attributable to these factors and the remaining 60% can only be explained by direct discrimination or unconscious bias (Fitzgerald, n.d.).

Another aspect of the gender pay gap is the parenthood pay gap. Even though the gender pay gap has been decreasing in recent years, the pay gap related to parenthood has been widening. Having children is associated with lower wages among women and higher wages among men (Budwig, 2014). This phenomenon may be due to the fact that men with children are seen as more committed, stable, and deserving of higher wages. In contrast, women with children are considered less committed to their work and have to pay a motherhood wage penalty (World Health Organization, 2019; Budwig, 2014). It is estimated that on average, each child can lead to a 4% wage penalty for women, and this is further exacerbated in lower-paying jobs such as community health workers, leading to an even wider pay gap (Budwig, 2014).

While the data is limited on the gender pay gap specifically for health systems, there is ample evidence that ignoring the gender pay gap leads to an exacerbation of other gendered inequities, such as a lower accumulated wealth over the lifetime for women, leading to poverty in older women, as well as diminishing their access to pay-related health and social benefits (World Health Organization, 2019; Fitzgerald, n.d.; Sen & Östlin, 2008). Furthermore, women not only receive less pay for a similar job but they face more job insecurity as well (Langer et al., 2015). Health systems employ a considerable proportion of the population. Addressing these inequities in working conditions and pay in health systems can lead to progress in achieving not only gender equity in society but also improved health outcomes for women employed in the health systems, and a more economically prosperous future in the healthcare sector which is projected to account for 40 million new jobs by 2030 (World Health Organization, 2019; Siddons, 2019).

Dual Burdens of Professional Work and Childcare and Household Chores

The pervasive global gender stereotype that assigns men the role of breadwinner and women the role of homemaker and primary caregiver for children (Reskin, 1993) is a significant limiting factor for women's full participation in the workforce and their ascent to higher positions.

When recalling enabling factors for reaching leadership positions, men tend to mention their merits, mentors, training programs, and other institutional factors. Women in the same positions of power often cite additional factors such as having a supportive family and spouse, having domestic help, division of domestic responsibilities, marrying late, or staying single (Dhatt et al., 2017). These types of statements underline the defining role of domestic responsibilities in how women approach work.

Women's participation in health systems as well as their domestic responsibilities leaves them with little time to invest in their health and wellbeing (Langer et al., 2015) or pursue leadership training or other resources enabling them to advance in their career. In fact, women have been penalized for tending to their family and professional duties at the same time. A paradigm shift would ensure that women in the workforce can enjoy full-time work and career breaks, career advancement, further education, as well as a family life (Langer et al., 2015). Additionally, men tend to relocate more easily for their jobs while their wives would follow them and lose accrued years of work in their institution and the associated promotion opportunities (Dhatt et al., 2017).

In the absence of institutional support, women overextend themselves to balance their personal and professional lives, plan pregnancies and manage childcare, develop professionally, and support their spouse's professional advancement as well (George, 2007). A retrospective study in the United States found that 85% of female physicians made career changes for the benefit of their children and family, while only 35% of male physicians did so (Warde et al., 1996).

Division of family care responsibilities allows women to balance work and home life more effectively. This division of responsibilities can be improved by adoption of gender-responsive policies that ensure this double burden of work can be alleviated so that women can enjoy flexible career trajectories and have equal resources and access to leadership roles within health systems (Langer et al., 2015). Such policies promote shared parenthood and subsidized childcare and preserve women's connection to their job market during their childbearing years (Langer et al., 2015). Health systems' governance is improved by designing and implementing policies that allow both men and women to contribute to their sector, in their best capacity, throughout their life course, while integrating their different social, biological, and occupational roles (Langer et al., 2015). Studies have proven that in fact having more women in leadership positions promotes adoption and implementation of these gender-responsive policies (Langer et al., 2015).

"Male" and "Female" Leadership Styles

Equating leadership to masculinity and attributing traits such as autonomy and being result-driven to masculinity and other forms of gender-labeling of leadership and management practices have reproduced stereotypes and reinforced the traditional gendered division of labor (Due Billing & Alvesson, 2000). This phenomenon has assigned everything that is socially perceived as non-masculine to the margins and outside of the organization and made it more difficult for women, often with responsibilities toward their family and children, to be recruited and promoted to positions of power within organizations (Due Billing & Alvesson, 2000).

Studies suggest that while the leadership styles between men and women differ, effective leadership is not exclusively in the domain of any gender, and both can learn from each other in that regard (Appelbaum et al., 2003; Eagly & Carli, n.d.). Women's style of participatory, people-oriented, and socio-expressive leadership, often classified as transformational, can actually yield better results in building coalitions and reaching consensus (Appelbaum et al., 2003; Eagly & Carli, n.d.; Eagly & Johnson, 1990). Women in positions of power and influence have demonstrated more collaborative and democratic work as compared to men's autocratic style of leadership, often classified as transactional. As a result, women are more effective in gaining trust and confidence of their colleagues and subordinates and, in the process, empowering them (Eagly & Johnson, 1990). Health systems are a perfect example of team-based, collaborative organizations that would benefit from more women in managerial positions and higher up in the hierarchy who are able to instill a sense of trust and cooperation in their team.

Stereotypes attributed to women often pose as a strong barrier to their advancement to leadership positions. This is based on both organizational psychology theories and women leaders' anecdotal experience (Koenig et al., 2011). These stereotypes often pertain to women's roles and abilities and are overwhelmingly negative in the work context given that they are incongruous with the common stereotypes of leadership (Eagly & Karau, 2002). In a model dubbed the "lack-of-fit" model, the more a workplace role is inconsistent with the attributes seen in an individual, the higher the expectation of failure for that individual in the role (Koenig et al., 2011). Even if performance is desirable, the unfavorable performance expectation will lead to biased judgments and less favorable performance evaluation. Discrimination is the organization's behavioral outcome of these processes (Koenig et al., 2011).

There is also some evidence that men and women tend to believe good leaders have masculine qualities. Men's collective group interest favors retaining leadership roles for their group (Koenig et al., 2011), contributing to the resistance women face and the increasingly narrow bottleneck they have to navigate to rise to leadership positions. It has been argued that leadership may in fact be more masculine in domains where fewer women are in leadership roles (Koenig et al., 2011).

The general perception is that for women to be accepted as leaders, they need to "behave *like men*," but in doing so they risk losing their "feminine traits" (Kodagoda,

2018) of being caring and kind. However, if women try to take on leadership roles, and more generally, access power of any kind, it can be seen as challenging the "right of men" to hold positions of power. At the same time, women leaders using those "feminine traits" might be undermined for an apparent incapability to do the job and this double standard does not work in their favor (Bourdieu, 2001). Overall, it seems that society is concerned with people who defy gender stereotypes or expectations, such as male nurses and female surgeons, and scrutinizes them to the point that the substance of their work goes unnoticed against their style of leadership and conduct (Eagly & Carli, 2007).

Women's Differential and Relative Lack of Access to Resources That Improve Career Development

Two essential institutional practices that invest in women's career advancement are mentorship and sponsorship. Cultivating mentorship opportunities throughout women's career trajectories in health systems, with a focus on mid-career level when women leaders have a greater risk of leaving the pipeline, provides them with guidance on career advancement, work-life balance, and professional resilience (Dhatt et al., 2017). Sponsorship is a more visible and active form of professional support, a relationship capital, in which women are either underinvested or have less access to. A sponsor would proactively advocate, open doors, and create opportunities for exposure, to demonstrate talent and hard work to a higher-level audience in the system and make a quantifiable difference in career success (Hewlett et al., 2010). Women would benefit additionally from sponsorship as it would allow them to surmount certain gender inequities and biases they face in the workforce (Hewlett et al., 2010). The aforementioned underinvestment is said to be partly due to the fact that women do not intentionally cultivate such relationships to cash out on further along, sometimes due to an underestimation of the crucial role a sponsor can play in one's career. But even women who understand a sponsor's crucial role may view it negatively based on a viewpoint that hard work alone is enough to advance in one's career and getting ahead based on who you know may be an inherently unfair approach. Additionally, a sponsor-protégé relationship might be avoided by highly placed men and highly qualified women to avoid misinterpretations of sexual interest (Hewlett et al., 2010). Moreover, women seem to have less access to sponsors and mentors through networking, owing to the fact that these networks are traditionally dominated by men and breaking into these circles requires spending substantial time after work to engage in activities. This time is seen better spent on family activities by women, not to mention that some of the after-work activities may be fairly undesirable to women (Eagly & Carli, n.d.).

It is worth iterating that mentoring done to fit women into male working models and male norms, without challenging the basis of these models, can lead to an exacerbation of these problematic forms of discrimination that often understand equality as conforming to male norms (George, 2007). This is observed when health workers are treated as being interchangeable within the system under the premise of "gender neutrality," but in fact it is a disguise for the prevalence of male norms, leadership, and the expectation from female health workers to conform to those norms (George, 2007).

Leadership Trajectories

When exploring leadership as a professional concept and examining the gendered experiences in this context, studies highlight that within a broad pattern of women getting fewer leadership opportunities than men, there is also a phenomenon evolving of women being offered particularly difficult opportunities, referred to as the "glass cliff." This term is used to describe a situation where it is more likely to put women into leadership positions when the odds of success are low and circumstances are risky and precarious. This sets them up for failure (Tominc et al., 2017). The glass cliff can have adverse implications for external views about women's abilities as leaders and managers, as well as women's own internal view about their abilities, potentially discouraging women from taking up leadership positions.

On the other hand the "glass escalator" concept is defined as the advantages men receive in so-called women's professions such as nursing, allowing them to progress toward leadership levels more easily and quickly as compared to their female colleagues who are the majority in the profession (Williams, 2013). This is particularly tangible in the health sector, given that women make up the majority of health workers but men ascend to leadership positions more easily and quickly, having the advantage of both the vertical and horizontal segregation.

Conclusion

To have more equitable, gender-responsive, and inclusive health systems that reflect these values at all hierarchical levels, gender biases, as part of an intersectional framework, should be documented and their influence on women's representation within health system leadership should be assessed.

Neutralizing gender stereotypes, improving access to family leave and childcare provisions in a gender equitable manner, assuring equitable access to opportunities at different levels and for different professional cadres, creating enabling environments of success for women and marginalized groups, investment in mentorship of women moving upward in the health system hierarchy, and finally, increased flexibility to accommodate personal, domestic, and family obligations are some recommendations to create an equitable structure for women to have fair representation in health systems leadership (Dhatt et al., 2017; George, 2007).

Although gender biases are widely prevalent at structural and subjective levels, they are not static nor universal, but actively debated, discussed, and adapted at the individual level. These individual attempts must be collectively and systematically expanded through improved policies and programs in health systems to be effective more comprehensively (George, 2007).

Health systems that allow flexible work schedules, shared parenthood benefits, career development, mentoring programs for women with the ambition to reach leadership positions, and increased promotion of competent women to leadership positions will benefit from improved performance, increased productivity, and higher retention of health workers (Langer et al., 2015). Addressing women's leadership in health systems is particularly important given the direct effect it has on reducing inequities in health outcomes for women (Dhatt et al., 2017; Downs et al., 2014). In fact, by addressing gender inequity in the health workforce, disruption of the gender bias in the health systems, affecting both the patients and providers, can be achieved (Gupta et al., 2019).

Health systems should be held accountable to address gender inequities (Hay et al., 2019). Reaching a higher representation of women in health systems leadership requires transformation of the discriminatory institutions, systems, and norms that are currently in place. Achieving gender equity in health systems leadership at all levels is fundamental to tapping into all the potential of the diverse human resources for health in the global community (Dhatt et al., 2017). The result of this effort is not only more gender equity in the human resources for health, but more equity in general, improving health systems' functioning and outcomes, more broadly, including achieving the United Nations Sustainable Development Goals and Universal Health Coverage (Hay et al., 2019).

References

Advisory Board Daily Briefing. (n.d.). *The 10 jobs with the biggest gender pay gaps. (Hint: 3 are in health care.).* Retrieved August 13, 2019, from https://www.advisory.com/daily-briefing/2018/11/28/pay-gap

Appelbaum, S. H., Audet, L., & Miller, J. C. (2003). Gender and leadership? Leadership and gender? A journey through the landscape of theories. *Leadership and Organization Development Journal, 24*(1), 43–51. https://doi.org/10.1108/01437730310457320

Bourdieu, P. (2001). *Masculine domination.* Stanford University Press. https://doi.org/10.2307/3089075

Budwig, M. (2014). *The fatherhood bonus and the motherhood penalty. Parenthood and the gender gap in pay,* Washington (DC). Retrieved August 14, 2019, from https://www.west-info.eu/children-boost-fathers-career-but-damage-mothers/next_-_fatherhood_motherhood/

Chunharas, S., & Davies, D. S. C. (2016). Leadership in health systems: A new agenda for interactive leadership. *Health Systems & Reform, 2*(3), 176–178. https://doi.org/10.1080/23288604.2016.1222794

Commission on Social Determinants of Health (2008). *Closing the gap in a generation health equity through action on the social determinants of health.* Retrieved April 7, 2019, from https://apps.who.int/iris/bitstream/handle/10665/43943/9789241563703_eng.pdf?sequence=1

Dhatt, R., Theobald, S., Buzuzi, S., et al. (2017). The role of women's leadership and gender equity in leadership and health system strengthening. *Global Health, Epidemiology, and Genomics, 2,* e8. https://doi.org/10.1017/gheg.2016.22

Downs, J. A., Reif, L. K., Hokororo, A., & Fitzgerald, D. W. (2014). Increasing women in leadership in global health. *Academic Medicine, 89*(8), 1103–1107. https://doi.org/10.1097/ACM.0000000000000369

Dr. Richard Anker MHMM. (n.d.). Gender-based occupational segregation in the 1990's. Retrieved April 8, 2019, from https://www.ilo.org/declaration/info/publications/eliminationofdiscrimination/WCMS_DECL_WP_18_EN/lang%2D%2Den/index.htm

Due Billing, Y., & Alvesson, M. (2000). Questioning the notion of feminine leadership: A critical perspective on the gender labelling of leadership. *Gender, Work and Organization, 7*(3), 144–157. https://doi.org/10.1111/1468-0432.00103

Eagly, A. H., & Carli, L. L. (2007). *Through the labyrinth: The truth about how women become leaders. PsycNET.* Retrieved April 10, 2019, from https://psycnet.apa.org/record/2008-01900-000

Eagly, A. H., & Carli, L. L. (n.d.). *Women and the labyrinth of leadership.* Retrieved January 1, 2020, from https://hbr.org/2007/09/women-and-the-labyrinth-of-leadership

Eagly, A. H., & Johnson, B. T. (1990). *Gender and leadership style: A meta-analysis; (1990). CHIP Documents.* Retrieved April 8, 2019, from http://digitalcommons.uconn.edu/chip_docs, http://digitalcommons.uconn.edu/chip_docs/11

Eagly, A. H., & Karau, S. J. (2002). Role congruity theory of prejudice toward female leaders. *Psychological Review, 109*(3), 573–598. Retrieved April 10, 2019, from http://www.ncbi.nlm.nih.gov/pubmed/12088246.

Fitzgerald, G. (n.d.). *The gender pay gap.* Retrieved August 13, 2019, from http://levelmedicine.org.au/wp-content/uploads/2017/12/Gender-Pay-Gap.pdf

Gender Equality Glossary and Thesaurus. (n.d.). *European Institute for Gender Equality.* Retrieved April 8, 2019, from https://eige.europa.eu/thesaurus/browse

George, A. 2007. *Human resources for health: A gender analysis background paper prepared for the women and gender equity knowledge network and the health systems knowledge network of the WHO commission on social determinants of health background to the women and gender equity knowledge network.* Retrieved April 7, 2019, from https://www.who.int/social_determinants/resources/human_resources_for_health_wgkn_2007.pdf.

GHWA. (2013). The recife political declaration on human resources for health. *WHO.* Retrieved April 7, 2019, from http://www.who.int/workforcealliance/forum/2013/3gf_finaldeclaration/en/. .

Gilson, L. (2003). Trust and the development of health care as a social institution. *Social Science & Medicine, 56*(7), 1453–1468. Retrieved May 13, 2019, from http://www.ncbi.nlm.nih.gov/pubmed/12614697

Gilson L. *Health policy and systems research—A methodology reader.* World Health Organization; 2017. Retrieved August 15, 2019, from https://www.who.int/alliance-hpsr/resources/reader/en/

Gilson, L., Lehmann, U., & Schneider, H. (2017). Practicing governance towards equity in health systems: LMIC perspectives and experience. *International Journal for Equity in Health, 16*(1), 171. https://doi.org/10.1186/s12939-017-0665-0

Global Health U. (2015). *USAID's vision for health systems strengthening 2015–2019.* Retrieved April 19, 2019, from https://www.usaid.gov/sites/default/files/documents/1864/HSS-Vision.pdf

Gupta, G. R., Oomman, N., Grown, C., et al. (2019). Gender equality and gender norms: framing the opportunities for health. *Lancet (London, England), 393*(10,190), 2550–2562. https://doi.org/10.1016/S0140-6736(19)30651-8

Hawkes, S., & Buse, K. (2019). *Equality works. The global health 50/50 2019 Report.* Retrieved April 7, 2019, from https://globalhealth5050.org/2019-report/

Hay, K., McDougal, L., Percival, V., et al. (2019). Disrupting gender norms in health systems: making the case for change. *Lancet (London, England), 393*(10,190), 2535–2549. https://doi.org/10.1016/S0140-6736(19)30648-8

Hewlett, S. A., Peraino, K., Sherbin, L., & Sumberg, K. (2010). *The sponsor effect: Breaking through the last glass ceiling*. Retrieved April 21, 2019, from http://30percentclub.org/wp-content/uploads/2014/08/The-Sponsor-Effect.pdf

High-Level Commission on Health Employment and Economic Growth. (2016). *Working for health and growth: Investing in the health workforce. Report of the high-level commission on health employment and economic growth*. Retrieved form April 7, 2019, from https://apps.who.int/iris/bitstream/handle/10665/250047/9789241511308-eng.pdf?sequence=1

Kodagoda, T. (2018). Working long hours and its impact on family life: Experiences of women professionals and managers in Sri Lanka. *Indian Journal of Gender Studies, 25*(1), 108–126. https://doi.org/10.1177/0971521517738432

Koenig, A. M., Eagly, A. H., Mitchell, A. A., & Ristikari, T. (2011). Are leader stereotypes masculine? A meta-analysis of three research paradigms. *Psychological Bulletin, 137*(4), 616–642. https://doi.org/10.1037/a0023557

Langer, A., Meleis, A., Knaul, F. M., et al. (2015). Women and health: The key for sustainable development. *Lancet, 386*(9999), 1165–1210. https://doi.org/10.1016/S0140-6736(15)60497-4

Librarian, I. (2018). Resource spotlight: Gender and health workforce statistics. Retrieved April 7, 2019, from https://www.hrhresourcecenter.org/gender_stats.html

Newman, C. (2014). Time to address gender discrimination and inequality in the health workforce. *Human Resources for Health, 12*(1), 25. https://doi.org/10.1186/1478-4491-12-25

Newman, C. J., Fogarty, L., Makoae, L. N., & Reavely, E. (2011). Occupational segregation, gender essentialism and male primacy as major barriers to equity in HIV/AIDS caregiving: Findings from Lesotho. *International Journal for Equity in Health, 10*, 24. https://doi.org/10.1186/1475-9276-10-24

Northouse, P. G. (2015). *Leadership: theory and practice* (7th ed.). Sage Publications.

Project Implicit: Frequently Asked Questions. (2011). Retrieved August 17, 2019, from https://implicit.harvard.edu/implicit/faqs.html

Reskin, B. (1993). Sex segregation in the workplace. *Annual Review of Sociology, 19*(1), 241–270. https://doi.org/10.1146/annurev.so.19.080193.001325

Robinson, D. (1998). *Differences in occupational earnings by sex* (Vol. 137). Macpherson and Hirsch. Retrieved April 23, 2019, from http://www.ilo.int/public/english/revue/download/pdf/robinson.pdf

Rytina, N. F. (1982). *Earnings of men and women: A look at specific Occupations*.Retrieved April 23, 2019, from https://pdfs.semanticscholar.org/db59/0dc3ac3b3458cac317a775645 3e071c79729.pdf

Sen, G., & Östlin, P. (2008). Gender inequity in health: why it exists and how we can change it. *Global Public Health, 3*(suppl 1), 1–12. https://doi.org/10.1080/17441690801900795

Sheikh, K., Gilson, L., Agyepong, I. A., Hanson, K., Ssengooba, F., & Bennett, S. (2011). Building the field of health policy and systems research: Framing the questions. *PLoS Medicine, 8*(8), e1001073. https://doi.org/10.1371/journal.pmed.1001073

Siddons, E. (2019). *Why health's gender pay gap is a problem for everyone*. Apolitical. Retrieved August 14, 2019, from https://apolitical.co/solution_article/why-healths-gender-pay-gap-is-a-problem-for-everyone/

The American Association of University Women. (2016). *Barriers and bias: The status of women in leadership*. Retrieved August 17, 2019, from https://www.aauw.org/app/uploads/2020/03/Barriers-and-Bias-nsa.pdf

Tominc, P., Šebjan, U., & Širec, K. (2017). Perceived gender equality in managerial positions in organizations. *Organizacija, 50*(2), 132–149. Retrieved April 7, 2019, from http://organizacija. fov.uni-mb.si/index.php/organizacija/article/viewFile/758/1155

U.S. Bureau of Labor Statistics (2018). *The Gender Wage Gap by Occupation 2017 and by Race and Ethnicity The Gender Wage Gap Between Occupations*. Retrieved April 23, 2019, from http://www.bls.gov/cps/cpsaat39.htm

Warde, C., Allen, W., & Gelberg, L. (1996). Physician role conflict and resulting career changes. Gender and generational differences. *Journal of General Internal Medicine, 11*(12), 729–735. Retrieved April 24, 2019, from http://www.ncbi.nlm.nih.gov/pubmed/9016419.

WHO. (2014a). Monitoring the building blocks of health systems: a handbook of indicators and their measurement strategies. Retrieved April 23, 2019, from https://www.who.int/healthinfo/systems/monitoring/en/.

WHO. (2014b). *A universal truth report—No health without a workforce.* Retrieved April 6, 2019 from https://www.who.int/workforcealliance/knowledge/resources/hrhreport2013/en/

Williams, C. L. (2013). The glass escalator, Revisited. *Gender and Society, 27*(5), 609–629. https://doi.org/10.1177/0891243213490232

Williams, J. C. (2006). Deconstructing Gender. *Michigan Law Review, 87*(4), 797. https://doi.org/10.2307/1289293

Women in Global Health. (n.d.). *Women in global health in 2018.*

World Health Organization. (2019). *Delivered by women, led by men: A gender analysis of the global health and social workforce.* Retrieved April 7, 2019, from https://apps.who.int/iris/bitstream/handle/10665/311322/9789241515467-eng.pdf?ua=1

Zeinali, Z., Muraya, K., Govender, V., Molyneux, S., & Morgan, R. (2019). Intersectionality and global health leadership: Parity is not enough. *Human Resources for Health, 17*(1), 29. https://doi.org/10.1186/s12960-019-0367-3

Interview with Penina Ochola Odhiambo, Former Dean of the School of Nursing and Midwifery and Current Principal of the College of Health Sciences at the Great Lakes University of Kisumu, Kenya

Rosemary Morgan and Kate Hawkins

"It is an achievement for all when we win, and when we fail, it is everyone's failure".

Dr. Penina Ochola Odhiambo has over 30 years of extensive cross-cultural public health experience in Eastern and Southern Africa working in diverse sociocultural settings. She holds a diploma in advanced nursing from the University of Nairobi and a Master of Public Health degree from the Harvard T.H. Chan School of Public Health and has received a PhD from Great Lakes University of Kisumu, Kenya. She is a founding member of the Tropical Institute of Community Health and Development in Kisumu (TICH) and the Kisumu Medical and Education Trust. In addition, she was previously the country director of African Medical and Research Foundation (AMREF) in South Africa, regional health advisor for PLAN International for Eastern and Southern Africa, and country director for FHI/AIDSCAP in Tanzania and worked for AMREF for 15 years as director of Primary Health Care, a role that extensively exposed her to global health. She was also the dean of the School of Nursing at the Great Lakes University Kisumu. Despite being retired, she continues to do short-term consultancies. She recently coordinated a collaborative research partnership on adolescent sexual and reproductive health between TICH and the University of Hull and conducted a Service Availability and Readiness Assessment for the COVID-19 response in Siaya county, Kenya. She is currently a member of the task force for Universal Health Coverage in Kisumu county, Kenya.

R. Morgan (✉)
Department of International Health, Johns Hopkins Bloomberg School of Public Health, Baltimore, MD, USA
e-mail: Rosemary.morgan@jhu.edu

K. Hawkins
Pamoja Communications Ltd., Research in Gender and Ethics (RinGs), Brighton, East Sussex, UK
e-mail: kate@pamoja.uk.com

© Springer Nature Switzerland AG 2022
R. Morgan et al. (eds.), *Women and Global Health Leadership*,
https://doi.org/10.1007/978-3-030-84498-1_19

Early Years

I am the firstborn child in a family of 11 children. We were eight girls and three boys. My father believed that girls should be given equal opportunities in education as boys, so all the girls and boys in the family are well educated. My father worked for the then East African Railways and Harbours which included Kenya, Uganda, and Tanzania. His work with the railways provided opportunity for the family to travel and live in the three countries, exposing us to people of different sociocultural backgrounds at an early age.

This exposure later became a pillar that helped me particularly to develop a deeper understanding of the way of life of the people, and the issues that affect their lives in health and development. This later added immense value to my professional development. As the firstborn child, I took up a leadership role at a very tender age, supporting my parents in bringing up my siblings, particularly making sure that we all adhered to the standards and values that my father and mother had set for our growing up. It is this earlier exposure to a stimulating environment and adherence to the core values of life that shaped the leadership insight that I have practised over the years.

The exposure instilled a sense of confidence and high levels of performance both at school and at the workplace. This overwhelming support came not only from my loving parents but also from the extended family, especially my paternal grandfather as well as maternal and paternal uncles and aunties. My father was always available to coach us at home. He reviewed our books and helped us to improve in our schoolwork; I owe it to my father and mother who made me and my siblings become what we are today. *Thank you Mama and Baba for a job well done.* Both my parents passed on in their midyears of life at 69 and 57 years, respectively, but I remained a strong pillar of strength for the family.

As I was growing up, I was influenced by a cousin of mine who had gone to the UK to study nursing. Each time she came back home for holidays, I admired her stories about nursing as a career; she became my professional role model and I decided to take up nursing as a career. I studied nursing up to the highest level which was the diploma in advanced nursing at the University of Nairobi, a qualification that prepared me well to take leadership in nursing education and nursing administration. I later went to Harvard T.H. Chan School of Public Health to study for a Master of Public Health degree. This was a multidisciplinary class that helped me to mingle with people from diverse social and professional backgrounds coming from different parts of the world. The Harvard experience was an eye opener; it gave me the worldview of health and development and facilitated my professional growth in public health. I am currently completing my PhD at Great Lakes University of Kisumu. My leadership was nurtured by an enabling environment at home, at school, and at the workplace and a wide range of role models, mentors, and well-wishers.

A Wealth of Experiences

In 1978 at Alma-Ata, primary health care (PHC) was born; the whole world was thrilled about "Health for All" by the year 2000, a slogan that was popularized by Dr Halfdan Mahler who was then director-general of the World Health Organization (WHO). During that period, I was a young professional nurse, teaching undergraduate nurses; I was also the chairperson for the National Nurses Association of Kenya (NNAK), the Rift Valley Branch. The Alma-Ata Declaration was expected to bring change where the voiceless members of communities, like women, would participate in matters that affected their lives. Consultation and participation by all and self-reliance were the ultimate goals. All sectors had a role to play, and the Chief Nursing Officer at that time, Dr Muringo Kiriaini, gave a directive that all nurses be given orientation on PHC to help them understand their role.

As the chair of NNAK, I was tasked with the responsibility of rolling out the concept for nurses in the Rift Valley region of Kenya. PHC was getting popularized in Kenya and other countries of the developing world; it was like wildfire! The assignment was enormous since I had no idea what the concept was all about, but I took it with courage and searched for information about the Alma-Ata Declaration and its implementation strategy. The information was readily available in the library; it was particularly well articulated in a journal called *MEDICOM* (the African journal of hospital and scientific medicine). The information was detailed and very exciting; it later influenced my interest in primary health care. The assignment was an eye opener, a turning point that enriched my career. I never looked back as I developed interest in PHC and public health as a whole. The experience opened doors to other opportunities for leadership in public health.

My subsequent career progression was full of exciting challenges that made me grow even better in my leadership role. The most exciting experience was my 15 years working with the African Medical and Research Foundation (AMREF) where I headed the division of primary care/community-based health care (PHC/CBHC), a position that exposed me further into global health. Presenting papers at scientific conferences on best practices from the field, I participated in technical working groups to contribute and add value to the strategy of PHC/CBH. For example, as a temporary advisor to WHO, I contributed to issues on community participation in PHC, the role of community health workers in the health system, and health centers in the context of the district health system. I was familiar with the vast health issues of the region of Eastern and Southern Africa and sub-Saharan Africa as a whole. The experience enabled me to train and equip mid-level managers of health with skills to design and implement PHC/CBHC programs in the countries of Eastern and Southern African countries, as well as supporting the development of strategic plans, evaluating and designing community-based primary health-care programs with NGOs and faith-based organizations in partnership with the government health sectors where AMREF worked.

The wealth of experience at AMREF was valuable as it provided opportunities to contribute to global health agendas, particularly around maternal, newborn, and child health; HIV/AIDS and adolescent sexual health; and malaria and other communicable diseases. Interaction with people from diverse professional and sociocultural backgrounds enriched my worldview and understanding of global health issues. AMREF was like a school—it sharpened my professional and leadership skills that subsequently earned me positions as country director with FHI (AIDSCAP program), funded by USAID in Tanzania; regional health advisor with Plan International providing technical guidance to 13 countries of the regions of Eastern and Southern Africa; country director in Pretoria, South Africa with AMREF; and finally going back to academia as the dean of the School of Nursing at the Great Lakes University of Kisumu. I have retired, but as they say—I am not tired! I still find time to contribute as a member of the board of trustees of the Tropical Institute of Community Health (TICH) in Kisumu where I am also a founder member, a board member and treasurer of the Kisumu Medical and Education Trust (KMET), and as one of the founders of the Great Lakes University of Kisumu. In addition, I am still doing short-term consultancy in health.

What Makes a Good Leader?

Leadership is about getting the best out of people, creating a friendly working environment that allows people to make mistakes and explore possible solutions at the workplace. After all, making mistakes is also part of the learning process. This kind of leadership builds confidence and makes people open to discussions around gaps and remedies, allowing them to make changes without feeling intimidated. This requires a leader who is not threatened by colleagues who excel in their work; he or she embraces excellence from team members and pats them on the shoulders when an excellent job is accomplished. A good leader is consultative and applies the principle of collective responsibility, nurturing both hidden talents and professional aptitudes. A good leader creates an enabling environment which is friendly and allows for creative thinking to harness the potential that people possess. A good leader is tolerant and able to resolve conflicts at the workplace. He or she is knowledgeable, competent, and people centered.

Leading from the Front

A good leader also leads from the front, not from behind, exuding confidence and understanding of the context and direction to be followed toward the set goal. Leading from the front means that the leader is constantly scanning the environment, looking at factors that influence success or failure; a visionary leader is aware of competitors and the comparative advantages that her organization brings to the table. A leader who leads from the front is on top of her game, passionate about the work of the team, constantly providing timely and clear direction. That kind of a leader has people management skills. A leader with poor interpersonal skills often destroys the team spirit, resulting in chaos at the workplace.

A leader who leads from the front understands the tasks of each team member and has the ability to coach staff toward the desired results. They regularly hold dialogue to harmonize the team's efforts toward the goal. Leading from the front helps the leader to understand characteristics of team members and the overall capability of the organization. It helps a leader to learn from the people they are leading as they become conversant with global and local issues which are shared from time to time to improve performance and visibility of the organization. Democratic leadership is good, but caution must be applied to control its abuse; some degree of firmness is required to make it work better. Steering the team toward the vision means that team capacity is built, and that team members are motivated to work for the good of their own personal growth and excellence of the organization. An enabling environment is key, as it provides freedom and space for people to actively participate and share experiences. It is about collective responsibility and a consultative leadership that respects and values contributions from every member.

Throughout my leadership, whether as a country director, regional health advisor, trainer, or even as the dean of the School of Nursing, I recognized potentials that people brought to the workplace. Harnessing the innate attributes and expertise helped to harmonize efforts to achieve the set standards and goals.

A Woman Leader in an Organization Run by Men

Working in a male-led organization can be challenging for women leaders, and one has to devise tactics of survival. The organizations I worked for were male led, but as the country director or regional health advisor I also led multidisciplinary teams of men and women. They included PhD holders, social scientists, nurses, teachers, and medical doctors. The executive directors at AMREF, FHI, and Plan International were pro gender, gender mainstreaming in programming was embraced as a strategy, and opportunities were provided for both men and women to excel equally in their roles.

What makes me happy is that I have earned respect from both the men and women that I have worked with. However, my worst experience is when I competed for a consultancy to lead a strategic plan development on PHC in Namibia. I was competing with a very high-ranking medical doctor in the country. I nearly missed the job! Why? Probably because my competitor was a male executive. I felt intimidated by the impressions that the assignment gave in relation to needing an experienced senior person. However, that was not the case, all the Namibia government needed was someone with experience in PHC/CBHC, period! My CV met the criteria and I was ultimately the preferred consultant. The Health Ministry in Namibia was male dominated comprising returnees from exile, who were already exposed to public health matters from the countries where they had resided, but I simply had to put my best foot forward and perform to the best of my ability. The national strategy for PHC/CBHC was finally completed and was launched by His Excellency, the President of the Republic of Namibia Sam Nujoma; it was a colorful occasion held in a stadium in the presence of dignitaries. I later went back to Namibia to help roll out the strategy in the whole country. A successful mission which put me on the map and contributed to my growth immensely.

My determination carried me through to win the hearts of both men and women. I proved my worth, and one has to overcome such challenges or else you end up with a crashed self-esteem, leading to worthlessness. Cultivating a team spirit, a good working environment where people feel equal and empowered, can defuse male dominance. As the workplace is the second home where people spend long hours, it has to be friendly, enjoyable, empowering, and comfortable for all to be productive. Teamwork is all about winning or losing together, success is for everyone—whether man or woman, it is an achievement for all when we win, and when we fail it is everyone's failure. A woman leader can feel threatened, intimidated, and worthless if confronted by these negative challenges, making her confused and disorganized. Women must be strong and focused in whatever they do despite the challenges they may face. A woman has to work hard to prove herself in a male-dominated environment. I always had a strong voice within my heart that continuously encouraged me to be strong; this inner voice encouraged me to do my best to overcome obstacles in life.

It's a Man's World

Even to get one woman who has a voice, to get the voices of other ordinary women out there is a struggle. In Kenya, the policy is very clear, they talk about the one-third gender rule, but Parliament can't pass it. Nobody is really serious about women's participation in leadership. Yes, it is written but it is not executed. Women have fought in this country for that particular policy to be passed, but men gang up and they make sure that it doesn't go through. It tells you that we still have issues to deal with. Why would men feel uncomfortable with that policy which is simply saying "one-third gender rule" to allow more women to participate in nation building? A policy like that must be supported by political leadership. The few women that are already in leadership positions are still fighting to make sure that the voices of women, even those at the grassroots, are heard and to contribute to matters that affect their health and economic empowerment.

Policies and strategies often do not consult a wide spectrum of women; the policymakers are not cognizant of women's role in health and development. And a lot of development projects fail because they are top down, omitting the voices of the silent majority in the society, the women! Particularly those in remote poor settings. Who will speak for them if policies like the one-third gender rule are not taken seriously? It means that men still hold the keys to economic empowerment. Poor women are the wearers of the shoe and they know where the shoe is pinching; therefore, more women leaders are required to reach out for the majority of women left out of the health and development agenda. Women who struggle to make ends meet, the women of this world—where are their voices? Who will speak for them on matters that affect their lives? Encouraging women to have a voice on matters that affect their lives at every level in every country from the grassroots to global level is the direction to go if the world is serious about achieving lasting change in health and development. It is retrogressive not to endorse a policy that empowers women leaders, who should themselves reach and empower the voiceless mothers. And not to endorse a policy is an indication that major issues affecting women will go unattended, that the voices of women are lost at the top decision-making table. What do men fear about more women participating in leadership? Women are the workers in every front; we need more of them at the policy and decision-making tables. We have a long way to go. It is still a tough world; it is still a man's world!

Balancing Work and Home Life

There were challenges along the way. I had two children: a girl and a boy ages 14 and 7 years who needed very close parental guidance. My job was demanding. As I travelled extensively overseas, within Africa, and locally within Kenya, it was tough for them, but I constantly explained why I had to travel. I remember my late son Jim would draw a graph showing the days I was in or out of the house—"mummy in, mummy out"—and he would diligently count the number of nights I was away. It was definitely a great challenge which made me occasionally take them along with me. That was the balancing act that I employed to make sure they grew up well and were not challenged by the nature of my job. Oh! They always looked forward to the travel away from home with mummy. I think the challenges had some indirect positive influence in their lives later. My son passed on when he was at fourth year at the university—he was a strong leader who was very popular among his peers and a great basketball player, who was celebrated by his colleagues even after he had long gone. My daughter worked with the World Health Organization (WHO) where she travelled extensively in West Africa and Europe. It was a tough growing up, but I was a role model at the same time.

The Importance of Women Role Models

AMREF as an organization was home to me. I interacted with experienced leaders who coached me to become a good leader; I worked there for 15 years. My potential was discovered and nurtured. I was surrounded by people who were highly experienced. Leaders who got the best out of people. I emulated their style of leadership and put it into practice. The numerous interactions with people from diverse cultures and experiences enriched my overall leadership abilities. The period of growing up can be tricky and young people, particularly girls, who face numerous challenges as they grow up needing a conducive environment that helps them to discover themselves.

Role modeling for girls by older experienced women is transformative as they emulate some characteristics that can influence their behavior to become responsible women leaders. Role modeling prepares them for their future roles as mothers as well as contributors to the workforce. In the African traditional society, girls and boys were coached by older women and men like grandmothers and grandfathers or aunties or uncles. They had a variety of skills, which helped them to face their different roles in life. Role modeling is still very relevant today, particularly when young people are exposed to numerous information that can cause confusion in their lives and distract them from achieving their full potential.

I admired some women in my life; they were women that one would call "women of substance," women with outstanding characteristics—brilliant, confident, people-centered, and all together. These women were supportive of women's affairs. I interacted with them directly or admired them from afar. A good example is Maya Angelou whose books I enjoyed reading; each book of Maya had important life lessons. Some of my role models were within the extended family—they influenced my decision to go into nursing. At my young age, I was a great admirer of Honorable Dr Phoebe Asiyo, a woman politician in Kenya who is about 87 years to date. She was a member of parliament who was never intimidated to speak her mind on gender issues even when challenged by male politicians during her political campaigns and during debates in parliament—she is always very articulate, intelligent, confident, and brave. She pushed gender issues boldly amidst objections from men, but the debate continued over the years culminating into the policy of the one-third gender rule that has not been implemented to date.

Dr Asiyo, together with other outstanding women of the world, organized the 1985 UN World Conference on Women that was held in Nairobi, Kenya. I had just arrived from Harvard after completing my master's degree in public health and was in good time to participate in this conference. I admired Phoebe and her team; they articulated women's issues, demonstrating their organizational skills and exuding confidence in facilitating the conference proceedings. There was always something to learn from them. I got inspired and I said to myself quietly: "one day I hope I will be like these ladies." I was being mentored from afar.

I have met Phoebe several times after that and I still admire her intellect, dignity, and beauty. Phoebe has remained focused on women's issues. She was one of the earlier women politicians when Kenya had only three women in parliament. A strong voice that echoed loud and clear on behalf of the majority of the voiceless women. She was never threatened by her male counterparts in politics. When she came back from the Beijing women conference, she was fiery and tabled gender issues for debate in Parliament, men shouted at her, but she was not intimidated at all. She fought with dignity and courage, not losing her integrity and focus, a politician who has held the hands of many young women to grow to their full potential. These attributes make her my role model.

Dame Nita Barrow was also among the women that I admired. Nita Barrow was already renowned in her nursing and midwifery career—she was the first woman governor-general in her country, Barbados. She is a very strong and intelligent woman.

Young girls must admire qualities and virtues of a role model who can influence and make a difference in their lives. As a young woman, admire and interact with someone whose character appeals and adds value to your life, and emulate the characteristics that appeal to you. Such people can be found from reading books, or people who surround you in media, or physically in the community where you live.

The Importance of Women in Leadership

Putting more women in leadership at various levels from grassroots to global platforms can influence realistic policies that are sometimes written without consciousness about issues that women go through. We need women leaders who are conscious of what is happening at the grassroots level. We need women leaders who will represent poor women at various levels up to the global level to talk on behalf of those at the grassroots, to talk for women whose voices cannot been heard in policymaking. That woman must be well versed with issues affecting fellow women at all levels of development, a woman passionate on women's issues, and have the zeal to articulate these issues. She can deal with challenges often faced by women in leadership. There are many brilliant women out there in the communities, at the country level, and at the global level, women facilitators who can join hands to transform this world and help women unleash their capabilities and contribute to the development of this world, whose voices could be brought to the fore to transform this world and make it a better place for all to live in.

Systemic Barriers to Career Growth: Women Outreach Workers of India

Manasee Mishra, Barun Kanjilal, and Dilip Ghosh

Background

Women in contemporary India are engaged in a wide range of health careers. They are in various health-related occupations in the formal sector of the country's economy, pursuing conventional professions (e.g. physicians and nurses) as well as new age careers such as those of medical transcriptionists and healthcare managers. Historically, women have been midwives in the country, assisting pregnant women during childbirth. Mavalankar and colleagues note that India had well-trained European and indigenous midwives during the period of British colonial rule (Mavalankar et al., 2011). The widespread presence of women in India's health workforce in recent decades is due to several reasons. These include the spread of modern education in Indian society during the period of British colonialism, the continued emphasis on girls' education in independent India, and affirmative action by the Indian state. The country has also transitioned to becoming a fast-growing partner in the global modern economy, offering numerous careers in health. Women are at the frontline of community health programming in the country, consciously mobilized by the Indian state and non-governmental organizations (NGOs) for this work. This chapter is an elucidation of India's feminized outreach workforce and its limited presence in the country's health bureaucracy. It concludes with suggestions on how its health systems could be more accommodative of such talent, enabling women outreach workers to assume leadership positions in the health bureaucracy.

M. Mishra (✉)
IIHMR University, Jaipur, India

B. Kanjilal
Retired, IIHMR University, Jaipur, India

D. Ghosh
Retired, Department of Health and Family Welfare, Government of West Bengal, Kolkata, India

© Springer Nature Switzerland AG 2022
R. Morgan et al. (eds.), *Women and Global Health Leadership*,
https://doi.org/10.1007/978-3-030-84498-1_20

207

India has several states and centrally administered union territories (Government of India, n.d.-a). Health is on the "State List" of the Indian Constitution with "public health and sanitation; hospitals and dispensaries" being the domain of the constituent states (Government of India, n.d.-b). Nevertheless, the central government formulates policies on health for the country. It often designs and rolls out centrally funded programmes and schemes which are then implemented by the states and the union territories within their respective administrative boundaries. The state governments formulate their policies on health, and design and implement programmes. The public healthcare delivery system in urban India is not well defined. Local municipalities may run different types of healthcare facilities that include hospitals, clinics, dispensaries, and health units. Some such facilities date back to the colonial era. Consequently, the state-run urban health infrastructure differs considerably across cities of India. The National Urban Health Mission (NUHM) is recent, having been launched in 2013. It lays down norms for setting up an Urban Primary Health Centre (1 per population of 50,000–60,000) and an Urban Community Health Centre (1 per 5 to 6 Urban Primary Health Centres) in big cities (Government of India, n.d.-c). The states and union territories are currently in the process of setting up such healthcare facilities in their urban areas. In contrast, the state-run public healthcare delivery system in rural India is decades old, standardized, and guided by defined population norms. The Indian Public Health Standards (IPHS)—formulated in 2007 and revised in 2012—sets the standards for the different tiers of healthcare facilities in rural India, with an objective of meeting the dynamic public health challenges facing the country. As per IPHS, there should be one Sub-Centre per 5000 population in the plains, and 3000 population in hilly and tribal areas. IPHS envisages the Sub-Centre as the "first contact point with the community", serving as an "interface with the community at the grass-root level, providing all the primary health care services" (Government of India, n.d.-d). There needs to be a Primary Health Centre (PHC) per 30,000 population in the plains and 20,000 population in the hilly and tribal areas. A Rural Hospital/Community Health Centre is the next level healthcare facility, catering to a population of 100,000. A sub-district/sub-divisional hospital is an important link in the chain, being a referral destination for the lower-level state-run healthcare facilities (Government of India, n.d.-e). The District Hospital is at the apex of the rural public healthcare delivery system in a district. The profile of the required human resources at each level of facility is defined as well. Outreach workers provide preventive, promotive, and curative services at the Sub-Centre level, as well as implement "all" national health programmes. The PHC is a bedded facility with qualified medical practitioners at the helm. The higher-level facilities in the district are focused on curative care and have several specialist doctors.

India's Feminized Outreach Workforce

Women dominate the health workforce in the world. It is estimated that 67% of the health workforce in 104 countries are women (WHO, 2019). It is a gendered pattern though. In most countries, men tend to be physicians, dentists, and pharmacists, while women concentrate in nursing and midwifery jobs. However, the share of women in conventionally men-dominated careers has been increasing in recent times (WHO, 2019). Women are particularly valued in some health careers. A "gender-balanced" health workforce is considered to be critical to securing the health of women and children across countries in the world (WHO, 2010a). Notwithstanding the numerical preponderance of women in the health workforce, their limited representation in leadership positions and the gender pay gap are telling statements on gender inequity in the sector. Gender transformative policies are therefore being mooted in order "to address inequities and eliminate gender-based discrimination in earnings, remove barriers to access to full-time employment, and support access to professional development and leadership roles" (WHO, 2019).

There is a wide variety of community health workers (CHWs) in low- and middle-income countries (Olaniran et al., 2019). In their study of ten different cadres of CHWs in five countries in Asia and Africa, Olaniran and colleagues find that, irrespective of their training duration and characteristics, "all CHWs identify pregnant women, provide health education and screen for maternal health conditions" (Olaniran et al., 2019). India is one of the countries in the study. The authors observe that CHWs across the study countries are "under pressure to provide" maternal and newborn health services "beyond their scope of practice and there was a tendency for CHWs in some settings to take on a healthcare facility-based role at the expense of a more traditional community-based role" (Olaniran et al., 2019).

The association of women outreach workers with maternal and child healthcare is a gendered one. They are accessible to women who would otherwise not confide in male health workers. The cultural norm of secluding women from (unrelated) men has been in practice in many societies, both historically and during contemporary times (Esposito, 2003). Moreover, pregnancy and childbirth are exclusively experienced by women and the profession of midwifery continues to be dominated by women in modern times.

Maternal and child health issues have dominated the public health agenda of India. Women constitute a large and visible workforce engaged in it. Historically, there have been several cadres of women outreach workers in rural India. In 1951, there were 578 women health visitors in the country, the number increasing to 4283 in 1970 (Government of India, 1974). The Auxiliary Nurse Midwife (ANM) has been an important actor in India's public healthcare delivery system. Typically, an ANM is a high school-educated woman who undergoes a 2-year course on nursing and midwifery. She is posted in a Sub-Centre/PHC and is primarily responsible for outreach work in the community. This includes generating awareness on wide-ranging issues, identifying cases, and providing services. She has a varied job description with community-based outreach services in maternal and child health forming the core of her job function. She is "squarely responsible" for maintaining and updating the registers on couples eligible for contraception (Government of India, n.d.-d). Over the years, the capacities of the ANMs have been stretched with increases in population and workload without a commensurate expansion of public healthcare facilities in rural India. There has been a change in the work profile of an ANM too. It has been observed that, in the 1960s, an ANM used to provide services pertaining to assistance during childbirth and basic curative care. Over time, her work has changed to the promotion of contraception and preventive services (Mavalankar & Vora, 2008).

The post of the second ANM was created under India's flagship programme, National Rural Health Mission (NRHM). The second ANM was to complement the ANM, who was found to be deficient in attending "to the complete needs of maternal and child care in any village" (Government of India, n.d.-f). The second ANM is appointed on contract and should be a woman residing in a village that falls under the jurisdiction of the Sub-Centre (Government of India, n.d.-f). IPHS recommends that two ANMs (one essential and one desirable) be posted in those Sub-Centres where childbirths are not carried out. Two ANMs (essential) are recommended for those Sub-Centres where childbirths are conducted. If the number of childbirths is 20 or more in a month, then a Staff Nurse needs to be posted in such Sub-Centres. An ANM is to be posted there in the event of the non-availability of a Staff Nurse (Government of India, n.d.-d). In the year 2005, there were 133,194 Female Health Workers/ANMs in position. The cadre has grown in the last decade, the corresponding figure being 219,980 in the year 2016 (Government of India, n.d.-g). There may be other posts such as those of the Lady Health Visitor or Health Supervisor (Female) in public healthcare facilities—the gendered terminology being telling.

Another development has led to the augmentation of the ranks of women outreach workers in rural India. The cadre of Accredited Social Health Activist (ASHA) was created under the NRHM as a part of "architectural correction" of India's healthcare system. ASHAs are locally resident volunteers who cater to a population of 1000 persons. They need to be educated at least till Class Eight. A core strategy of the NRHM is to "promote access to improved healthcare at household level" through ASHAs (Government of India, n.d.-f). Their work includes motivating pregnant women to opt for childbirth in healthcare facilities, promoting immunization, encouraging the adoption of contraceptive methods, and carrying out village-level health education activities. Their work profile has expanded over the years. They are now provided with a drug kit containing medicines for minor ailments, and testing kits for pregnancy and malaria. ASHAs are provided an honorarium of INR (Indian National Rupee) 2000 per month, and receive several task-linked incentives. The ANMs act as facilitators so that ASHAs may discharge their roles well. They also monitor the activities of ASHAs (Government of India, n.d.-h). Initially 400,000 ASHAs were to be recruited upon the launch of NRHM in the last decade (Government of India, n.d.-f). As of September 2018, a total of 1,031,751 ASHAs had been selected in states and union territories of India (Government of India, n.d.-i).

Outreach workers in urban India tend to be women as well. They are unevenly spread due to the amorphous nature of the state-run urban healthcare facilities that are run by municipal bodies in the country. The NUHM seeks to secure public health in the rapidly urbanizing country by strengthening its urban health infrastructure. It stipulates 1 ANM per 10,000 population. An ASHA is to function as a community link worker per 200–500 households in urban areas (Government of India, n.d.-c). Often, female volunteers play a supplementary role in community-based outreach activities in urban India. The NUHM (as well as the NRHM) have since been subsumed under the overarching National Health Mission. Given the recency of the urban component, it will take time for the programme to mature on the ground, offering careers in health for its personnel.

There is another large cadre of women outreach workers in India. The *Anganwadi* Workers (AWWs) are women providing a host of services to women and children at the hamlet level. They are a part of India's Integrated Child Development Services (ICDS), a mammoth country-wide scheme aimed at providing wide-ranging services to young children, pregnant and lactating women, and adolescents. The services include pre-school education and supplementary nutrition. AWWs are attached to *Anganwadi* Centres (AWCs) which are hamlet-based centres functioning as sites for community-based outreach activities on health and nutrition. As of December 2018, there were 1,370,457 operational AWCs spread across rural and urban India (Government of India, n.d.-j). The number of AWWs stood at 1,307,576 as per recent records (Government of India, n.d.-k).

In contrast to the burgeoning women outreach workers, there is a dying cadre of Male Health Workers in the country. The cadre was created in 1974 and typically provides outreach services in areas that fall beyond the remit of maternal and child health. The IPHS recommends that one Male Health Worker is essential in every Sub-Centre, irrespective of whether childbirths are conducted there or not (Government of India, n.d.-d). It also recommends that Male Health Workers should be posted "on priority" in areas where vector-borne diseases are endemic (Government of India, n.d.-d). Such workers are particularly expected to be engaged with various grassroots-level activities of the National Vector Borne Disease Control Programme of India (Government of India, n.d.-d). They are expected to take a lead in carrying out surveys in the area in order to identify and refer, inter alia, persons with skin lesions or other symptoms indicative of leprosy, visual and hearing impairments, mental health problems and epilepsy, and those affected by fluorosis (Government of India, n.d.-d). As per recent reports, there are 56,263 Male Health Workers in position at the Sub-Centres, as against the sanctioned strength of 89,296. The required number of Male Health Workers at the Sub-Centres is considerably higher at 156,231 (Government of India, n.d.-l). Thus, Male Health Workers occupy far fewer posts than what is required, leading to a large shortfall. Even the number of posts that are sanctioned to be filled is about 57% of the required strength. As Male Health Workers retire, states in India have either not been able to get the posts filled by suitable candidates, or have stopped filling the vacant posts due to resource constraints (Government of India, 2010). Consequently, the number of Male Health Workers shows a declining trend in recent decades (Government of India, 2010). The recent National Health Policy of India recommends the "revival and strengthening" of this cadre of outreach workers so that the emerging challenges of infectious and non-communicable diseases could be "effectively" managed at the community level (Government of India, n.d.-m).

Systemic Barriers to Career Growth

Across the world, women of different social groups have different career trajectories in health. Women from the advantaged social groups are more likely to be in well-paying, professional jobs, having benefitted from socio-political developments resulting in their improved social status (Mishra, 2016). Owing to better opportunities, they have been ahead of their less privileged sisters in matters of professional education and employment. In India, women physicians and bureaucrats usually hail from the upper castes and the upper/middle classes residing in the urban areas. They are college educated and are more likely to acquire professional qualifications and pursue respectable and well-paying careers. They are well versed in English—the language of professional communication in the country.

Bureaucracy is a "specific form of organization defined by complexity, division of labour, permanence, professional management, hierarchical coordination and control, strict chain of command, and legal authority" (Rockman, 2019). The health bureaucracy of the governments at the central and state levels in India comprises techno-managerial personnel responsible for securing population health. Members of India's coveted civil services—Indian Administrative Service (IAS)—occupy the highest echelons of the health bureaucracy at the central and the state levels in the country. They are responsible for policy making and providing programmatic directions. They are a part of the permanent executive, which has been historically elitist in its character, and vested with immense powers. The cadre has been reflective of a colonial state and, subsequently, a newly independent country engaged in nation building. Career bureaucrats are aided by technocrats who are typically physicians or nurses.

There is an increasing visibility of women at different levels of the health bureaucracy at the central and state levels in the country. About 50 years ago, there were 6.1 women physicians and surgeons per hundred men (Government of India, 1974). Women had begun to specialize in disciplines that were non-conventional for them then, such as radiology and anaesthesia. They were beginning to hold positions such as administrators of hospitals and public health programmes. Decades later, retired women career bureaucrats and physicians constitute a part of the country's upper classes who have served distinguished careers. There is a prominent representation of upper caste, urban women hailing from upper/middle classes in various professions in India today, including those in the health sector.

But the career paths of ANMs, ASHAs, and AWWs are markedly different. They constitute the subaltern in a context where leaders are drawn from the permanent executive which hails from a different social milieu. The leadership possesses techno-managerial skills that are distinct from those of the women outreach workers. A senior ANM may become a Public Health Nurse, which is a district-level position responsible for outreach activities in the area. At the pinnacle of her career, she would be in a *mofussil* town overseeing the implementation of community health activities in the surrounding (rural) areas. Opportunities remain limited for her in the existing career progression pathways. Postings in the state capitals are unlikely since state-run healthcare facilities are usually located in rural India. Nor does she enjoy a position with a structured and definite mandate to participate in, and meaningfully contribute to, policies and programmes, drawing from her decades of rich experience in community-based outreach work. She participates limitedly in consultation meetings on health policies and planning at the state or the central levels. Her representation at the central level is non-existent too. Institutional arrangements do not exist wherein her rich knowledge of the field could be systematically tapped into during policy and programme formulation. (ANMs may occasionally be a part of consultation meetings, though. For instance, ANMs have been a part of consultation meetings during the revision of IPHS guidelines.) With her non-representation at the senior levels of the health bureaucracy, and her limited participation in the formulation of policies and programmes, decades-long experience of working with local communities is not leveraged systemically.

The career paths of AWWs are just as limited. A senior AWW may be promoted to the position of an ICDS Supervisor and thus, become a part of the supervisory cadre that monitors the work of *Anganwadi* workers. Despite the ICDS being women dominated, systemic barriers exist in it that limit the participation of AWWs and ICDS Supervisors in deliberations on policy and programme formulation. Senior levels in the ICDS are occupied by college-educated professionals whose socio-demographic backgrounds are at variance from that of the school-educated AWWs. The AWWs remain largely restricted to their hamlets, responsible for community-based outreach work. They are subalterns like the ANMs, socio-demographically distinct and with expertise and experience that is not institutionally tapped into during policy and programme formulation. Thus, there are structural impediments to the growth of the AWWs within the system.

ASHAs and other volunteers are usually not considered to be a part of the health systems. Volunteerism has often been a characteristic feature of CHWs across countries of the world (WHO, 2010b). CHWs are expected to be "posted in the areas that they belong to so to assure maximal local engagement and ownership" (WHO, 2010b). CHW programmes need to be "driven, owned by, and firmly embedded in communities" or risk being on the "geographical and organizational periphery of the formal health system" (WHO, 2007). Moreover, ASHAs are new and ad hoc, indispensable though they may be. It has been commented that they are overworked, undervalued, and undercompensated (Kammowanee, 2019). It may however be mentioned here that the National Health Policy of India "supports certification programme for ASHAs for their preferential selection into ANM, nursing, and paramedical courses" (Government of India, n.d.-m). It concedes that most ASHAs would continue to provide voluntary services in the community. However, "those who obtain qualifications for career opportunities could be given more regular terms of engagement" (Government of India, n.d.-m).

Climbing the Health Bureaucracy

There are systemic barriers to the professional growth of women outreach workers in India. The higher levels of its health bureaucracy—at both the central and the state levels—are structurally distinct from the cadres of outreach workers that constitute the frontlines. There is limited organic growth for the latter within the bureaucracy. The health systems in India present a microcosm of the widespread socio-demographic inequities prevalent in the country. Personnel at different levels hail from different social backgrounds and experience the associated privileges or disadvantages. The structural distinctions become more pronounced for women due to the historical neglect they have faced in terms of education, employment, and participation in the public sphere.

Another systemic reason is the bifurcation of health and nutrition services in India. Usually, separate departments oversee health and the ICDS at both the state and the central levels in the country. At the state level, ANMs and ASHAs are with the Department of Health and Family Welfare, while AWWs work for the Department of Women and Child Development. The two departments are under separate ministries at the central level, viz. Ministry of Health and Family Welfare, and the Ministry of Women and Child Development, respectively. ANMs, ASHAs, and AWWs do work jointly in reaching out to local communities. Active dialogue takes place between the two departments and their respective ministries too. However, the distinct organizational hierarchies and lines of management limit career opportunities for the women outreach workers across the allied fields of health and nutrition. This presents a systemic barrier to their growth. As it is, their participation is limited in forums hosted by senior levels in their respective departments/ministries. Participation in high-level deliberations on policy and programme formulation in the non-parent department/ministry is systemically blocked. Restricted career growth and limited opportunities to share their rich knowledge of the field are, thus, further constricted by the bifurcation.

A few years ago, a proposal to augment the clinical skills and autonomy of nurses was mooted in India. It envisaged their career progression through the acquisition of academic degrees, on- the- job skill enhancement, and the shouldering of managerial responsibilities (Government of India, n.d.-n). If realized, it would have led to strengthened health systems in a country where there is a shortage of doctors in its public healthcare facilities. More recently, it has been recognized in the draft National Education Policy that there is "severe under-capacity" in many professions in India, including the nursing profession (Government of India, 2019). There is a commitment in the policy to the creation of "professional development pathways for nurses with different levels of qualifications" (Government of India, 2019). It is considered important to develop the capacities of nurses so that they can "compensate in part for the non-availability of doctors" (Government of India, 2019). However, there is no mention in the draft policy document of the capacity building of outreach workers in the health sector. This is in spite of its recognition of "a more holistic approach to healthcare that balances wellness, prevention, and cure" and calls for reforms in healthcare education aiming to improve the quality of infrastructure for primary and secondary healthcare, especially in rural India (Government of India, 2019).

The country is witnessing major public health challenges. Historically, India's public health orientation has had a medical bias with a strong focus on doctors. The focus is misplaced in a country where many social determinants are compromised, and medical professionals are scarce and concentrated in its urban areas. Therefore, the recent policy commitment to the development of mid-level service providers in India for providing comprehensive primary care is welcome. It envisages the building of the capacities of such professionals through undergraduate courses in community health and/or competency-based bridge courses and short courses (Government of India, n.d.-m). A career progression pathway for Nurse Practitioners in Midwifery has been contemplated too (Government of India, 2018). However, a considered strategy for developing leaders by providing opportunities to women outreach workers to contribute to health policies and programmes through well-articulated career progression pathways is necessary as much for advancing public health goals as it is about building equitable health systems.

Currently, there are limited career ladder opportunities available to CHWs in countries across the world. The World Health Organization observes that "providing health workers with a career ladder (that is, opportunities for progressive advancement to higher-level positions in a health system, or upgrading skills and expanding roles) is universally seen as a good practice to reinforce both motivation and retention" (WHO, 2018). There have been calls for the coherent insertion of such CHW cadres into the health systems and their explicit inclusion in strategic planning for human resources in health at the country and local levels (WHO, 2010b). The matter has not attracted much attention in India though. The skills and opportunities provided to India's feminized outreach workforce need to be significantly enhanced for them to be in higher positions in the country's health systems. Health and nutrition services need to be more fully integrated too. Promoting in-service acquisition of undergraduate and post-graduate degrees (such as a Master of Public Health), and providing opportunities for lateral entry in the health bureaucracy would lead to higher representation and participation of women outreach workers. Their conscious inclusion in institutionalized platforms for policy making and programme formulation would significantly enhance their exposure and build their capacities. Task shifting is a global challenge and health systems are grappling with rationalization of their human resources. Reallocation of tasks to new entrants in a well-entrenched health bureaucracy can be challenging and unsettling. However, if the rich knowledge and the vast experience of women outreach workers are to be harnessed, then their organic integration with India's health bureaucracy is called for. Growth within the organizational hierarchy needs to be actively promoted for such a large, feminized, skilled, and experienced workforce.

References

Esposito, J. L. (Ed.). (2003). Seclusion. In *The Oxford dictionary of Islam*. Oxford Islamic Studies Online. Retrieved September 6, 2019, fromhttp://www.oxfordislamicstudies.com/article/opr/t125/e2128

Government of India. (1974). *Towards equality: Report of the committee on the status of women in India*. Ministry of Education and Social Welfare.

Government of India. (2010). *Guidelines for multipurpose health worker (male)*. Ministry of Health and Family Welfare.

Government of India. (2018). *Guidelines on midwifery services in India*. Retrieved September 2, 2019, from https://nhm.gov.in/New_Updates_2018/NHM_Components/RMNCHA/MH/Guidelines/Guidelines_on_Midwifery_Services_in_India.pdf

Government of India. (2019). *Draft national education policy 2019*. Retrieved September 7, 2019, from https://mhrd.gov.in/sites/upload_files/mhrd/files/Draft_NEP_2019_EN_Revised.pdf

Government of India. (n.d.-a). *States and union territories*. Retrieved July 29, 2019, from https://knowindia.gov.in/states-uts/

Government of India. (n.d.-b). *Seventh schedule (article 246)*. Retrieved July 29, 2019, from https://www.mea.gov.in/Images/pdf1/S7.pdf

Government of India. (n.d.-c). *National Urban Health Mission (NUHM) as a sub-mission under the National Health Mission*. Retrieved July 31, 2019, from http://pib.nic.in/newsite/PrintRelease.aspx

Government of India. (n.d.-d). *Indian Public Health Standards (IPHS): Guidelines for sub-centres (Revised 2012)*. Retrieved July 29, 2019, from https://nhm.gov.in/images/pdf/guidelines/iphs/iphs-revised-guidlines-2012/sub-centers.pdf

Government of India. (n.d.-e). *Indian Public Health Standards (IPHS): Guidelines for sub-district/sub-divisional hospitals (31 to 100 bedded) (Revised 2012)*. Retrieved July 29, 2019, from https://nhm.gov.in/images/pdf/guidelines/iphs/iphs-revised-guidlines-2012/sub-district-sub-divisional-hospital.pdf

Government of India. (n.d.-f). *National Rural Health Mission: Meeting people's health needs in rural areas (Framework for implementation: 2005-2012)*. Ministry of Health and Family Welfare.

Government of India. (n.d.-g). *Health and family welfare statistics in India 2017*. Ministry of Health and Family Welfare.

Government of India. (n.d.-h). *Indian Public Health Standards (IPHS): Guidelines for primary health centres (Revised 2012)*. Retrieved July 29, 2019, from https://nhm.gov.in/images/pdf/guidelines/iphs/iphs-revised-guidlines-2012/primay-health-centres.pdf

Government of India. (n.d.-i). *State/UT-wise details of ASHAs selected under NHM as on September 2018*. Retrieved July 31, 2019, from https://data.gov.in/node/6649821/download

Government of India. (n.d.-j). *State/UT-wise number of Anganwadi Centres across the country as on December 2018*. Retrieved July 31, 2019, from https://data.gov.in/resources/stateut-wise-number-anganwadi-centres-across-country-december-2018-ministry-women-and

Government of India. (n.d.-k). *State/UT-wise number of Anganwadi workers (AWWs)/Anganwadi helpers (AWHs) sanctioned, in-position as on 31.12.2018*. Retrieved July 31, 2019, from https://data.gov.in/node/6649820/download

Government of India. (n.d.-l). *State/UT-wise male health worker at sub centres as on 31-03-2017*. Retrieved July 31, 2019, from https://data.gov.in/node/4220481/download

Government of India. (n.d.-m). *National health policy 2017*.

Government of India. (n.d.-n). *Seeking comments/feedback from stakeholders on "Recommendations on Clinical Autonomy for Nurse Practitioner in Midwifery (NPM)"*. Retrieved July 31, 2019, from https://mohfw.gov.in/sites/default/files/5383642421448971338_0.pdf

Kammowanee, R. (2019). ASHAs' health services: Social service or care work? *Economic and Political Weekly, 54*(49), 12–15.

Mavalankar, D., Raman, P. S., & Vora, K. (2011). Midwives of India: Missing in action. *Midwifery, 27*, 700–706.

Mavalankar, D., & Vora, K. S. (2008). *The changing role of Auxiliary Nurse Midwife (ANM) in India: Implications for Maternal and Child Health (MCH)*. Indian Institute of Management.

Mishra, M. (2016). Health careers. In N. A. Naples (Ed.), *The Wiley Blackwell encyclopedia of gender and sexuality studies* (1st ed.). John Wiley & Sons, Ltd. https://doi.org/10.1002/9781118663219.wbegss520

Olaniran, A., Madaj, B., Bar-Zev, S., & van den Broek, N. (2019). The roles of community health workers who provide maternal and newborn health services: Case studies from Africa and Asia. *BMJ Global Health, 4*, e001388. https://doi.org/10.1136/bmjgh-2019-001388

Rockman, B. (2019). *Bureaucracy. Encyclopaedia Britannica*. Retrieved May 22, 2021, from https://www.britannica.com/topic/bureaucracy

WHO. (2007). *Community health workers: What do we know about them?* Retrieved September 7, 2019, from https://www.who.int/hrh/documents/community_health_workers.pdf

WHO. (2010a). *Access for all to skilled, motivated, and supported health workers: Global strategy for women's and children's health*. Retrieved March 2, 2018, from http://www.who.int/workforcealliance/knowledge/resources/UNstrategypaper_skilledworkers.pdf

WHO. (2010b). *Global experience of community health workers for delivery of health related millennium development goals: A systematic review, country case studies, and recommendations for integration into national health systems*. Retrieved July 22, 2019, from https://www.who.int/workforcealliance/knowledge/publications/CHW_FullReport_2010.pdf

WHO. (2018). *WHO guideline on health policy and system support to optimize community health worker programmes*. World Health Organization.

WHO. (2019). *Gender equity in the health workforce: Analysis of 104 countries* (Health Workforce Working Paper 1). Retrieved March 26, 2019, from https://apps.who.int/iris/bitstream/handle/10665/311314/WHO-HIS-HWF-Gender-WP1-2019.1-eng.pdf

Interview with Poonam Khetrapal Singh, Regional Director of the WHO South-East Asia Region

Sulzhan Bali and Roopa Dhatt

"Be determined and move on. Don't give up."

Poonam Khetrapal Singh is the Regional Director of the WHO South-East Asia Region (SEARO). She is currently serving her second 5-year term in office following unanimous reelection by SEARO's 11 member states in September 2018. Dr. Khetrapal Singh is an Indian national and the first woman to hold the post. She served as WHO Deputy Regional Director for SEARO from 2000 to 2013 and prior to that was a civil servant in India as a member of the Indian Administrative Services. This included roles as both joint Secretary and Secretary of Health in the state of Punjab. She has also served as the WHO Executive Director, Sustainable Development and Healthy Environments Cluster, and a member of the Director-General's Cabinet, as well as worked with the World Bank as part of the Health, Population and Nutrition Practice.

Could You Share with Us Your Global Health Journey?

I studied in a convent which was run by German missionaries—St. Mary's Convent. Then I was in a college called Christ Church College where I studied and did my undergrad. I did my post-grad in three subjects—English literature, political science, and population studies—then I took the Indian Administrative Service (IAS) examination and joined the IAS. In the IAS, which is the government civil service of India, there is a career path already worked out for you. As a civil servant, I moved to Chandigarh as the Joint Secretary of Health, and that is where my deep interest in health commenced. I enjoyed working for people, I enjoyed going out and talking to women, I enjoyed solving women's problems, and I then got an offer from the World Bank and so I joined the World Bank. After three or so years at the World Bank, I was called back by my government, and the option for me was either to resign from the IAS and continue in the World Bank or to give up the World Bank and come back to my government, and I chose the latter.

S. Bali (✉) · R. Dhatt
Women in Global Health, Washington, DC, USA
e-mail: roopa.dhatt@womeningh.org

© Springer Nature Switzerland AG 2022
R. Morgan et al. (eds.), *Women and Global Health Leadership*,
https://doi.org/10.1007/978-3-030-84498-1_21

219

I decided to come back and work in Punjab, again in Chandigarh, where my career really was between the Ministry of Finance and the Ministry of Health, so I was Managing Director of the Punjab Financial Corporation and the Punjab Industrial Development Corporation, which were basically financing institutions, and in that capacity I was also director of the Industrial Development Bank of India (IDBI), which gives large-scale loans to the industrial sector. I also served as the Special Secretary of Health, then I became Secretary of Health, so it was like one tenure in health and one tenure in finance, that's the way it worked until I took one sabbatical in England to do a Master of Health Management degree.

I did my dissertation on user fees in Punjab, and based on that I was invited by WHO to give a presentation. The Director-General of WHO, Gro Harlem Brundtland, thereafter offered me a job in her cabinet. She was starting afresh in WHO as Director-General in 1998, and I was offered the post of Executive Director. I was to look after healthy environments and sustainable development, as well as nutrition, so it was really a cluster which took care of environment, water, sanitation, food safety. I worked there with her, and then my parents fell very ill, so I came here to India, because we have a regional office of WHO here, and I joined as number two here, because the number one, which is the Regional Director, which is my present post, is an elected post, so you are elected by all the Health Ministers of the region.

Then in 2013, I won my first election, and joined as Regional Director of SEARO in February of 2014, and after my first term, which was five years, I won a second election, because we're allowed two terms, and I got reelected unopposed from my region, and now my second term is on, so my second term started on the first of February of 2019, and it will go on for five years. That's been my career path.

Do You See Other Women Like You in Global Health?

I do see some of them, but not as many as I would like to see. In the South-East Asia Region, they have women who've done very well, if you see that leaders and Prime Ministers and Presidents, you will find it; and yet I feel that there is a lot of disparity among those who've made it to the top level and those who are still struggling below.

What Are Some of the Obstacles Women Face, Especially in South-East Asia?

I do feel that, in some parts of the world, such as South-East Asia, women are very hesitant to come out and to work. When we advertise for posts and positions, even though I go out of my way to encourage women to apply, there are few who apply. Sometimes it's cultural—they don't like to go out of their own known territory. Sometimes it's the demands of home, where they feel that when their husband is working they need to be at home, they need to take care of the kids.

Women carry a double burden as well. When I was in Chandigarh as the Secretary of Health, I used to find that many women who used to come to work would tell me that they have to get up in the morning to prepare food for the entire family, then go to work, then rush back in the evenings, cook again. So, they carry a double burden that way. They are working and earning, plus they're taking care of the kids, plus very often they're taking care of their in-laws or older people in the family, and they are also doing household chores like cooking, so it becomes so difficult for them.

In many countries like mine, there is a strong son preference right from the beginning, and this preference is so apparent, and it's related a lot to cultural issues. This strong son preference becomes a big barrier and a challenge to women who are growing up, which leads to a very difficult mindset, as far as the men go, because they assume that they have a certain role which is superior to women. I do believe very strongly that it's not only women but also men and young boys who need to be sensitized; it should start very early in life.

Not just global leadership, but I also feel local leadership is very important, because when you're growing up all this matters. You see a woman in a local area in a position of authority, and you feel it is possible and it can be done. But if you only see men around you, then you do not think you'll be able to break that barrier or that you'll be able to assume that kind of position. Certain things are happening in countries like India which are good, for example, representation at the local level, and in village-level governance, one-third representation goes to women. I think it's a very healthy, important step, because when women are in a position of local leadership, then it makes a huge difference.

What Promotes Women's Careers in Institutions? How Can Institutions Empower Women?

First of all, I feel that women have to be given an opportunity, and they have to know that they will have an opportunity after they attain their education. We have to see that they are empowered enough to be able to take the competitive process of recruitment, so that they do get an opportunity to join the workforce. When they join the workforce, that itself gives encouragement to those around them, the younger set of women. I think that has a very good multiplier effect, because seeing women in high-level positions, or even in positions which are mid-level, gives an impetus to those who are younger to try to attain that.

Coaching classes help. In my organization, we don't discriminate between men and women, we have them for all, but we see that when we let women come out of their shells, they are empowered enough to be able to compete in a process where they can then be in a leadership position. It's very important to build their confidence.

Sexual harassment is also an issue to address. We need to be very strict about it. I think these cases don't come to the fore, and they don't come to the fore because women are very often hesitant to bring them up, thinking that nothing would happen. They must be given the confidence to be able to come and complain, and then, if they complain, we must see that the person who has transgressed is given the punishment that he deserves. I think one must make it very clear to everybody that there will be zero tolerance for it. I do feel that it's very important to take some corrective measures immediately. Once you send that strong message, and there are a few people we take to task for doing it, it declines. I've noticed that in my own organization.

I've also seen that what really helps is to have a woman at a senior level there who they can go to and complain, because when a woman is facing these kinds of advancements from male colleagues, she's not very comfortable going to a supervisor who is a male and who may not look at it the way a woman would. Therefore, I think it's very important to have a woman at a senior level where your workforce consists of at least 30%, 40%, or 50% women, which is the target we have in WHO, to have at least 50% women. In my organization now, I try very hard to empower women. If a junior of mine asks me for time, there's no way I won't see them. I may not see them the day they ask me, I may see them after three days or a week, but I will see them. Then they feel that they can go and approach someone who would have a sympathetic ear to them.

How Did You Address Obstacles in Your Own Career?

When I joined the service I was very fortunate, because when you join the IAS in India, you are not discriminated against on basis of gender. My first posting was in a very backward district in Punjab, and I was very apprehensive when I went there, but I realized very quickly that a lot depends on how you project yourself. Somehow, when women work they really have to prove themselves, and once you've done that, then it's better, but the initial part is very important. You need to set the stage, conduct yourself such that you don't seem hesitant to take bold decisions. You don't appear to dilly-dally, you just take your decisions and move on with them, and they may be harsh sometimes but that's what your job requires of you.

How Did Your Family Influence Your Career?

I was born in a family where there was total equity between my brothers and me. No discrimination of any sort. My mother was very encouraging. She would want me to learn a lot of things and achieve excellence. I don't remember a single incident where I was second in class, be it a big test, be it a math test, be it a yearly test. That, I think, endeared me a lot to my mother, who had high ambitions for me, and she wanted me to become a doctor. I was not interested in that at all, though I did join some of the classes. I realized after one dissection that it was not something I was cut out for, and I would not be able to really do justice to that kind of role. Instead, I was very interested in reading and writing, and I wanted to really write books. That is what inspired me to get into humanities rather than medicine.

My parents encouraged me but were also not very keen that I should work. I grew up in an environment where, even though equal opportunities were given to me for education, there was always this thought behind that I would get married early. When I wanted to work and got into the service and I didn't want to give it up, there was some struggle at home and my father finally said, "Okay, go through the training, but don't join." So, I agreed. I said okay. But once I was there, then I was empowered enough, economically I was empowered, and I was in a situation where I could say I am enjoying it very much and I want to do it.

Having said that, there was a lot of support from them afterward. I remember when I had my daughter, my mother helped out and supported me. You do need somebody, you can't be sitting in an office and thinking if your child's been given milk at the right time or has eaten at the right time, because that's really going to distract you from your work. I was fortunate there, again, that I had that kind of support, so if my child was ill, my mother would take her to the hospital. If my child had to do her studies, it was my mother who would supervise that, but I had worked out her schedule in such a way that I would drop her to school in the morning and then she would get picked up by my mom, and then I would come home for lunch, so I would have lunch with her always.

How Did Your Peer Network Influence Your Career?

I decided to take the IAS exam because a friend of mine in school came to me for some advice and wanted some books from me because she was taking the IAS exam. In our generation, this was considered the best you could do because now there are so many opportunities to try many professions, many careers for women, but at that time, this was considered one of the respectable careers for a woman.

She came to me and she asked me for some help with books, and then I thought to myself that if she's taking this and she was a mediocre kind of student, a good friend of mine, maybe I too should do that. Really the inspiration came from her; in fact, she asked me, "Why don't you also prepare for this and we can prepare together?" So, we both started preparing together for this exam, we had about three or four months left untill the exam, and we took it. That was how my career got influenced, and I just joined the IAS, not after a lot of careful thought. It was not something that I planned to do. It just happened because a friend of mine encouraged me and I thought that it would be a good career for me.

In Every Career, People Make Mistakes or Experience Success and Failure. How Do You Address Those?

I faced a few failures in my life, of course there were some. When I joined my service, there was a movie hall I crossed, and I went with a friend to see a movie that I really wanted to watch. When I went there to see the movie, I realized that they had written "house full" outside, but inside half or maybe three-fourths of the hall were empty. So very quickly I realized that they were selling tickets at a premium, much more than what the price was. When I came to office the next day, I was very worked up, and I was very upset that all this was going on and there's nothing we could do about. My boss, who was like a mentor, asked me "What exactly do you want to do?" I said, "I'd like to raid this movie hall." He said, "These are very dangerous people and I don't think you should do that," but I was very insistent, and I said, "No, I think we should do that." He didn't want to discourage me. He laid a caveat. He said, "Okay, go, but take a senior (aged) subordinate person with you."

So I went, and I found at least 20 violations there and I already typed up a report and next morning told my boss that the "movie hall should be closed because there are so many violations." He said, "Okay, we'll close it but this man is very well-connected, so tomorrow we may face trouble." So, he closed the movie hall, and I was very happy that I'd spent so many hours reading the act and going there, looking at everything, preparing the report. The next morning, when I was coming to work, I realized that the hall was open, and I realized that the same thing was going on. I was really very upset, so I went to him and I said, "Why is that hall open today?" He said, "Because I've been overruled by the Home Secretary, who has the authority to overrule me, and he has decided that we should open the hall." I was totally upset. Then he said to me, "I told you earlier that this belongs to somebody who can do these kinds of things, but I didn't want you to just go by my opinion. I wanted you to see it for yourself." This is where I learned that not everything is always in your control. What you can do is what your job requires of you. You cannot control the behavior of those who are your supervisors, or supervisor's supervisors or whatever. They may be having their own challenges and compulsions to deal with, so don't take it personally. You've done what you had to do in the course of your duty.

It was the first lesson I learned in life that sometimes you may try to do things which are correct, and yet you may not be able to take that all the way. There may be others who may not perceive it the way you perceive it, and they may take decisions which are not the kind of decisions you would take, and you would feel very let down. All you can do is what you think is right, and then don't be hesitant to do what you think is right.

Failures help you grow, and they also empower you, and most importantly, you become wiser as you go along. You learn to pick your battles; you learn to see whether your decision is going to be sustained or not.

Were There Any Mentors That Influenced Your Career Trajectory?

I think it's very important that you meet people early in your life, even in school, who are going to shape you and who are going to encourage you to take on these kinds of responsibilities later, and I was blessed to have a teacher like that. I will never forget her. She used to be a nun, Mother Mary. She really took a lot of interest in me, and my growth and my development, including encouraging me to do things which I thought were not possible. With her encouragement, I realized nothing is impossible if you really set your heart on it, if you're determined to achieve it, and if you're disciplined enough to be able to get there. With her, she played a very important part in my life. That is when I think I realized the potential I had. That set the tone for me, because your last years of school become very important. So, she was one person who I think played a very important part in my life.

I've already mentioned my mother to you. She also played a very important part in my life because I can't remember a single incident where I was not given encouragement from her, which is very important when you're trying to decide on your future, the kind of things you're going to do. Somebody has to hold your hand and tell you that what you're doing is the right thing.

What Advice Would You Give to Young Women Who Are Aspiring to Be Global Health Leaders?

My advice to them would be to be determined in what they're trying to do, and not to get deterred by minor disturbances or minor things or obstacles that come their way. Obstacles will come. There is no way you're going to have a career or a lifetime of work where you're not going to face obstacles. You'll have good supervisors, you'll have bad supervisors, you'll have people who will help you to grow. There will be people who will not be bothered about that. Be prepared for that, but that should not let you lose your determination. Just be focused on what you really want to achieve. Don't let haters or bullies bother you. Keep your own discipline, keep your own determination, and keep going. That is the only way to achieve what you've set out to achieve in life.

I would also like to advise them that it's important to have a healthy work/life balance. They must have some other interests besides just work, and that also adds a lot to the kind of contribution they will make to their work. It will help them to relax, to reduce stress. I think these are some of the things which are very important when women go out into the world and when they face challenges.

If You Could Have a Billboard for Other Women Leaders, What Would It Say?

It would say, "Be determined and move on. Don't give up."

The Glass Ceiling: Gender Segregation Within Health Workforce Leadership with Matriarchal and Patriarchal Societies in Indonesia

Nuzulul Kusuma Putri

Despite women's increased participation in leadership within the health system, equal participation of men and women in decision-making is not guaranteed. This is the result of embedded patriarchal norms which favour masculine leadership structures and characteristics. While the number of women leaders in health organizations is increasing, this has revealed what is known as the glass ceiling. The glass ceiling, first introduced by Gay Bryant in 1984, is the presence of invisible barriers that impede the career advancement of women (Barreto et al., 2009). It is called a brass ceiling in military organizations and the celluloid ceiling in the cinematic industry. Since the healthcare workforce is dominated by a significant number of women, there is an urgent need to systemically describe how the glass ceiling in health care has occurred and its impact.

This chapter discusses gender leadership succession and gender segregation in the context of the health workforce within matriarchal and patriarchal societies in Indonesia, demonstrating how the increasing number of women as leaders at the top of the health system does not guarantee that women at lower levels have an equal opportunity to obtain leadership positions compared to men. In the last 15 years, the Indonesian health system has been led by women ministers; the chapter describes how even though the health system within Indonesia was led by women, gender segregation still occurs in its lower structural and technical levels. The chapter finishes by presenting recommendations for researchers and practitioners in analysing gender segregation in health care.

N. K. Putri (✉)
Research Group for Health and Well-being of Women and Children, Faculty of Public Health, Universitas Airlangga, Surabaya, Indonesia
e-mail: nuzululkusuma@fkm.unair.ac.id

© Springer Nature Switzerland AG 2022
R. Morgan et al. (eds.), *Women and Global Health Leadership*,
https://doi.org/10.1007/978-3-030-84498-1_22

Women at the Top

The health workforce in Indonesia is composed mostly of women. Many studies have found that female leaders in the health sector lag considerably behind their male counterparts in advancing into strategic decision-making positions (Elwér et al., 2012; Paoloni & Demartini, 2016; Rincón et al., 2017; Wanigasekara, 2016). Since becoming an independent country in 1945, Indonesia has had 20 Health Ministers, and only 4 of them were women. However, women have started to occupy strategic positions in the health sector.

Since 2004, presidents of the Republic of Indonesia chose women to act as Ministers of Health, even though the number of female ministers is always much fewer than male ministers in the cabinet. In his first 5-year term of office, President Susilo Bambang Yudhoyono appointed a senior female cardiologist as the Minister of Health. She was the very first woman who served as Minister of Health in Indonesia and was 1 of 4 female ministers among all 34 ministers at the time. President Yudhoyono appointed another female as Minister of Health in his second presidential run, a doctor with expertise in public health. She was 1 of 5 female ministers of 34 ministers at the time. Unfortunately, she passed away in her third year of service due to lung cancer and was replaced by her male Vice Minister. After only 2 months in this position, President Yudhoyono replaced him with a female paediatrician. President Joko Widodo, the following president, also chose a woman as Minister of Health, who was 1 of 8 female ministers among 34 ministers at the time. A senior ophthalmologist, who was also the wife of a former Health Minister, was appointed as the fourth female Minister of Health in Indonesia. The trend of having female Health Ministers in Indonesia, however, ended after the second presidential run of President Joko Widodo at the end of 2019 when he assigned a male military doctor. After 15 years of being led by a woman, the Indonesian Ministry of Health was officially led by a man. President Joko Widodo's agenda to counter-terrorism and radicalism in Indonesia is one of his reasons for assigning a male Health Minister with military background.

Even though there is no research that focuses on the impact of women leaders on public health in Indonesia, the leadership of four women had other effects within the country. The first female Minister of Health demonstrated that women could also be good leaders. She persistently fought for the non-commercialization of the avian influenza vaccine. The second woman health minister proved that women in leadership result in more woman-sensitive policy in health care. Even though she served as minister for only 2 and a half years, she placed a strong emphasis on maternal and child health care. She was the first Indonesian Minister of Health to legally regulate exclusive breastfeeding and banned health workers from promoting formula milk, obligating the existence of a breastfeeding room in all government offices. The third female minister also advocated for woman-sensitive policy. Based on her experience as Deputy Chair of the National Commission on Violence Against Women, she initiated the establishment of the National Commission for Indonesian Children Protection. The final female minister initiated a social innovation movement that advocated for team-based health workers as opposed to individual medical workers to solve high maternal and neonatal mortality. While women had attained leadership at the summit of the system, it is unclear how their leadership had been accommodated at the lower levels of the system in Indonesia, and whether it allowed for greater opportunities for women to be leaders in the lower levels of the health system.

Leadership in Decentralized Matriarchal and Patriarchal Systems

Indonesia has embraced decentralization and is comprised of 34 autonomous provinces that contain districts. The districts are the local government who manage and perform their public services independently. District Health Offices are coordinated by local government as a result of decentralization. Civil servants in the District Health Office get promoted only by the recommendation of an advisory board at the district level that is responsible for suggesting the name of expectant structural officers to the regent or major as district head. Besides considering the fulfilment of basic qualifications regulated nationally, this board takes into account the work performance of the individual. The promoted officers will either become the top-level, middle-level, or low-level manager in the District Health Office.

A series of position reviews of the organizational structure of District Health Offices (Fig. 1) were conducted to analyse the glass ceiling in leadership succession. Position reviews, or position analysis, is a systematic process that is commonly used in human resource management. It identifies the set of knowledge, skills, and abilities required to perform the responsibilities and duties of a specific

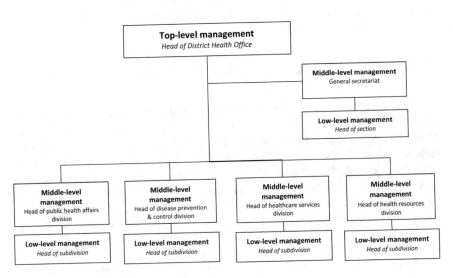

Fig. 1 Organizational structure of the District Health Office

job position through job analysis (Mathis & Jackson, 2008). Human resource specialists execute this activity to review the job description which determines the value of the job (Griffin, 1978). The position analysis was conducted in Minangkabau, one of the biggest matriarchal societies in the world (Stark, 2013). Minangkabau tribes are the only matriarchal society in Indonesia. They live at the West Sumatra province where every child born to the Minangkabau tribe follows his mother's tribe.

The analysis was compared to the patriarchal society of East Java. Various books and studies are still debating whether matriarchy should be considered the opposite of patriarchy (Eisenstein, 1979; Murray, 2005; Walby, 1991; Witz, 2004). Patriarchy is defined as a social system where men predominate above women in the roles of political leadership, moral authority, social privilege, and control of the property. It is not the result of sex differences between men and women, but the gender roles which are constructed for each gender by society. A matriarchy accommodates women as a maternal symbol, which has a significant influence on the next generation of both men and women. It emphasizes the central role of women in all social practices. Women in matriarchal societies are placed in positions with the highest control and power over men. On the other hand, matriarchy has been described as equal power-sharing between men and women with an egalitarian perspective (Leacock, 1978). Minangkabau is a non-class-based society and the women are autonomous; Minangkabau women do not depend on their husbands; moreover, their brothers are responsible for their children rather than their husbands (Stark, 2013).

The position reviews were held in 6 districts of West Sumatra province and 11 districts of East Java province. These districts were chosen based on the District Health Office transparency (publishing its organizational structure along with the officer's names on the official website). 338 health managers in both District Health Offices were observed in this position review: 110 managers in the matriarchal setting (West Sumatra) and 228 managers in the patriarchal setting (East Java).

Glass Ceilings Within Matriarchal and Patriarchal Societies

Surprisingly, even in the District Health Offices within the matriarchal setting, there was evidence of the glass ceiling at work. There was a wide gap in promotion probability between male and female health officers. The promotion probability between male and female health officers is presented in Figs. 2 and 3. There were double the number of female officers as heads of subdivision in the matriarchal society, but only 30.6% of these were successfully promoted to become head of the division (see Fig. 2). This was lower than the probability of male officers getting promoted. In the patriarchal setting, the probability of male officers being promoted was higher than for female officers (see Fig. 3). A female low-level manager in matriarchal society has only 30.6% probability of being promoted into middle-level manager. This probability is much lower when compared to the probability of male low-level manager to be promoted to the middle-level. A male low-level manager in matriarchal

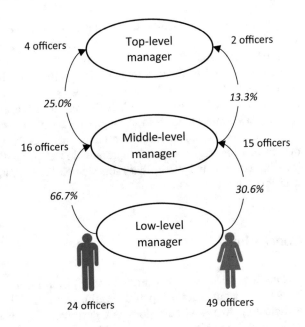

Fig. 2 Promotion probability in the matriarchal sample

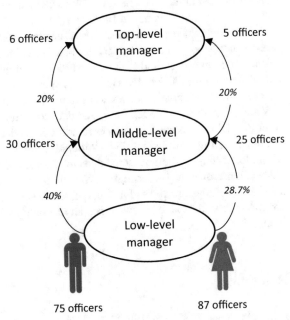

Fig. 3 Promotion probability in the patriarchal sample

society has a 66.7% probability of being promoted into middle-level manager. This glass ceiling reportedly not only happened among healthcare workforce but also in various aspects of public affairs in the matriarchal society (Idris, 2011; Mutolib et al., 2016; Rohman, 2014).

Women who successfully became an elite manager often need to apply extra effort to reach their position compared to men (Davies-Netzley, 1998). For this reason, the educational background of each health manager was analysed and compared to the job specification required for promotion. All of the health managers, both male and female, possessed a bachelor's degree in accordance with the job specification. In fact, more than half the female managers had a master's degree. This is 10% higher than male managers with a master's degree. This reveals that greater technical competence or merit is not necessarily a determinant that leads to men having higher proportional representation in managerial positions. Likely, it is invisible barriers, not merit, that limit women being promoted to higher levels of decision-making.

Conclusion

Our findings uncover gender differences in governmental offices in Indonesia. The existence of women at the top of the health system and the large number of women participating in the system does not guarantee that women are represented as decision-makers at its technical level. The glass ceiling still occurs both in matriarchal and patriarchal societies in Indonesia.

To overcome this issue in the setting of health workforce leadership, more transparent succession plans for leaders in district health offices are needed. Gender-sensitive instruments should be used to evaluate any indication of gender stereotyping and segregation in the job description and specification. Mainstreaming gender in the context of leadership succession plans in Indonesia is still underperformed, which leads to inadequate reporting and data collection about gender inequality. In order to establish policy frameworks to address gender-related differences in organizational settings in Indonesia, additional evidence related to gender equality within leadership in the government sector is needed. Future research should provide evidence on how gender segregation within governmental settings happens and how glass ceilings are formed and perpetuated. By uncovering these mechanisms, governments will be able to reduce gender inequality within leadership structures in Indonesia.

References

Barreto, M., Ryan, M. K., & Schmitt, M. T. (2009). Introduction: Is the glass ceiling still relevant in the 21st century? In *The glass ceiling in the 21st century: Understanding barriers to gender equality.* (pp. 3–18). doi: https://doi.org/10.1037/11863-001

Davies-Netzley, S. A. (1998). Women above the glass ceiling: Perceptions on corporate mobility and strategies for success. *Gender and Society, 12*(3), 339–355. https://doi.org/10.1177/0891243298012003006

Eisenstein, Z. (1979). Developing a theory of capitalist patriarchy and socialist feminism. In E. Zillah (Ed.), *Capitalist patriarchy and the case for socialist feminism* (pp. 5–40). doi: https://doi.org/10.2307/3177483

Elwér, S., Aléx, L., & Hammarström, A. (2012). Gender (in) equality among employees in elder care: implications for health. *International Journal for Equity in Health, 11*(1), 1. https://doi.org/10.1186/1475-9276-11-1

Griffin, H. R. (1978). Human resources practice in the public sector. In L. Shi (Ed.), *Managing human resources in health care organizations* (Vol. 8, pp. 73–98). doi: https://doi.org/10.1097/00005110-197812000-00007

Idris, N. (2011). The external and internal barriers to the political leadership for Minangkabau women in West Sumatera. *Masyarakat, Kebudayaan, Dan Politik, 24*(2), 130–141.

Leacock, E. (1978). Women's status in Egalitarian society: Implications for social evolution. *Current Anthropology, 19*(2), 247–275.

Mathis, R. L., & Jackson, J. H. (2008). *Human resource management* (Vol. 15, 12th ed.). Mason.

Murray, M. (2005). The law of the father? In *The law of the father?* doi: https://doi.org/10.4324/9780203993859

Mutolib, A., Yonariza, & Mahdi. (2016). Gender inequality and the oppression of women within Minangkabau matrilineal society : a case study of the management of Ulayat Forest land in Nagari Bonjol, Dharmasraya District, West Sumatra Province, Indonesia. *Asian Women, 32*(3), 23–49.

Paoloni, P., & Demartini, P. (2016). Women in management: Perspectives on a decade of research (2005–2015). *Palgrave Communications, 2.* https://doi.org/10.1057/palcomms.2016.94

Rincón, V., González, M., & Barrero, K. (2017). Women and leadership: Gender barriers to senior management positions. *Intangible Capital, 13*(2), 319. https://doi.org/10.3926/ic.889

Rohman, A. (2014). The comparison of power and authority of women in China and Minangkabau societies. *The International Journal of Humanities and Social Studies, 1*(12), 141–145.

Stark, A. (2013). The matrilineal system of the Minangkabau and its persistence throughout history: A structural perspective. *Southeast Asia: A Multidisciplinary Journal, 13*(January 2013), 1–13.

Walby, S. (1991). *Theorizing patriarchy.* Basil Blackwell Ltd..

Wanigasekara, W. M. S. K. (2016). Women's networking and career development: A systematic analysis of the literature. *International Journal of Business and Management, 11*(11), 231. https://doi.org/10.5539/ijbm.v11n11p231

Witz, A. (2004). *Professions and patriarchy (J. Urry, ed.).* Taylor & Francis.

Interview with Senait Fisseha, Clinical Professor of Obstetrics and Gynecology, University of Michigan Medical School, and Director of International Programs at the Susan T. Buffett Foundation

Sulzhan Bali and Roopa Dhatt

"Make your own rules. Don't be bound by societal rules!"

Born in Ethiopia, Senait Fisseha is a leading global health advocate, a reproductive endocrinology and infertility academic at the University of Michigan, and the Director of International Programs at the Susan T. Buffett Foundation. Dr. Fisseha is known for her work as an advocate for global reproductive health, rights, and gender equality. She is the founder of the Center for International Reproductive Health Training (CIRHT) at the University of Michigan, and she chaired and led the election campaign of Tedros Adhanom, the first African director-general of the World Health Organization, from 2016 to 2017.

Early Career

I was born in Ethiopia and moved to the United States right after high school for undergraduate studies. I studied my undergraduate degree in Chicago, at a small Catholic college called Rosary College, now called Dominican University. Then I went to medical school and law school at Southern Illinois University.

I came to the University of Michigan to do my residency in obstetrics and gynecology and did a fellowship in reproductive endocrinology and infertility. It was the year when Bill Clinton was running for office. Hillary Clinton was in the news every day talking about healthcare reform. There was a lot in the news about medical malpractice and the need for reform, particularly how medical malpractice in the southern United States was affecting OB/GYNs' and neurosurgeons' ability to provide care. It was a time when National Institutes of Health (NIH) grant money was

S. Bali (✉) · R. Dhatt
Women in Global Health, Washington, DC, USA
e-mail: roopa.dhatt@womeningh.org

© Springer Nature Switzerland AG 2022
R. Morgan et al. (eds.), *Women and Global Health Leadership*,
https://doi.org/10.1007/978-3-030-84498-1_23

235

drying up, and there was enormous pressure on scientists to produce data. I saw a lot of unethical practices and pressures. Then came the Beijing conference on women's rights. There were many things happening that led me to also be interested in the law.

I've always been interested in women, human rights, and women's rights and women's health. I studied abroad in Oxford—international and human rights and comparative civil liberties. I stayed as faculty at the University of Michigan as an assistant professor, doing teaching and research, as well as clinical services. I ran our center for reproductive health and our IVF unit. By the time I finished, I had become a full professor. I took my current job at the Buffett Foundation around five years ago to head their global programs for reproductive health.

Are There Any Mentors That You Credit for Your Success?

When I look at pivotal moments in my life that made a difference, it's always due to someone guiding me, someone who has made their experience and their path become a reflection for me, so that I don't make the same mistakes they have. I did not have a lot of women mentors, not because I wasn't interested, just because there weren't that many that I could access. There were some mentors who helped me in medical school and the laboratory. Later, when I started venturing into global health, I had a remarkable mentor, Tim Johnson, who was a professor. When I was interviewing for a residency spot at Michigan, I was pretty set on going to Johns Hopkins and they were interested in me but he encouraged me not to chase glamour and the next shiny thing and to come to Michigan. For me, that was so pivotal in figuring out the landscape. Not every global health intervention is created equal, and all of the things that we publicly now debate around power and shifting the rules of engagement were ingrained in me very, very early on. For example, our collaboration with the University of Ghana, which they call MichiGhana, taught me a lot about equity and power sharing.

A Supportive Spouse

My husband has been an incredible mentor throughout my life. If I had to pick a single person who's shaped who I am today, both as a person and a professional, it's my husband. When I began studying at the University of Michigan, my husband was a resident and someone introduced us. I reached out to him for career advice. At that time, he was a third year and he laid out to me why it would be helpful to me to have a deeper understanding of law and medicine. So that's how I switched paths from pursuing a career in research and decided to add law. We started dating a year later.

As a person who did not grow up in the United States and did not go to school there, I would not have been able to navigate my career and my education had it not been for his mentorship. At the beginning it was not like he was interested in me romantically. He invests in a lot of young people, especially Ethiopians, because he feels like he did not fulfill his own dreams and potential. He always jokes that he was living vicariously through me. I met my husband at such a critical moment in my life. I was 20 and he was ten years older than me and at that time it was so embarrassing. Because I felt, "Oh my gosh, I'm dating a very old man!" Now, at 49 and 59, we have no difference. But at that time, it was tough for me to even acknowledge to my family I was dating a person who was older.

It was incredible because he's from Ethiopia and we come from such a patriarchal and such a misogynistic culture. To find a partner who not only looked at me in adulation but was also so supportive and saw my potential, it was incredible. At his core he is a feminist. If I say that I learned feminism from him, it would not be an exaggeration. For example, at one point I got this urgent need to get married and settle down. He said, "If you want a ring, I'll give it to you. But I'm just worried that just the pressure from society will distract you from achieving your goals. So, let's postpone getting married." This is completely foreign to the culture I come from, to the experience of my immediate siblings and in my community.

When I wanted an experience like studying in Oxford, and I couldn't afford it, he supported me. He always said he didn't want anything in return from me, but he saw in me the potential to effectuate larger change in a way that he couldn't. Later, he said if somehow your career takes off and you can bring financial security to the household, I will stay home and raise the kids. I thought it was a joke but when I got the opportunity to take the job with the Buffett Foundation, without rubbing his eyes, he packed and moved, literally with no job, and he stayed at home until he figured out a job here. He left a very robust private practice that he'd established over 15 years. I can't tell you how many women miss opportunities for growth and for their career because they don't have that spousal support.

Informal Peer Networks—Helping Each Other?

I had a nanny at home and I had a husband who was in private practice. But it wasn't as easy for many of my colleagues who were very young and up and coming residents or junior faculty who are still paying loans and whose husbands were in the same boat that they were. So, I used to host our network at my house, and I would say, I have a nanny, bring your kids. That way, not having a babysitter would not be an issue for women to participate.

Although I had enormous support from my husband, at times it became frustrating because he's not an academic and doesn't understand the extent to which colleagues can be undermining. When you have a bad experience, you need somebody to validate it. Is it real? Am I paranoid? My informal networks of peers served this purpose. They took the weight off me. I am grateful for that. Every time I see a WhatsApp message now from Women and Global Health saying "here's an opportunity," it pretty much takes me to how we coped through the early challenges.

Challenging Cultural and Gender Norms as a Couple—A Woman Leader and a Feminist Husband

My family are predominantly girls, and to them he became the hero: the ideal husband, the ideal brother-in-law. But my very misogynistic brothers used to mock us and say, "How can you do this? You're creating a different standard in the household and our wives are going to have expectations." Or they would mock him saying, "Who's the man in the house, who wears the pants?" Because it was outside our cultural norm. His side of the family were also not happy that he put his wife on a pedestal.

A lot of the men in his professional circle were male African American physicians. They also couldn't relate to the way he behaved. The stereotype was not just within the Ethiopian culture. During my residency I traveled all the time and he was the primary caretaker of our children. He couldn't go and hang out at night or go to the clubs, and he had to modify his schedule and his meetings. He received a lot of flak for accommodating me. This was from American men as well, who define manhood and being the head of a household a certain way. He would always defend my style of motherhood when people would try and cut me down as not being available for my children. And that is my sore spot, because I constantly get reminded. But he's always reassured me saying, "Listen, I know stay-at-home moms and you're a better mom than them."

Dealing with Obstacles

I think in a way I've been very fortunate to have a career where I have had a lot of good people along the way. Having said that, it doesn't mean that there were no bumps in the road. In general, I'm a person who takes those things as a challenge and sees if I can work around them as opposed to having them defeat me or break me. My early career at the University of Michigan was quite challenging. I had a department chair who absolutely believed in me and started giving me leadership roles. That was not very well received by colleagues who were not used to a person of color, of short stature, who has an accent, in a leadership position. My directness was not taken well. They just did not see me as what they have historically accepted as a leader.

But because I had enormous support from up above and incredible support at home and then also who I am, I have overcome a lot of challenges as a child. I come from Ethiopia. Most women don't get the opportunities I have. How am I going to whine about this, right, when I've been given this enormous opportunity that I cannot afford to squander. I always find a way to deal with it and move forward. So, for me, I contextualized challenges and became good at convincing myself that in the grand scheme of things, these are not very relevant. I was the only black faculty in the entire department of 110 people and an immigrant. At the University of

Michigan, at the beginning, I really thought I was the only one struggling. The tragedy of racism in the United States is the first thing you would say is, "It's because I'm different from them, because I'm Black." It was an almost entirely male faculty, except for one woman who had been with them for 15 years by appeasing everyone. Tenured professors, who'd been there for a long time, engaged in this constant mocking. It was a very backhanded way of making my life difficult.

So, I hired a critical mass of new people who were aligned to my thinking, who took pride in clinical care as opposed to just getting an NIH grant. Very early on I started bringing resources. In academia money brings you power and freedom. Informal networks were also critical to propelling me and having something to fall back on. I started meeting other young faculty who were American women, who were facing enormous challenges being leaders. I had the most unlikely alliance with a PhD researcher and a rheumatology clinician and one other woman. We created a network to make sure we were publishing, pulling each other up, and sharing opportunities. We literally started putting each other on our grants. We pushed the medical school to have more of a focus on global health. We were organizing around women's promotion, women's access to resources, faculty development. I, and many of my colleagues, were serving on so many committees and walking into rooms and shocking men, white men with gray hair, with our very unorthodox and unusual style.

How Has Leadership Changed in the Last Few Decades?

I saw someone tweet the other day saying how global health is all being led by men. For me leadership is defined in so many incredible ways and we have come a long way. But if you look at formal leadership we have a long way to go. There is an enormous opportunity for people to identify themselves as a leader and find voices without getting formal authority to be called a leader. I have zero formal authority, frankly. A lot of the work I do is through my informal authority.

We are all leaders. We are global health leaders, we are inspiring, we're shaping. I think part of the push we need to make is a recognition that we do not need to be a head of an entity to be a leader. We do not need to be endorsed by someone to be a leader. We must figure out our own space and voice. When you create more space and become more collaborative and more inclusive, you create a constituency and a movement that will have its own rules and its own energy. Sooner or later, you will force those traditional institutions to respond to the demands that you are creating through your own informal channels.

Thirty years ago, when I was younger all the women leaders in medicine had attained that position by acting like men. They had done it by wearing gray suits and short hair, talking like men, sacrificing marriages and children, or getting married late and not by choice. And there weren't that many women to emulate. I remember how many people frowned when I decided to have four kids, in residency, in fellowship. Now it's becoming the norm. Style is changing there is more diversity.

Is the Perception of Leadership and Failures Different Because of Their Gender

We all know when you fail as a woman, it gets exaggerated that much more. It's the intersection of race and gender. A woman's mistakes tend to be amplified both in terms of social norms and societal expectation. You are under the microscope, you are scrutinized, your statements are exaggerated. I can make the same statement on social media as a male colleague, and the consequence or the response is very different. However, women also tend to be highly critical of themselves. We tend to stew a lot more over things that we feel are failures or mistakes, more so than our male colleagues.

Dealing with Failure

Of course, I have made mistakes along the way. There was a time in my life where I was absolutely absent from my family. I was gone from my house. I would come on a weekend, but there was an intense year and a half period where I was probably gone 90% of the time. This was around the time of Dr. Tedros's campaign. I was so consumed by the vision of having a person of color at the WHO, I really did not weigh up what the impact of my absence would be on my boys, who were shifting from middle school to high school. Although I'm happy with the outcome of the WHO campaign, it is time you cannot gain back. You just don't get a second chance to do parenting right. When you talk about failures and guilt, a lot of it for women, whether it's perceived or real, revolves around work-life balance.

My path to leadership was also an uphill battle, but I did get over it. Because I had support from up above, from the home, and because of the type of person I am. I overcame a lot of challenges as a child. I developed a skillset very early on that allowed me to deal with pushback and trauma. I always tend to focus on the positive, because if we harp on the negative we can get incapacitated. I come from Ethiopia where survival is low. Most women don't get the opportunities I have. How am I going to whine about this, when I've been given this enormous opportunity that I cannot afford to squander.

How Likely Are You on a Scale of 1 to 7 to See Other Women Leaders?

I would say six. We've come a long way. We have a long way to go.

What Measures Can Institutions Take to Inculcate Greater Representation of Women in Leadership Positions?

We need accountability mechanisms. People are not just going to change; they have to have a reason to change. WHO is trying, Dr. Tedros is trying, but institutions are not easy to change. By the time institutions change their policies, it is often too late for women. It literally breaks my heart but relying on institutions alone to bring the change that we want, that's going to take us a lifetime. That's what the evidence supports. If you are putting women in a toxic environment, without support, without an enabling environment, without the tools they need to succeed, representation alone doesn't mean anything.

So how do we support each other? How do we pull each other up? How do we learn to rely on each other and not undermine each other? These are the questions women need to figure out. So, I think some of the tools that we need to be women are how do they organize, how do they demand, how do they assert their rights? Because again, it literally breaks my heart, but relying on institutions alone to bring the change that we want, that's going to take us a lifetime.

You Don't Need Gray Hair to Be a Leader. Find Your Voice

For me, what is changing is one, we're seeing diversity, we're seeing diversity in age, we are accepting young leaders. Leadership is not related to gray hair, gender, skin color, language, right? So, use your voice and different skills and styles to reach out and not always looking up, but also looking down, and how do you mobilize people who don't have platforms and who don't have voices? And you don't necessarily do it to become a leader. But when you actually do those things to create more space and become more collaborative and more inclusive, you do emerge in creating a constituency and a movement that will have its own rules and its own energy to galvanize the movement and not necessarily wait for endorsement of an existing traditional leadership institute that will recognize you. And then sooner or later, you will force those institutions to respond to the demand that you are creating through your own informal channels.

What Advice Would You Give to Young Women Who Are Aspiring to Be Global Health Leaders?

First, I think having mentors is important. Mentors on all aspects of their lives, not just for our professional careers, but spiritual mentors. Mentors for wherever you need growth.

Second, young women have to be willing to cause a disruption. You don't make gains and progress by playing nice all the time. You must be willing to speak up. There is an art and science to doing that without creating havoc and reputational risk. But you need to be willing to use your voice when appropriate to challenge the status quo.

Third, women in general tend to invest in communities and not themselves. We spend a lot more time negotiating for the collective than for individuals. But I think the collective doesn't always look out for your interest. We need to teach young women to develop the ability to voice their own interests and advocate for themselves. Young women should identify a passion and purpose that will drive them and help them shape their opinion. If you have an issue that you deeply care about, the energy and effort you put into pushing that agenda will propel you and eventually will either force the institution to respond to your needs, or you will leave that institution in search of another one. I think finding purpose and passion instead of just fighting for mere leadership status is what's going to serve us all.

The challenge for the younger generation is how do you find your voice and space and influence outside institutions? For example, I think we have a long way to go in academic medicine. We are seeing some movement in UN entities and new global health organizations that respond to social media. But academic institutions are a place where you go, and the number of women deans and chairs is dismal. It is unbelievable how much work we have to do in that space.

If You Could Have a Billboard for Other Women Leaders, What Would It Say?

Make your own rules. Don't be bound by societal rules.

Health and Hierarchy: Exploring Workforce Inequalities in Uganda and Somaliland

Summer Simpson and Raquel Pérez Cañal

Ensuring the equal participation of women in the global health workforce—as in all spheres of public life—is an essential prerequisite to building more inclusive and equitable societies. While women comprise 70% of the global health workforce, contributing $3 trillion to global health annually, they remain critically underrepresented in health leadership and face significant barriers to promotional and professional advancement opportunities, with only 25% holding leadership positions (Devex, 2019; GHWN, 2018). On a global scale, systemic gender biases and inequities result in system inefficiencies, bottlenecks in health worker education and recruitment, and employment imbalances across the formal and informal health workforces (WHO, 2019). These challenges are hindering the contribution that women could make to effective leadership for health systems strengthening and, more broadly, are undermining our progress towards achieving Universal Health Coverage (UHC), particularly in low- and middle-income countries (LMICs) (Javadi et al., 2016; WHO, 2019).

In 2019, the Tropical Health and Education Trust (THET) conducted a qualitative participatory study in Uganda and Somaliland to deepen its organisational understanding of the main enabling factors and barriers posed to gender equality for health professionals in LMICs. Led by gender advocates from Uganda and Somaliland, the research approach was both diagnostic—seeking to identify how gender discrimination manifests, how it is experienced, and who it affects—and solution-oriented, seeking to identify trajectories of positive change and practical measures that can be introduced to address gender disparity. Through key informant interviews (KIIs) and focus group discussions (FGDs) with male and female health facility managers, clinical staff, academics, and policy-makers, a number of key themes were explored. These included gender discrimination and stereotypes, access to opportunities, flexible working patterns, the impact of unpaid care work,

S. Simpson · R. Pérez Cañal
THET (Tropical Health and Education Trust), London, UK
e-mail: summer.simpson@thet.org; raquel@iwpr.net

© Springer Nature Switzerland AG 2022
R. Morgan et al. (eds.), *Women and Global Health Leadership*,
https://doi.org/10.1007/978-3-030-84498-1_24

243

and representation and leadership. The peer-to-peer research approach and inclusion of gender advocates known to and active within their communities enabled an advanced level of access and insight.

Methodology

THET initially conducted a literature review on the role of women in health systems, focusing on the gendered enabling factors and barriers faced. This comprised over 30 publications, including international data from agencies such as the World Health Organization and the World Bank, as well as country-specific articles and publications from national governments and peer-reviewed journals focusing on gender and global health. The key themes identified through this review informed the development of the research framework.

The process which followed was highly collaborative and participatory. Within this, THET and a gender specialist worked with gender-focused academics and researchers in Uganda and Somaliland. The research framework and data collection tools were developed collectively to ensure the study posed questions which were relevant to each context and that these questions addressed both structural and agency-related factors. The in-country teams worked to identify target groups and to develop an appropriate structure for discussions.

The data collection methods employed were key informant interviews (KIIs) and focus group discussions (FGDs). KII participants included senior policy-makers, clinicians, managers, and academics, with the aim to gain detailed insights into the experiences of those in senior positions. A total of ten KIIs were carried out in Uganda and nine in Somaliland. The FGDs were facilitated by research assistants, who led discussions on the key themes identified in the research framework. FGDs ranged from 6 to 15 participants and were separated by gender to encourage open and honest discussions. This also helped to account for context-specific cultural norms. A total of 61 individuals participated in the FGDs in Uganda and 48 in Somaliland. Both data collection processes covered private and public sector health institutions, as well as academic and government bodies.

The collaborative approach to research design and the use of local teams for data collection were introduced as quality and relevance assurance mechanisms, ensuring the appropriate people were asking relevant questions, framed in the right way, to a representative group of participants. As the research was led by women and men active and well-connected within their communities, THET was able to gain a deeper level of access and insight than is often available.

While qualitative studies can at times incorporate reporting bias, the team worked to address this wherever possible through detailed and transparent recording and reporting structures. The main limitation of this study was therefore deemed to be the sample size. Due to time and resource constraints, the total number of participants was limited; however, the demographic composition of the participants was carefully assessed to ensure various aspects and levels of the health system were represented. We are confident that the sample is representative and can provide relevant and useful insights which can serve as a robust evidence base for further research and the development of gender-transformative tools.

Country Context: Uganda and Somaliland

The barriers posed to women in the health workforce cannot be understood in isolation. Many of these obstacles stem from the cultural, social, political, and economic context in which women are situated. As such, it is necessary to explore some key statistics at the national level before analysing progress towards gender equality.

Uganda

Despite a steady decline in the poverty rate over the past two decades (from 31.1% in 2006 to 21.4% in 2018), it is estimated that around seven million people are still affected by chronic poverty in Uganda (World Bank, 2016; PwC, 2018), and the country ranks 162nd of 189 countries in the 2017 Human Development Index. Uganda has an organised national health system comprised of both private and public providers. The private sector incorporates private not-for-profit institutions and private health practitioners, while the public sector includes government health facilities and ministry departments. The public sector, largely financed by government and international donor funding, is the main provider of decentralised health services at both national and district-based levels (Ssennyonjo et al., 2018). The burden of disease in the country is dominated by communicable diseases (including malaria, HIV/AIDS, tuberculosis, and respiratory diseases), accounting for over 50% of morbidity and mortality. Maternal and perinatal disorders are also a leading cause of illness and death among women (WHO, 2017), who represent 51% of the population (UBOS, 2019; UNDP, 2017).

As evidenced in the United Nations Development Programme (UNDP) Gender Inequality Index (GII), Uganda has made significant progress since the 1990s in addressing aspects of gender inequality, particularly through the introduction of legislation and policies. For example, the country has achieved gender parity in primary education, and almost 35% of parliamentary seats are held by women, 5% above the target set by the Beijing Platform of Action (Uganda MES, 2016; UNDP, 2020). Women are also economically active, with 67% of women over the age of 15 engaged in the labour force, compared to 74% of men (UNDP, 2020). However, significant gender inequalities persist in access to services and opportunities, particularly in relation to employment and financial services, meaning Uganda is ranked 131st of 162 countries in the GII (UNDP, 2020). More specifically, women's high rate of participation in the labour force has not translated into economic empowerment: there is still a 39% gender pay gap in the private sector, and, on average, women spend 7.5 hours per day on unpaid care work (UNDP, 2017).

Somaliland

Somaliland is estimated to have the fourth lowest gross domestic product (GDP) per capita in the world. According to the World Bank, the poverty rate in urban areas of Somaliland stands at 29%, compared to 38% in rural areas (World Bank, 2014).[1] More than half of the population is under the age of 20 years, with women comprising slightly less than half of the population.

Somaliland's dual healthcare system—comprising the private and public sectors—is dominated by private healthcare providers (Devi, 2015). The system is made up of a single national referral hospital, a single national mental health hospital, five regional referral hospitals, three district hospitals, and a number of mother and child healthcare centres (Issa et al., 2018). While limited data exists on health indicators in Somaliland, maternal mortality is identified as a leading cause of death among women of reproductive age (WHO-EMRO, 2014). The primary causes of mortality in Somalia include tuberculosis, lower respiratory infections, diarrheal diseases, and neonatal disorders (IHME, 2017).

In August 2017, Somaliland launched a new National Development Plan (NDPII). Despite not being an official signatory to the Sustainable Development Goals (SDGs), SDG targets are integrated within the NDPII, including SDG5: Gender Equality (Saferworld, 2018). While this represents positive progress, significant gender disparities persist across numerous indicators. Gender inequality exists at all levels of education, increasing at secondary and tertiary level. Women also have a lower labour force participation rate than men: 27% of women over the age of 10 are engaged in the labour force, compared to 48% of men. Of those women who are inactive in the labour force, 60% are unable to participate due to household duties. Additionally, of the 72 government ministers in Somaliland, only 2 are women (3%) (Somaliland MoPND, 2018).

Qualitative Research Findings

Drawing on personal accounts and analytical explorations at the institutional and system levels, the research identified a number of key insights. The findings of the qualitative study have been grouped into four areas: access to opportunities and promotion, gender discrimination and stereotypes, flexible working conditions and

---

[1] These figures are sourced from the most up-to-date data available in the public domain from a reliable source.

unpaid care work, and representation and leadership. The following section will explore each of these themes in turn.

Access to Opportunities and Promotion

In both Uganda and Somaliland, women's access to employment opportunities in the health sector is limited by a lack of transparency and inconsistency in hiring practices. This is particularly prevalent in Somaliland, where vacancies are shared informally through networks and private contacts, rather than through public advertisements, rendering "who you know" is more important than qualifications or experience. Men are more likely to benefit from these processes because the networks in which vacancies are circulated tend to be male-dominated. Women's predominance in the private spheres of home and community, dictated by religious and social norms, plays a significant role in limiting their exposure to informal networks. As stated by a female respondent from Somaliland: "Usually, jobs availability is passed on secretly, and women have no access to them". A female nurse from Somaliland similarly expressed: "people get employment opportunities because they know senior managers, or if you have someone who have links with them. The knowledge you have and whatever experience you retained is not relevant". In Uganda, women have greater access to vacancy information than their counterparts in Somaliland, with research respondents stating that jobs are frequently advertised through agencies and the media.

However, while women in Uganda may be able to access vacancy information more readily, they are less likely than their male counterparts to be invited to interview, with researchers identifying indications that some employers are allowing gender biases to influence the interview and selection process at the recruitment stage. A respondent based at a private hospital in Uganda stated that their institution implements an unofficial policy of not hiring female laboratory staff based on the assumption that women cannot withstand the demands of the role and the long hours incurred. However, further research would be needed to identify the extent to which gendered assumptions affect the transparency and fairness of hiring decisions in LMICs.

Gender biases also have a limiting effect on access to on-the-job training and promotion, posing a challenge to the career progression prospects of women. Female tutors in Somaliland noted that such opportunities are often shared by male managers with male doctors in informal situations such as tea breaks or social events after work. This informal system places women at a disadvantage, as women tend to spend less time in these spaces due to the additional responsibility of unpaid care work. In Somaliland, KII and FGD participants stated that in both public and private institutions, men are more likely to be promoted, even when they are competing against women with more experience and higher qualifications. Several female respondents stated that they had been actively discouraged from seeking promotional opportunities by senior colleagues and at times family members due to gendered cultural norms that assign unpaid care responsibilities to women. Taken together, gender bias in access to employment, training, and promotional opportunities significantly limits women's career progression and advancement to leadership positions.

Flexible Working Conditions and Unpaid Care Work

Unpaid care work, which includes caring for families, homes, children, and elderly relatives, directly correlates with "occupational downgrading"—a process through which women are restricted to part-time or precarious employment and are precluded from career advancement and leadership opportunities (WHO, 2019). The dual burden posed by unpaid domestic care obligations and professional responsibilities is a well-articulated challenge for women with families in both Uganda and Somaliland. The majority of respondents agreed that due to gendered cultural norms, unpaid care obligations are the responsibility of female health workers, with little or no shared responsibility. In both countries, female respondents stressed that this burden restricted the possibilities and opportunities available to them, especially in relation to their choice of specialisation and ability to progress to more senior positions or to undertake further medical training. For example, women are often precluded from working the long, unsociable hours—including night shifts—that are expected of junior doctors, placing their male counterparts at an advantage. A female Ugandan doctor explained that many women accept employment opportunities at health institutions that offer lower salaries to be closer to their families. A female medical academic from Uganda suggested that: "as a lady, every child you have is about ten publications that are lost". The dual burden is compounded by a lack of flexibility: with only the occasional exception, health employers were found to implement no flexible working policies that would allow women to work part-time or to limit the number of unsociable hours which they are expected to work.

Gender Discrimination and Stereotypes

Despite the existence of national laws and institutional regulations which promote gender equality, female respondents in Uganda and Somaliland cited numerous examples of latent and explicit gender discrimination in the workplace. This reveals a dissonance between accepted codes of conduct and gendered practices in health institutions. The majority of male respondents in both countries claimed that discrimination was not a prevalent issue in their institution, rendering it clear that men and women often experience and perceive discrimination differently. The researchers found that in many instances, biases and discriminatory attitudes derive from socially ingrained perceptions of male and female qualities, roles, capacities, and obligations. In both Uganda and Somaliland, a common assumption exists—reinforced through media representations and social narratives—that women entering the health profession will pursue nursing while men will become doctors. These associations are underpinned by gendered narratives—men as logical and capable, women as emotional and nurturing—which often go unquestioned. These narratives can affect women and girls at all stages of life. A senior Ugandan academic and doctor explained that as a child she had planned to become a nurse until her parents opened her eyes to the possibility of becoming a doctor: "My dad questioned why I wanted to be a nurse when I could become a doctor. I did not know that women could be doctors then. It is when I found this out, that I changed my dream career".

Further to this, a number of the male doctors interviewed in Uganda argued that paediatrics is more suitable for women than men. This was justified with reference to the traditional perception of women as nurturers, as well as to the more sociable working hours associated with the profession. A male Ugandan ophthalmologist noted that "Women are softer, and kids are calmer around them, so we encourage them to do paediatrics". A female Ugandan paediatrician expounded this assumption and explained that she had altered her aspiration of being a surgeon to become a paediatrician based on advice she received from a male supervisor during her third year of medical school: "the supervisor told me 'I know you are married and honestly is not fair for you to be a woman and a surgeon'". Respondents stated that such assertions are based on a normative assumption that men have more flexibility to respond to emergency calls and to spend long hours operating on patients. Within specialisations, the allocation of tasks is also gendered. In Uganda, for example, respondents noted that male nurses sometimes avoid certain tasks and procedures—such as wound dressing and drug dispensing—due to a perception that they are "feminine".

The implicit hierarchy of ascribed gender roles within the health profession was also reflected in patient biases towards male and female health professionals. In both countries, several instances were highlighted in which nurses were assumed to be significantly less knowledgeable than doctors, and in which female doctors had been exposed to the mistrust and abuse of patients. Several respondents reported occasions in which older male patients had been unwilling to accept the professional credibility of a female doctor, undermining their ability to examine and treat patients.

These perceptions of women's limited capabilities were found to extend beyond patients to colleagues within the health establishment. In both private and public sector hospitals in Uganda, respondents cited incidents in which male doctors or trainees had explicitly insisted on being assigned a male supervisor, revealing personal gender biases. Respondents also reported that female colleagues were failing to support or mentor young female interns. A female policy-maker in Uganda stated that female senior doctors were harsher in their treatment of female medical students, noting that senior female staff sometimes discriminated against other women both at the clinical and administrative levels. Young women were found to experience particularly harsh judgement by colleagues, with a young female medical professional from Somaliland recounting: "the men underestimate me and ignore me, and I am still struggling to prove that I can successfully do this work". She stressed that this made her feel obliged to constantly demonstrate her ability and resilience.

The male health professionals involved in the study acknowledged that gender biases largely work in their favour; however, a level of resentment was identified among males in Uganda towards affirmative action schemes designed to support women's participation in the health workforce. While women predominate in lower-level occupations in health institutions, significantly few occupy decision-making positions. Despite this, a male Ugandan doctor argued that due to affirmative action, recruitment in the health profession often worked in women's favour, to the detriment of male applicants. Several male doctors also stated that it was discriminatory for their female counterparts to be given 1.5 additional academic points to increase their chances of accessing university education (Kagoda, 2011).[2] They felt that this policy led to male students missing out on government sponsorship. These responses highlight the need to address the misperceptions surrounding affirmative action and to increase awareness among male health professionals about the gender inequalities that underpin such measures.

Representation and Leadership

Gender equality in leadership is an area in which progress is being made. While there was a consensus among the majority of respondents in both countries studied that leadership is male dominated, there are a number of positive exceptions to this rule. A senior doctor based in Uganda stated that women occupied four out of ten management positions in her institution. Similarly, the leadership of a Somaliland midwifery association involved in the study is made up largely of women, reflecting the growing number of leadership positions available to women in the countries studied. A number of the doctors and policy-makers interviewed in Uganda acknowledged their ability to utilise their seniority to make specific demands with regard to gender equality. A senior female doctor from Uganda, for example, lobbied management for the installation of a permanent breastfeeding room for new mothers. This said, women continue to face gendered barriers to leadership opportunities, and those who occupy positions of power face both passive and overt aggression and sexism from male colleagues. A female Ugandan doctor reflected on her experience as a woman in leadership within a government ministry, commenting that, while men in the organisation did not directly challenge her seniority, they actively undermined her authority as a decision-maker

---

[2] In the 1990s the government of Uganda introduced an affirmative action policy whereby an additional 1.5 points were allocated to all females qualified to enter public universities in Uganda to address the persistent gap in enrolment of women in higher institutions. The measure has substantially raised women's enrolment at university level (Kagoda, 2011; UNDP, 2012).

through their reluctance to take timely action on policies that required feedback and/or implementation. She was also subject to sexist jokes that undermined her reputation.

Female respondents in both public and private institutions in Uganda and Somaliland expressed a view that speaking up about their concerns is widely discouraged. A number of nurses in Somaliland stated that in public institutions, women's complaints are not listened to, and in some instances, individuals have been threatened by members of management for speaking out. Similarly, female members of a doctors' association in Somaliland explained that their concerns were not acknowledged because the majority of members are male and the men take responsibility for decision-making, "So most of the time they [men] don't consult us [women] and don't consider our decisions". This reality is mirrored at the government level, with a representative from a Somaliland government ministry stating that the ministry's overwhelmingly male leadership means that women have very little formal voice within the establishment–an inequity that is further compounded by the absence of a national gender policy. A similar situation exists in Uganda, where FGD participants noted that despite the existence of staff representatives through whom grievances can be raised, female staff are reluctant to voice concerns through fear of being reprimanded.

A positive example of women using their voice to affect change was provided by respondents in Uganda. A group of female respondents stated that in the past, motorcycles provided by their organisation for fieldwork and community outreach were often large, powerful ("macho") models better suited to men. Female staff raised complaints to the leaders of the organisation, who subsequently purchased smaller, user-friendly motorcycles suitable for all, enabling women to effectively participate in fieldwork.

Conclusion

This chapter has sought to identify the main enabling factors and barriers posed to gender equality for health professionals in Uganda and Somaliland. While the researchers identified some positive examples of women disrupting stereotypes, these cases are still in the minority, and the day-to-day reality of discrimination and imbalance remains the norm in Uganda and Somaliland. As a female doctor in Uganda made clear:

> *"until we get to a point where it is normal to see 50% or more of women on the board or at senior management, women are still not going to aspire for these positions and men will not accept that women can take these roles...You know how they say equality is giving everyone the same size of ladder to climb, sometimes you need to give the shorter person the taller ladder to climb to be able to see overboard".*

Gender bias and inequity in access to employment, training, and promotional opportunities has significant implications both for the health workforce and for patients in Uganda and Somaliland. On a global scale, women experience a dispro-portionate burden of morbidity and mortality due to inequities in access to basic healthcare, nutrition, and education. Increasing the representation of women in health leadership is a necessary step towards addressing this burden (Downs et al., 2014). Evidence shows that elevating women to positions of leadership instigates a ripple effect that has positive impacts on families, communities, and countries (Downs et al., 2016). Research also suggests that advancing women's leadership can "create stronger, fairer and more resilient health systems" through the develop-ment of gender-responsive and effective solutions at all levels of the health system (Dhatt et al., 2017; RinGs, 2018: 2).

To enhance women's access to employment opportunities and promotion, we recommend that health facilities institutionalise transparent recruitment criteria, use a wide range of channels to disseminate promotional opportunities to all relevant staff members, and establish objective selection processes based on comparative knowledge and experience. To help minimise the burden of unpaid care work, we recommend that health institutions facilitate flexible working arrangements—such as part-time or flexi-time contracts—and standardise the provision of affordable childcare near or in health workspaces. To dismantle gender stereotypes and mini-mise discrimination, we recommend launching gender awareness and sensitisation activities for male and female health professionals, patients, and members of local communities. This could take place through various media channels, including social and traditional media, and through mandatory gender training for all staff. At the institutional level, we recommend introducing formal, discrete channels for staff to raise complaints about discriminatory behaviour and for appropriate disciplinary action to be taken. To improve the representation of women in health leadership, we recommend setting quotas at the national level to offset institutional gender biases and ensure that women are represented in middle- and top-level management. Research has shown that quotas can provide a useful starting point for ensuring that an initial critical mass of women are represented in leadership, helping to normalise gender equality in health leadership (Rohini & Ford, 2012). To support this process, we recommend that a gender audit be carried out in both Uganda and Somaliland to map progress towards female leadership targets.

It is important to note that inequality experienced on the basis of gender is often compounded by other factors such as age, socioeconomic status, and access to edu-cation. Such nuances and overlapping cleavages need to be given appropriate con-sideration when approaching gender equality. As such, the findings put forward in this chapter should contribute to the existing evidence base on gender equality in LMICs, aiming to stimulate further research and greater gender awareness across the health and international development communities and to support the advance-ment of cross-sectoral gender equality.

Acknowledgements Alyson Brody, Dr Lydia Namatende Sakwa, and Roda Ali Ahmed contrib-uted to the research which informed this chapter. The chapter was submitted on behalf the Tropical Health and Education Trust (THET), which works to create a world where everyone, everywhere, has access to quality healthcare. We achieve this by training and educating health workers in low-

and middle-income countries (LMICs) in partnership with volunteers from across the UK health community. In 2019, we sought to strengthen our approach to gender equality, building on previous studies in Uganda and with a new focus on Somaliland, two countries where THET has a longstanding footprint and track record.

References

Devex. (2019). *Q&A: Nurse leadership and tackling health workforce shortages.* Retrieved from https://www.devex.com/news/sponsored/q-a-nurse-leadership-and-tackling-health-workforce-shortages-94242.

Devi, S. (2015). Slowly and steadily, Somaliland builds its health system. *The Lancet World Report, 358,* 2139–2140.

Dhatt, R., Theobald, S., Buzuzi, S., Ros, B., Vong, S., Muraya, K., & Jackson, C. (2017). The role of women's leadership and gender equity in leadership and health system strengthening. *Global Health, Epidemiology and Genomics, 2*(8).

Downs, J., Reif, L., Hokororo, A., & Fitzgerald, D. (2014). Increasing women in leadership in global health. *Academic Medicine, 89*(8), 1103–1107.

Downs, J. A., Mathad, J. S., Reif, L. K., McNairy, M. L., Celum, C., Boutin-Foster, C., & Fitzgerald, D. W. (2016). The ripple effect: Why promoting female leadership in global health matters. *Public Health Action, 6*(4), 210–211.

Health Workforce Network. (2018). *Gender Equity Hub.* Retrieved from https://www.who.int/hrh/network/GEH2018-overview.pdf.

IHME. (2017). *Somalia.* Retrieved from http://www.healthdata.org/somalia.

Issa, H., Harris, M., & Darzi, A. (2018). The international community needs to help reconstruct Somaliland's healthcare system, *The BMJ Opinion.* Retrieved from https://blogs.bmj.com/bmj/2018/01/26/the-international-community-needs-to-help-reconstruct-somalilands-healthcare-system/.

Javadi, D., Vega, J., Etienne, C., Wandira, S., Doyle, Y., & Nishtar, S. (2016). Women who lead: Successes and challenges of five health leaders. *Health Systems & Reform, 2*(3), 229–240.

Kagoda, A. M. (2011). *Assessing the effectiveness of affirmative action on women's leadership and participation in education sector in Uganda.* International Institute of Educational Planning, UNESCO. Retrieved from http://cees.mak.ac.ug/sites/default/files/publications/SEM313_20_eng.pdf

PwC. (2018). *Uganda economic outlook 2018.* Retrieved from https://www.pwc.com/ug/en/assets/pdf/ug-economic-outlook-2018.pdf.

RinGs. (2018). *The role of women's leadership in health system strengthening.* Retrieved from https://ringsgenderresearch.org/wp-content/uploads/2018/07/The-role-of-womens-leadership-and-gender-equity-in-leadership-and-health-system-strengthening-1.pdf.

Rohini, P., & Ford, D. (2012). *Gender quotas and female leadership.* Retrieved from https://siteresources.worldbank.org/INTWDR2012/Resources/7778105-1299699968583/7786210-1322671773271/Pande-Gender-Quotas-April-2011.pdf.

Saferworld. (2018). *Building a peaceful, just and inclusive Somaliland: SDG16+ priorities for action.* Retrieved from https://www.saferworld.org.uk/resources/publications/1173-building-a-peaceful-just-and-inclusive-somaliland-sdg16-priorities-for-actioon.

Somaliland Ministry of Planning and National Development (MoPND). (2018). *Women and men in Somaliland: Facts and figures 2018.* Retrieved from http://www.somalilandcsd.org/wp-content/uploads/2018/11/Gender-Booklet-05.pdf.

Ssennyonjo, A., Namakula, J., Kasyaba, R., Orach, S., Bennett, S., & Ssengooba, F. (2018). Government resource contributions to the private-not-for-profit sector in Uganda: Evolution, adaptations and implications for universal health coverage. *International Journal for Equity in Health, 17*(130), 1–12.

Uganda Bureau of Statistics. (2019). *Population clock*. Retrieved from https://www.ubos.org/

Uganda Ministry of Education and Sports (MES). (2016). *Gender in education section policy*. Retrieved from https://www.education.go.ug/files/downloads/GENDER%20IN%20EDUCATION%20SECTOR%20POLICY.pdf.

UNDP. (2012). *Gender equality and women's empowerment in public administration: Uganda case study*. Retrieved from https://www.undp.org/content/dam/undp/library/Democratic%20Governance/Women-s%20Empowerment/UgandaFinal%20-%20HiRes.pdf.

UNDP. (2017). *Promoting gender equality and women's empowerment: Our journey*. Retrieved from http://www.ug.undp.org/content/uganda/en/home/library/womens_empowerment/UNDPUgandaGenderJourney1988-2017.html.

UNDP. (2020). Human Development Report 2020. Retrieved from https://report.hdr.undp.org/

World Bank. (2014). *New World Bank GDP and poverty estimates for Somaliland*. Retrieved from http://www.worldbank.org/en/news/press-release/2014/01/29/new-world-bank-gdp-and-poverty-estimates-for-somaliland.

World Bank. (2016). *Uganda poverty assessment 2016: Fact sheet*. Retrieved from http://www.worldbank.org/en/country/uganda/brief/uganda-poverty-assessment-2016-fact-sheet.

World Health Organization Regional Office. (2014). *Somaliland women of reproductive age mortality survey 2014*. Retrieved from http://www.emro.who.int/images/stories/somalia/Somaliland_WRA_mortality_survey_Final_report-1_Dec.pdf?ua=1.

World Health Organization. (2017). *Country cooperation strategy: Uganda*. Retrieved from https://apps.who.int/iris/bitstream/handle/10665/136975/ccsbrief_uga_en.pdf?sequence=1.

World Health Organization. (2019). *Global health: Delivered by women, led by men. A gender and equity analysis of the global health and social workforce. A literature review*. Geneva.

Interview with Cheryl Overs of the Michael Kirby Centre for Public Health and Human Rights, Co-founder of the Global Network of Sex Work Projects and Internationally Renowned Expert on HIV

Kate Hawkins

"Leadership has always been a difficult issue for me because I didn't set out to lead anything and I think of myself as more committed to disrupting hierarchies than creating them".

Cheryl Overs is a Senior Research Fellow at the Michael Kirby Centre for Public Health and Human Rights at Monash University in Melbourne, Australia. She is known for her work in promoting sex workers' rights. She founded the Prostitutes Collective of Victoria, Scarlet Alliance Australia, and the Global Network of Sex Work Projects. She worked as an early advisor to the Global Program on AIDS at the World Health Organization. In 2011–2012 she was a member of the Technical Advisory Group of the Global Commission on HIV and the Law, and in 2012 she delivered a plenary speech at the International AIDS Conference in Washington, DC.

How Did You Get into Health Activism?

The short version of my pathway to advocacy for sex workers' health is that I was already involved in sex worker activism at a time when the right to health unexpectedly shot to the top of the rights agenda. That was the early 1980s. The HIV pandemic had begun.

The longer version of my story is like most people's—a tale of circumstances, predisposition, opportunities, choices, and luck. If my story is of interest, it is because it is about a young, working-class woman in the Melbourne sex industry who was able to play a role in mobilising sex workers from around the world to influence law and policy.

K. Hawkins (✉)
Pamoja Communications Ltd., Research in Gender and Ethics (RinGs),
Brighton, East Sussex, UK
e-mail: kate@pamoja.uk.com

© Springer Nature Switzerland AG 2022
R. Morgan et al. (eds.), *Women and Global Health Leadership*,
https://doi.org/10.1007/978-3-030-84498-1_25

255

When I was a teenager, I moved from my happy but dull suburban home to a shared house in Melbourne's hip inner city where I could better focus on my social life. I worked as a waitress, nightclub door girl, and then, at the invitation of a friend, as receptionist in a massage parlour. By massage parlour I mean "happy endings" massage, which was prostitution under the Victorian law at the time. This made the inoffensive massage shop technically a brothel which meant that I encountered the absurd and terrifying game of "cops and hookers" that plays out wherever sex work is illegal. Everyone knows the drill for busting sex workers: cops posing as clients, staff avoiding mentioning "extras" till the client is undressed, female cops wired for sound posing as job seekers, booking sheets and condoms collected as evidence, and so on. What I didn't encounter was violence, drugs, or exploitation. I am sure they were about, but the place I worked was routine and uneventful. Tame even. I was outraged the first time I saw two friendly "clients" pull out badges before dragging two university students out sobbing in shock and horror at being arrested. This remained with me and even intensified when I realised that the methods of the 1970s Melbourne vice squad were benign by global standards.

The outrage was soon channelled into joining a campaign to decriminalise prostitution which was driven by a feminist lawyer, Bebe Loff. With a small group of women, both sex workers and not, we formed a lobby group. I was a spokesperson and I was pretty dreadful. Bebe managed to suggest, without offending me, that if I was going to advocate for legal change, I needed to know something about law which would involve a university. I was able to act on that great advice because it came at a moment in Australian history when there was a socialist government providing free university places to thousands of people who would not otherwise have had that access.

I remember the first time I read about AIDS. Before it was AIDS. In *Rolling Stone*. To the credit of the state government of the time, the period between when I read that article and our lobby group the Prostitutes Collective of Victoria opening its first drop-in centre in Melbourne's red-light district was very short. This was because HIV had caught the medical establishment totally off guard. The usual tools for preventing the spread of infectious disease—screening, vaccines, treatments, and quarantines—couldn't address the new retrovirus. The only things society had to throw at HIV was education, condoms, clean syringes, and social support.

At the time the only people officially interacting with sex workers were police and maybe nuns but that was to punish sex workers or save their souls. The fact that both were failing dismally wasn't a concern to officials until HIV arrived. A new way had to be found, urgently. At the Prostitutes Collective of Victoria (PCV) where I was now director, we were already forging that new way. The PCV would train sex workers to provide information, condoms, clean needles, and sexual health referrals in Melbourne's brothels, escort agencies, and to street workers at all hours of the day or night. We mobilised health workers, held safe sex and self-defence workshops, produced a newsletter, and pressured the police to treat sex workers properly. We negotiated with brothel owners about sexual health and, as often as possible, about broader working conditions. It was such a learning curve. It was so new. There was no body of literature or evidence, and terms like "peer education" and "harm reduction" that are so familiar now hadn't been invented. But neither did we have donors telling us what to do or imposing the complicated activity LogFrames and monitoring protocols that my successors understandably complain about. I remember making up what we would say in the car on the way to meetings.

One of the things we made up was the Ugly Mugs list. The list described violent or abusive men with descriptions of their appearance, modus operandi, and often their car including licence plate numbers. It was updated by both male and female sex workers each day and put on display at the drop-in centre for sex workers to consult while collecting condoms before going out to work. As a list of crimes that were either unreported or not prioritised, it was very embarrassing to police, which made it a valuable negotiation tool as well as a source of potentially lifesaving information for sex workers. It has since been replicated in several other countries, including the UK, where it is extremely successful.

The PCV continued to push for law reform, with our case now enhanced by the argument that criminalisation meant that sex workers had reduced ability to protect themselves from HIV. I pushed this in my role as sex industry representative in the consultation that led to the 1994 Prostitution Act. Although I don't attribute this success to my work, it is true to say that since few jurisdictions have liberalised sex work law, I am one of few sex workers' rights activists lucky enough to lead a successful law reform campaign. This early victory empowered (or emboldened) me in ways that led to other right times and places.

Can You Tell Us About Your Time in Leadership of Different Sex Worker Organisations?

Leadership has always been a difficult issue for me because I didn't set out to lead anything and I think of myself as more committed to disrupting hierarchies than creating them. I more or less stumbled into it because I wanted to get certain things done, and setting up organisations to do them was the way to go at the time. Having said that, I suppose that the willingness to put in huge amounts of unpaid work and be exposed to public scrutiny while being sufficiently thick skinned to withstand the consequences of "speaking truth to power" could be seen as leadership qualities. Making that leadership authentic, ethical, and inclusive is a complex challenge. A measure of successful leadership in social movements, as in government, is that leaders leave and are replaced. So that's what I did.

The second organisation I founded and led was the Global Network of Sex Work Projects. I was sure from the outset that bad public health policy was a serious threat to sex workers' rights. My experience at the PCV made me realise that those worst affected would be women of colour, trans, and male sex workers living in poverty and without the rule of law. That is, outside Australia.

In those pre-Internet days, I was aware of sex workers' groups in other countries but I didn't meet other sex worker and HIV activists until the 1989 Montreal AIDS

Conference. Several of the very first sex workers' groups, concerned about HIV, were there from North America, Latin America, and Europe. It was a crash course in global sex work issues. Gloria Lockett from California described the dynamics of health and law in the lives of cis and trans African American women. Gabriela Leite, the Brazilian sex worker leader, explained that decriminalisation should look different in countries where sex workers are excluded from health, justice, welfare, and finance systems. If sex work is not recognised as an occupation, then sex workers are non-citizens, she said. I remember thinking, "Oh, like an undocumented migrant, but in your own country", my main frame of reference at the time for systematic exclusion. Danny Cockerline, a Canadian porn actor and sex worker, argued that sex work is a skill and that sex workers should be seen as an asset, not a liability, in the HIV response. Carol Leigh, the San Francisco performance artist Scarlot Harlot, who had recently invented the term sex worker, was also there providing musical and theatrical direction to our noisy activism.

In fact, we were united in outrage and anger. Until I recently saw footage of ACT UP demonstrations at that conference (https://plri.wordpress.com/2016/12/27/our-bodies-our-business-1989-reflections-on-a-film/), I had forgotten the depth of the despair and open grief of the early HIV epidemic. Sex workers' outrage was also focused on the stigmatising discourses underlying the epidemiological information that was being presented by panels of male researchers. Female sex workers, they said, won't use condoms and were vectors of HIV to clients and their innocent wives and children. One of them showed an "AIDS education" poster showing a sex worker as the grim reaper stalking unsuspecting men. We went ballistic.

It was clear to me that as valuable (and fun) as protesting was, to really influence this new dimension of public health, we needed to organise in a way that policy makers could engage with, hence the creation of the Global Network of Sex Work Projects. Thanks to the director of the World Health Organization's Global Program on AIDS, Jonathan Mann, we had a hope of being listened to. Mann is remembered for recognising the role that the human rights of drug users and sexual minorities would play in responses to HIV. Now it's unremarkable, or even routine, for sex workers to address UN meetings—but back then it was revolutionary.

When Mann invited me to join discussions about HIV with some of the world's foremost epidemiologists and infectious disease researchers in Geneva, I worked very hard to learn enough about the nuts and bolts of public health to take part. Bebe probably popped up again to tell me to do a Master of Public Health degree but I must have ignored her. Rather, my focus was on building solidarity and opportunities for sex work activists around the world to speak out. Crucially, this meant expanding the sex workers' rights movement to include the many emerging activists and allies from the Global South that would be participating in the HIV response.

I knew that the dynamics of local community organising in privileged Melbourne—with its hometown contacts and support—were very different to international organising with its complex terrain of different politics, languages, laws, cultures, and very different institutions. But I am not sure I knew how different, and I certainly didn't appreciate the complex issues of colonisation and co-option that worry me so much these days. At the time, such concerns were insignificant compared to the value of bringing together sex workers from countries as different as Mongolia and Madagascar or Ukraine and Uganda. The information, issues, and strategies they bought to the space were so consistent they seamlessly formed an authentic and coherent global agenda for public health and sex work—decriminalisation; recognition of labour and civil rights; equal access to appropriate, affordable health care; information; condoms; and needles. In retrospect, I think naivety played an important role in my leadership of the Global Network of Sex Work Projects, but it enabled me to focus entirely on building solidarity and on pushing the demands it produced, which remain unchanged today and continue to be pushed by my successors.

What Were the Gendered/Intersectional Challenges That You Faced?

A colleague recently described the hallmarks of stigma as "prurience, titillation, outrage, and disgust", which is an apt description of the minefield around all women's sexual and reproductive health work. Stigma, including self-stigma, is the most powerful tool for controlling sexuality and enforcing gender conformity, and of all areas of women's health, sex work is one of the most stigmatised. This both makes it interesting and puts it at the pointy end of women's health advocacy.

Sex workers' rights advocacy involves constantly interacting with people who see sex work as a problem of one kind or another to be solved. It means being seen and often treated as criminal, crazy, or both for defending the indefensible. This applies not only to conservatives and religious people who are opposed to improving sex workers' lives for moral reasons but also to many feminists and otherwise liberal thinkers. Many feminist and human rights organisations define sex work as violence against women, while public health agencies typically define selling sex as a "risky behaviour", which can be just as damaging because it considers female sex workers as vectors of infection. The first challenge around leadership on sex work issues is the lack of a substantial or reliable network of support to help deal with prejudice, disrespect, misconceptions, and suspicion.

Organisational discrimination against sex work organising was also severe. While all the other organisations of people affected by HIV were up and running, sex workers found it almost impossible to get funding. Where they did it was for local projects limited to core public health activities of distributing condoms and information, and motivated by the idea that peers could "reach" this "hidden population". Money for global sex work advocacy only came later when the Network of Sex Work Projects changed its membership criteria from sex workers to NGOs concerned with sex work.

Volunteerism and underpayment are high on the list of any woman's challenges in global health work. So much of the work I and other sex work movement leaders did in the 1990s to establish a space for sex workers in the HIV response was done for free, which meant putting aside our own needs and other opportunities.

Stigma becomes unbearable and undeniable when it converts to personal discrimination. Although I have been luckier than some of my counterparts who have faced unemployment as a result of their activism, I look back aghast at the trail of personal discrimination I survived. Every woman who puts her head above the parapet is immediately and continually assessed—is she the right woman with the right demeanour, background, skin colour, affiliations, clothes, etc.? Is her tone pitched at the right place between aggressive and humble? Does she represent the right balance of empowerment and victimhood? As a working-class Australian at the vanguard of a very stigmatised cause, "no" was always going to be available as a response for anyone who wanted it when the question was asked about me.

The feminist philosopher Sara Ahmed says that "when you expose a problem you pose a problem"; that is, through the process of complaint, the woman herself becomes the problem that needs to be "dealt with" by officialdom. At the beginning, exposing multi-level, institutional failures to protect cis and trans sex workers from abuse and disease certainly made me a low-level problem. But as time went by and I began to suggest that the official solution—education, STI checks, condoms, and [maybe] social support—not only can't solve the problem but also might make it worse, I became a higher-level problem. This view about sex work and health programmes, which I still hold and can credibly defend, took me into the dangerous territory of the difficult, uncooperative, and ungrateful woman.

In retrospect, although my daily work was all about stigma, for the first couple of decades I was oblivious to its accumulative impact and to the lifetime of discrimination I was buying into. That's youth for you.

Where Are You Now and What Advice Do You Have for Other Women Working in This Area?

First and foremost, I'm dedicated to self-care and my only concern about that is that it may be too little, too late. This speaks to the question of what advice I would give young women in health advocacy. To those for whom women's rights and health are a passion rather than a career, I think the most important advice is to find out what self-protection mechanisms work for you, put them into practice, and stick to them. Bulls can get a lot done in a china shop, but it's a costly way of operating.

For the last few years, I have been working in broader human rights research and supporting sex workers who are studying gender and sexuality. I am also involved in advocacy around the rollout of pre-exposure prophylaxis for HIV prevention to cis and trans women who sell sex. I recently addressed a lifelong bugbear about lack of accurate and consistent information about sex work and the law by producing a map of laws that affect sex workers. At the same time, I have been slowly but surely archiving boxes of fascinating but chaotic documentation of the sex workers' rights movement in the HIV response. I try to share information that will strengthen the work of future activists from a seat at the back of the sex workers' rights bus. I frequently hop off entirely and I sometimes watch it go by, often with delight but sometimes not. What matters is that three decades after the first World Whores Congress in Brussels, that bus continues on its journey regardless of who's driving.

When I think about women's leadership in civil society, I think first about the advances in sexual and reproductive health rights achieved by social movements led by women. Campaigns for girls' education and against child and forced marriage, female genital mutilation, unsafe abortion, rape, and gender-based violence have all begun with grassroots movements of women and frequently by one or two women "at the kitchen table", as the media often characterises it. But soon after I think about the well-canvassed issues that affect women in all leadership roles—the glass ceiling, volunteerism, unpaid care, sexist attitudes towards women's behaviour and appearance, sexual harassment, heteronormativity, male-dominated management, patriarchal assumptions. Which leads me to worry about "civil society" itself. What is it? Who does it benefit? Who controls it? What voices does it privilege and silence?

Massive expansion of professional NGOs, supported by large grants from bilateral and national agencies such as the Gates and Soros foundations, has seen civil society generally and health NGOs specifically grow into what many have called an industrial complex. I am one of many feminists concerned that alongside the positive impact of money going to good causes and plugging gaps caused by states' failures, this "NGO industrial complex" suffocates social movements' transformative agendas through a process of instrumentalisation and de-politicisation.

A frequently cited quote by Lilla Watson perfectly encapsulates the problem of "help":

> If you have come here to help me, you are wasting your time. But if you have come because your liberation is bound up with mine, then let us work together.

Well-meaning "helpers" certainly have a challenge when it comes to sex work and health. Funding "sex work" organisations to provide medical services and recognising those services as speaking for sex workers has been a steady process of colonisation by public health agencies. Sex workers' assertion of the right to be free from state persecution and protected by the rule of law has been appropriated and repackaged as a recommendation that law reform is needed to stop the spread of HIV. Crucially, it is civil society that has laid this AstroTurf over the grassroots and it has ostensibly done it to "help".

Even where the colonisation of women's issues by civil society is recognised, there is a dearth of suggestions as to how women might address the problem. Clearly, intersecting systems of oppression mean that the way forward must be grounded in intersectional organising. Before we look "up" to philanthropists or humanitarian agencies for support, we should look "across" to each other in mutual solidarity.

Women's Leadership in Global Health: Evolution Will Not Bring Equality

Roopa Dhatt and Ann Keeling

For decades, women have been told that it is just a matter of time before they will have equal representation in leadership with men. If women can be patient, equality is just over the horizon. Armed with the right qualifications and training, women will, in time, burst out of the professional pipeline into the sunshine, standing shoulder to shoulder in leadership at all levels with men. First, however, like knuckle-walking primates evolving into *Homo sapiens*, women must learn how to walk standing up, learn how to use tools, and learn the coded language and behavior practiced in executive level boardrooms and parliaments. A woman can learn to be more like a man.

The paradox of global health is that there is no deficit of women in the health and social workforce. In a minority of countries, it is still critical that girls complete secondary school so they are able to train and enter the health and social workforce. But in most countries women are the majority in the pipeline, and globally they hold the majority (70%) of jobs in the sector. Despite this and the promise of equality by evolution, women hold only a minority (25%) of senior leadership roles in health (WHO, 2019), and strangely, it seems necessary to remind decision-makers that the default health and social care worker is a woman. Indeed, the first recommendation of the 2019 WHO report *Global Health: Delivered by Women, Led by Men. A Gender and Equity Analysis of the Global Health and Social Workforce* is that: "It is time to change the narrative. Women, as the majority of the global health and social care workforce, are the drivers of global health" (WHO, 2019).

It is as though women in the health and social health workforce have been hiding in plain sight.

R. Dhatt (✉) · A. Keeling
Women in Global Health, Washington, DC, USA
e-mail: roopa.dhatt@womeningh.org; ann.keeling@womeningh.org

© Springer Nature Switzerland AG 2022
R. Morgan et al. (eds.), *Women and Global Health Leadership*,
https://doi.org/10.1007/978-3-030-84498-1_26

Commitments Have Been Made

The year 2020 marks a quarter century since the landmark Fourth World Conference on Women in Beijing where 189 governments agreed:

> Women's empowerment and their full participation on the basis of equality in all spheres of society, including participation in the decision-making process and access to power, are fundamental for the achievement of equality, development and peace. (United Nations, 1995)

That principle and related commitments to action have been echoed in numerous global agreements made by the world's governments since the Beijing Conference, including the Sustainable Development Goals (SDGs) (United Nations, 2015) and the 2019 Political Declaration from the High-Level Meeting on Universal Health Coverage (United Nations, 2019). There is no need for additional commitments. We are not asking governments for anything that has not already been agreed.

Twenty-five years after Beijing, however, as the interviews in this book demonstrate, while there has been progress, global health is still delivered by women and led by men. In 2020, COVID-19 exposed fault lines in global health that have persisted because governments failed to deliver on commitments to achieve gender equality in health decision-making.

History Matters

Women have always been healers, made herbal remedies, cared for the sick, and assisted other women in childbirth. In traditional societies, women still play those roles in health. When medicine was formalized as a profession, however, it was established by men as an all-male profession with rules excluding women. Over centuries, women fought for the right to study and practice medicine, and their numbers in health have increased rapidly in the last 30 years, particularly in higher-wage healthcare occupations (Boniol et al., 2019). Women are now 90% of the world's nurses, midwives, frontline community health workers, and social care workers (WHO, 2019).

In some countries change has come relatively recently: the first female doctor graduated in El Salvador in 1945 (Tiempocultural, n.d.), and it took until 2011 for the first woman to qualify as a surgeon in Papua New Guinea. In 2018, three Japanese medical schools admitted to discriminating against female applicants by imposing a higher entry mark for women (McCurry, 2018). It is perhaps not surprising then that Japan has the lowest percentage of women in medicine in the OECD, at just over 20% (WHO, 2019). And for some groups of women, particularly women from racial and ethnic minorities and disadvantaged classes, it has taken much longer to break through the gendered, social, and economic barriers to gain entry to medicine and the higher status specialities.

As an illustration of progress, most physicians, dentists, and pharmacists aged under 40 today are female (Boniol et al., 2019). But women's past exclusion from medicine still has an impact today. In the USA, for example, women were only 20% of enrolled medical students in 1976 (Walsh, 2008). Women from that 1976 cohort are now in their 60s, and since women were just 20%, it is inevitable that their male counterparts will now be holding the majority of senior roles. As a result, younger professionals of all genders have not had the female leadership role models and mentors they would have had if women had been 50% of medical students in 1976. The absence of those women from decision-making leadership roles in health has further entrenched the gendered social norm that leadership has, and should have, a male face.

The United Nations Development Programme (UNDP)'s Gender Social Norms Index (UNDP, 2020) 2020 reports social attitudes toward gender equality in 75 countries, demonstrating that gendered social norms on leadership remain widespread today: 50% of people surveyed said men made better political leaders than women, while more than 40% felt that men made better business executives. This bias against women leaders, even by women themselves, continues to be a serious barrier to women's advancement into leadership in all sectors, including health, and perpetuates gender inequality. UNDP report that the world is not on track to achieve the SDG targets for gender equality by 2030 and note from their survey a small but growing backlash against gender equality (even though it has not yet been achieved in any country).

In the years since the Beijing Conference, there has been significant progress for women in almost all countries. Legal barriers to gender equality have been removed, women can and do vote, they have access to education, and increasingly, they participate in the economy with fewer formal restrictions. Women, however, face a glass ceiling accessing political leadership and other positions of power. The higher the power and responsibility of a role, the wider the gender gap. Women hold only 24% of parliamentary seats globally, and the number of female heads of government (10 out of 193 countries) has fallen in the last 5 years (from 15) (UN Women, 2019). On current trends, it will take 257 years to close the gender gap in economic opportunity (World Economic Forum, 2019). It is all the more alarming then that people in many countries feel gender equality has gone too far. This would, however, be consistent with a gendered social norm that it is appropriate for women to work as lower-status, lower-paid frontline health and social care workers, whereas leadership in health is a male domain. While these jobs are essential for a health system to function, they remain undervalued, especially as they are predominated by women. The UNDP concluded:

> ... Societies often tell their girls that they can become anything they want and are capable of, while investing in their education. But the same societies tend to block their access to power positions without giving them a fair chance. (UNDP, 2020)

A gender equitable society would ensure the important roles in our health systems that are often occupied by majority women are given both dignity and the financing that they deserve.

Seven Significant Shifts Since Beijing 1995

The Rise of Movements

One important change in the last 25 years has been the rise of virtual social movements organized across borders around a common objective, using social media. These movements can now reach people with power directly, including political and business leaders who are accessible on social media, as never before. In women's rights, the #MeToo movement brought women together to break the silence on sexual harassment and abuse. Women in Global Health is another example, formed in 2015, around gender equity and health leadership when its founders met on Twitter. Less than 5 years later, it has over 20 national chapters, 2 regional networks, and over 20,000 followers. Women in Global Health used its virtual network in 2020 to crowdsource data on gender and leadership of global and national task forces on COVID-19, demonstrating that around 80% of decision-makers were men. Before widespread use of social media, it would have been impossible to mobilize information on 87 countries at such speed. Such movements have provided opportunities for leadership outside traditional power hierarchies for younger leaders and others from minority groups and have provided an important means to work collectively on gender inequities, linking the national and the global.

Girls as Leaders

In the 25 years since Beijing, perceptions of girls have changed from viewing them as beneficiaries and dependents to potential global leaders. Girls such as Greta Thunberg and Malala Yousafzai have become respected political leaders of global movements with huge followings. A number of non-governmental organizations (NGOs) now focus on enabling girls and young women to network and lead. This change in social perceptions and support for girls and young women is building cadres of future female leaders who will have new routes into power and influence through social movements.

Intersectionality

The term "intersectionality" predates the Beijing Conference, coined by Kimberlé Crenshaw and emerged out of the Black feminist movement, but is now widely used to describe how a person's social and political identities (race, class, sexual identity, gender identity, nationality, etc.) can combine to amplify either discrimination or privilege. When analyzing who leads in global health, it is critical to take an intersectional approach to asking: who is not in power and has a contribution to make?

Since Beijing, there has also been greater acknowledgment that gender is not a masculine/feminine binary and it increased recognition of the rights and exclusion of people who are non-binary and otherwise transgender.

Fixing Systems of Privilege, not Women

For decades the emphasis has been on training women to fit into leadership. The implication was that women had deficiencies not shared by men that needed to be fixed for them to advance. The 1995 Beijing Platform for Action includes commitments (United Nations, 1995) to:

> Provide leadership and self-esteem training to assist women and girls, particularly those with special needs, women with disabilities, and women belonging to racial and ethnic minorities to strengthen their self-esteem and to encourage them to take decision-making positions;

and

> Create a system of mentoring for inexperienced women and, in particular, offer training, including training in leadership and decision-making, public speaking and self-assertion, as well as in political campaigning.

More recently, the focus has changed to fixing the systemic bias and discrimination in laws, policies, and organizational cultures that exclude women from leadership, rather than fixing women to fit into those systems.

Evidence on the Impact of Women's Leadership

There is a small but growing body of evidence on the positive impact of women's and diverse leadership that is important when persuading skeptics. To date this evidence has mostly centered on women's leadership in politics and business, and there is a dearth of evidence in the health sector. New centers for women's leadership have been launched in a number of countries to collect and disseminate the evidence which will support the role for women's participation in leadership at all levels.

Shared Language

Since Beijing, women have organized around new language which names and forges a shared understanding around unacceptable and discriminatory behavior. On social media, #MeToo and #TimesUp have been used as terms to label and call out sexual harassment. New words such as "mansplaining" describe a pattern of male behavior that is not new, but labeling it signals to both men and women that women find it discriminatory. The term "manel" to describe an all-male panel of speakers has been used to garner pledges from men not to participate and sparked a "manel watch" reporting mechanism on social media that publicizes bad practice. Developments in language signal social change.

COVID-19

Probably the most seismic shift in global health in the last 25 years, besides HIV/AIDS, has been the COVID-19 global pandemic. It is too soon to know whether the death and devastation caused by the pandemic will catalyze greater equality for women in the health and social sector. The pandemic has highlighted the critical role of women as frontline health and social care workers, has exposed the hidden burden of women's unpaid work both in the household and within health systems, and has brought praise for female political leaders who have managed the pandemic with low levels of mortality. One study indicated that countries with women leaders suffered six times fewer deaths from COVID-19 than countries with governments led by men, and much has been written about the positive impact of the leadership style of those women (Coscieme et al., 2020). It remains to be seen whether governments will recognize gender inequality in the health workforce, including in leadership, as a fatal flaw in health systems.

Beyond Gender Parity: Gender Transformative Leadership

Equal representation of women and men in health leadership needs no justification in a workforce with 70% women. Gender parity is a critical first step, but beyond parity the goal must be diversity in leaders of all genders. Health leaders should reflect the constituencies they serve. In addition, since gender equality is the foundation of strong, resilient health systems, it must be an imperative for all leaders. All health leaders therefore should be gender transformative leaders (Dhatt et al., 2018), enacting policies that challenge power and privilege, promote equity, and transform gender relations and gendered institutions.

Gender transformative leadership brings together the values of gender equality and transformative leadership. Transformative leadership is a leadership approach through which leaders and followers help each other identify needed change and create a vision to guide the change, while at the same time advancing a higher level of morale and motivation within workers (Burns, 1978). Transformative leadership's goal is to make members of an organization transformative leaders themselves. Gender transformative leadership seeks to cultivate individuals, including decision-makers, who empower themselves and their organizations "to pay close attention to gender power structures and discriminatory practices—both formal and informal—in order to advance gender equity within their organizations" as well as in the communities and constituencies they serve (UN Women, 2016).

Women in Global Health defines gender transformative leadership as:

- Grounded in a vision of gender equality and women's rights.
- Challenging privilege and imbalances in power to eliminate gendered inefficiencies and rights deficiencies that undermine global health.
- Intersectional, addressing social and personal characteristics that intersect with gender (race, ethnicity, etc.) to create multiple disadvantages. In global health, gender transformative leadership would drive equal participation of all genders from all geographies.
- An imperative for leaders from all genders, not a leadership approach for women only.
- Applying to leadership at all levels in global health from the community to the global.
- Recognizing different forms of leadership, such as thought leadership, which are not based on simple hierarchy and people management.
- Allowing for different starting points and contexts but prioritizing inclusion of the most marginalized and excluded.
- Assuming that gender equality = smarter global health and that gender transformative leadership is therefore necessary for the achievement of all global goals in health, including the SDGs.

Doing Things Differently in Gender Equality and Global Health

The interviews in this book indicate that there has been progress but that deliberate steps are needed to speed up the pace of change for gender equity in health leadership. These are things that can be done differently to catalyze change:

- **Change the narrative:** women in global health are change agents and drivers of health, not only service users and beneficiaries.
- **Shift the mind-set:** take advantage of 100% of the talent pool, especially women, all genders, marginalized groups, and people from diverse backgrounds; commit to diverse leadership because it fosters better decisions and better health outcomes.
- **Include voices from the Global South:** especially women, as central to global health decision-making.
- **Record and value unpaid health and social care work** by girls and women in order to move that work into the formal labor market.
- **Stop "fixing women":** adopt gender transformative strategies that change the gender-biased environments women work in, and stop "fixing women" to fit into unequal organizations and cultures.

- **Root out inequity:** address the power relations and structures that promote inequity in work and organizations, especially all forms of discrimination, harassment, and violence, which make toxic working environments for women.
- **Close all gender gaps** including the gender data gap, gender pay gap, and gender leadership gap—all are interconnected.
- **Customize policy solutions** to fit the societal and cultural context, but do not compromise on the goal.
- **Support collective action** through movements and partnerships, to accelerate progress; build coalitions across health professions and with political actors.
- **Commit to gender equality in global health as everyone's business:** this is not a "women's issue," it applies to all sectors, countries, genders, and people.

Final Word

The interviews in this book show it can be lonely for women fighting single-handed against systemic discrimination and organizational cultures designed to exclude them. The slow pace of progress in gender equality in global health leadership undermines both strong health systems and global health security. It is a serious concern that the targets of SDG 5 on Gender Equality are not on track, since gender inequality undermines human and economic development across the board and therefore threatens all 45 SDG targets.

In health specifically, there is a major opportunity to address the global shortage of health workers that impacts almost all countries, weakening health delivery and health security. Demographic changes and rising demand for health services are projected to drive the creation of 40 million new jobs by 2030 in the global health and social sector. At the same time, there is an estimated shortfall of the 18 million health workers in low- and middle-income countries required to achieve universal health coverage (WHO, 2019). Since women are 70% of the health and social care workforce, gaps in health worker supply will not be closed without addressing the gender inequities faced by women in the health and social workforce, including in health leadership.

Ensuring gender parity in health leadership, addressing power and discrimination through gender transformative leadership, and investing in decent work for the female health workforce together offer a "triple gender dividend":

- **Health dividend:** tens of millions of new jobs in health and social care needed to meet growing demand and deliver universal health coverage by 2030 can be filled.
- **Gender equality dividend:** investment in women and the education of girls to enter formal, paid work will increase gender equality as women gain income and greater autonomy. In turn, this will have positive spinoffs for family education, nutrition, and health.
- **Development dividend:** new jobs created in the health and social care sector will fuel economic growth.

As countries struggle to recover from the death and economic devastation of the COVID-19 pandemic, investment in decent work in health for women can be the game changer that finally delivers health security. The pandemic has highlighted the role of female frontline workers in health and social care and women's unpaid work. This is the time to capitalize on the increased awareness of women's work and advocate to #BuildBackBetter gender-responsive health systems based on equitable leadership.

References

Boniol, M., McIsaac, M., Xu, L., Wuliji, T., Diallo, K., & Campbell, J. (2019). Gender equity in the health workforce: Analysis of 104 countries. In *WHO*. World Health Organization. Retrieved from http://www.who.int/hrh/resources/gender_equity-health_workforce_analysis/en/

Burns, J. M. (1978). *Leadership*. Harper & Row.

Coscieme, L., Fioramonti, L., Mortensen, L. F., Pickett, K. E., Kubiszewski, I., Lovins, H., McGlade, J., Ragnarsdóttir, K. V., Roberts, D., Costanza, R., Vogli, R. D. E., & Wilkinson, R. (2020). Women in power: Female leadership and public health outcomes during the COVID-19 pandemic. *MedRxiv*, 2020.07.13.20152397. https://doi.org/10.1101/2020.07.13.20152397

Dhatt, R., Keeling, A., Thompson, K., & Manzoor, M. (2018). *Opinion: A new vision for global health leadership | Devex*. Devex. Retrieved from https://www.devex.com/news/opinion-a-new-vision-for-global-health-leadership-93772

McCurry, J. (2018, December 11). *Two more Japanese medical schools admit discriminating against women*. The Guardian. Retrieved from https://www.theguardian.com/world/2018/dec/12/two-more-japanese-medical-schools-admit-discriminating-against-women

Tiempocultural. (n.d.). *Al Día De La Mujer Salvadoreña*. Retrieved May 1, 2021, from http://revistatiempo.fullblog.com.ar/al-dia-de-la-mujer-salvadorena.html

UN Women. (2016). Transformative leadership: Leading for gender equality and women's rights. *Presentation at 2016 World Health Summit*.

UN Women. (2019). *Women in politics: 2019*. Retrieved from https://www.unwomen.org/en/digital-library/publications/2019/03/women-in-politics-2019-map

UNDP. (2020). *Human development perspectives tackling social norms: A game changer for gender inequalities*. Retrieved from http://hdr.undp.org/en/content/

United Nations. (1995). *Beijing declaration and platform for action*. Retrieved from https://www.un.org/en/events/pastevents/pdfs/Beijing_Declaration_and_Platform_for_Action.pdf

United Nations. (2015). *Goal 5: Achieve gender equality and empower all women and girls*. United Nations Department of Economic and Social Affairs. Retrieved from https://sdgs.un.org/goals/goal5

United Nations. (2019). *Political declaration of the high-level meeting on universal health coverage "universal health coverage: moving together to build a healthier world."* Retrieved from https://www.un.org/pga/73/wp-content/uploads/sites/53/2019/07/FINAL-draft-UHC-Political-Declaration.pdf

Walsh, J. J. (2008). *Old time makers of medicine*. Lethe Press.

WHO. (2019). *Delivered by women, led by men: A gender and equity analysis of the global health and social workforce*. World Health Organization. Retrieved from https://www.who.int/hrh/resources/health-observer24/en/

World Economic Forum. (2019). *Global gender gap report 2020*. Retrieved from https://www.weforum.org/reports/gender-gap-2020-report-100-years-pay-equality

Index

© Springer Nature Switzerland AG 2022
R. Morgan et al. (eds.), *Women and Global Health Leadership*,
https://doi.org/10.1007/978-3-030-84498-1

Printed in the United States
by Baker & Taylor Publisher Services